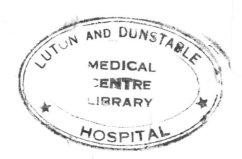

Medicines in the Elderly

**This book is to be returned on or before
the last date stamped below.** ✓

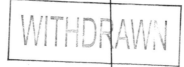

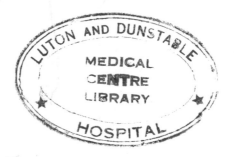
Medicines in the Elderly

Edited by

David Armour

MSc, MRPharmS

Senior Pharmacist
Pharmacy Department
Springfield University Hospital
London, UK

Chris Cairns

MSc, FRPharmS

Director of Pharmacy and Dietetics
University Hospital
Lewisham
London, UK

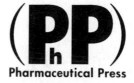
Pharmaceutical Press

Published by the Pharmaceutical Press
1 Lambeth High Street, London SE1 7JN, UK

© Pharmaceutical Press 2002

First published 2002

Text design by Barker/Hilsdon, Lyme Regis, Dorset
Typeset by MCS Ltd, Salisbury, Wiltshire
Printed in Great Britain by TJ International, Padstow, Cornwall

ISBN 0 85369 446 X

A catalogue record for this book is available from the British Library

Contents

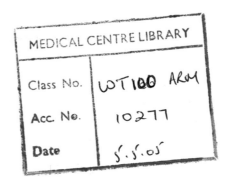

Preface

> ... the lean and slippered pantaloon ... his shrunk shank ... sans teeth, sans eyes, sans taste, sans everything.
>
> As You Like It II.vii.139 *et seq.*

William Shakespeare's sixth and seventh ages of man paint a rather gloomy picture of old age, a theme which has been echoed by many poets down the ages, including more recently T S Eliot with his 'cold friction of departing sense' and 'laceration of laughter at what ceases to amuse'. Such archetypes are still with us as representatives of typical old age.

In my view such pessimism sits badly with what actually constitutes old age for the majority of people in western society in the 21st century. Improvements in nutrition and housing in childhood, better availability of secondary and tertiary education and better prosperity have contributed to a cohort of ageing people who are, in general, healthier by far than previous generations. People in the UK can now expect to live longer and, in general, with a better quality of life in their later years than their forebears. The new archetype of old age is much more likely than hitherto to be physically sound and in full possession of his/her senses.

Medical or surgical problems in old age, however, can still carry a heavy burden of prolonged incapacity, delay in recovery and increased dependence. The medicines used may help to ameliorate these problems, but they all carry the potential for harm and this possibility may be greatly increased by any deterioration of liver or kidney function or by the adverse effects of multiple therapies which tend to be prescribed for some individuals; both these possibilities are more frequent in old age. This book is therefore partly about ways of dealing with such difficulties but it also takes a wider perspective in looking at how disease affects the major body systems, which are most likely to be adversely influenced in those of advanced years, and how drug therapy can best be directed to helping those people. Its content will be of interest to any health professional with an involvement in elderly care.

In the first chapter Peter Millard and I explore what is meant by old age and we reach a conclusion which some may find surprising. In Chapter 2 Alison Ewing looks into the factors in the ageing body which may change how the body distributes and eliminates a drug and how a drug influences bodily function. In Chapter 3 Anne and Moira Kinnear discuss the common disorders of the gastrointestinal tract and their treatment, especially as they affect the older patient. In Chapter 4 Andrzej Kostrzewski takes an illuminating look at the complexities of cardiovascular medicine and in Chapter 5 Anne Boyter and Kenneth Dagg discuss the major respiratory problems of the elderly. In Chapter 6 Barbara Baigent brings a professional lifetime's experience of medicine use in mental disorders to her chapter and in Chapter 7 Soraya Dhillon explores the fields of epilepsy and Parkinson's disease. There follow particularly extensive chapters on infections (8: Caroline Bradley) and endocrine disorders (9: Jayne Wood), both areas of particular importance in old age, as is osteoporosis (10: Marion Bennie, Janice Harris and Catherine Sedgeworth). In Chapter 11 Anne Watson, Fiona Thomson and Aileen Muir have dealt in depth with musculoskeletal disorders and in Chapter 12 Duncan Livingstone gives a useful perspective of eye and ear problems. Virginia Hill (Chapter 13) has cast an experienced eye over common skin disorders and Mahesh Sodha (Chapter 14) has written a particularly interesting chapter on palliative care. Then in Chapter 15 we have a most comprehensive review by Larry Goodyer of compliance, concordance and their relationship to polytherapy and the book concludes in Chapter 16 with a fascinating discussion by Alice Oborne about the main ethical issues affecting research in old age.

Many medicines-related aspects of care in the elderly are highlighted in the recently-published government policy document, the National Service Framework for Older People and its supplement, Medicines for Older People. The need for regular medication review and other medicines management issues in older people are highlighted and a specific milestone of the policy is that by 2004 schemes will be organized locally so that the elderly are able to get more help from pharmacists in using their medicines.

David Armour
July 2001

Acknowledgements

The editors are extremely grateful to the following people for assistance, advice or provision of resources in the process of preparing this book:
Professor Steve Hudson
Mr Roger Tredree
Professor Peter Millard
Ms Jean McQuade
Mr Roy Sinclair
The library staff at St George's Hospital Medical Library.

About the editors

David Armour qualified in pharmacy at the Liverpool School of Pharmacy (now part of Liverpool John Moores University) and spent his first professional years in community pharmacy. Since 1978 he has been working in hospital pharmacy in a variety of clinical and management posts.

Recently, Mr Armour has been working part-time in hospital pharmacy, where he has developed an interest in clinical audit. He has also been able to undertake project work, including studies in the pharmacoeconomics of the use of injectable antibiotics and of patient-controlled analgesia at St George's Hospital, Tooting. He has also organised and carried out for a local health authority an observational study in the relationship between prescribed medicines and hip fracture in the elderly. The latter project aroused his interest in the subject matter of this book.

David Armour is a member of the Royal Pharmaceutical Society of Great Britain and of its Hospital Pharmacy Group. He also holds membership of the United Kingdom Clinical Pharmacy Association, the College of Pharmacy Practice and the Institute of Health Service Management. *Medicines in the Elderly* is his first venture as editor.

Chris Cairns is the Director of Pharmacy and Dietetics at University Hospital Lewisham, London. Previously he was the Director of the Pharmacy Academic Practice Unit at St George's Hospital, London. Since qualifying in 1977, he has practised in a number of clinical pharmacy settings, including care of the elderly, clinical nutrition, cardiology and critical care. He has carried out pharmacy practice research in a number of areas, including drug utilisation, pharmaceutical outcomes, intravenous therapy and pharmacoeconomics. Chris was the recipient of the Guild of Healthcare Pharmacists Medeva Gold Medal for 1999.

Contributors

Barbara Baigent B Pharm, MRPharmS
Formerly Principal Pharmacist, Pharmacy Department, Springfield
Hospital, London, UK

Marion Bennie Ad Dip Clin Pharm, MRPharmS
Consultant in Pharmaceutical Public Health (Lothian/Fife),
Edinburgh, UK

Anne C Boyter MSc, MRPharmS
Lecturer in Clinical Practice, Department of Pharmaceutical Sciences,
University of Strathclyde, Glasgow, UK

Caroline Bradley MSc, MRPharmS
Principal Pharmacist, Pharmacy Department, St George's Hospital,
London, UK

Kenneth Dagg MBChB, MRCP
Consultant Physician, Respiratory Unit, Wishaw General Hospital,
Lanarkshire, UK

Soraya Dhillon BPharm, PhD, MRPharmS
Director Taught Postgraduate Studies, The School of Pharmacy,
University of London, London, UK

Alison B Ewing MSc, MRPharmS
Director of Pharmacy, Countess of Chester NHS Trust, Chester,
Cheshire, UK

Larry I Goodyer PhD, MRPharmS
Head of Pharmacy Practice Research, Department of Pharmacy,
King's College, London, UK

Janice Harris MSc, MRPharmS
Senior Pharmacist, Care of the Elderly, Lothian University
Hospitals NHS Trust, Edinburgh, UK

Virginia A Hill MRCP, MRCGP
Specialist Registrar in Dermatology, Great Ormond Street Hospital for
Sick Children, London, UK

Anne E Kinnear MSc, MRPharmS
Principal Pharmacist, Royal Infirmary of Edinburgh, Edinburgh, UK

Moira Kinnear MSc, ADCPT, MRPharmS
Principal Pharmacist, Western General Hospital, Edinburgh and
University of Strathclyde, Glasgow, UK

Andrzej Kostrzewski MSc, MMedEd, MRPharmS
Principal Pharmacist, Guy's and St Thomas' Hospital Trust, London, UK

Duncan Livingstone MSc, MRPharmS
Chief Pharmacist, Queen Victoria Hospital NHS Trust, West Sussex, UK

Peter H Millard MD, PhD, FRCP
Emeritus Professor, Division of Geriatric Medicine,
St George's Hospital Medical School, London, UK

Aileen Muir MSc, MRPharmS
Principal Pharmacist, Clinical Effectiveness, Fife Health Board, Scotland,
UK

C Alice Oborne MSc, Clin Pharm, MRPharmS
Research Pharmacist, Clinical Age Research Unit, Guy's, King's College
and St Thomas' School of Medicine, London, UK

Catherine Sedgeworth MSc, MRPharmS
Senior Pharmacist, Care of the Elderly, Lothian University
Hospitals NHS Trust, Edinburgh, UK

Mahesh Sodha MSc, MRPharmS
Community Pharmacist, Chelmsford, UK

Fiona C Thomson MSc, MRPharmS
Senior Pharmacist, Medicines Information, South Glasgow University
Hospitals NHS Trust, Glasgow, UK

Anne M Watson MSc, MEd, MRPharmS
Area Specialist Education and Training, Southern General Hospital,
Glasgow, UK

Jayne Wood MPhil, MRPharmS, MCPP
Head of Pharmaceutical Services, North Manchester Healthcare
NHS Trust, Manchester, UK

Abbreviations

ABPI	ankle–brachial pressure index
ACE	angiotensin-converting enzyme
ACTH	adrenocorticotrophin
ADAS-cog	Alzheimer's Disease Assessment Scale cognitive subscale
ADH	antidiuretic hormone
ADL	activities of daily living
ADR	adverse drug reaction
AF	atrial fibrillation
AIDS	acquired immune deficiency syndrome
AMI	acute myocardial infarction
APTT	activated partial thromboplastin time
ARA	American Rheumatism Association
BMD	bone mineral density
BMI	body mass index
BMUs	bone multicellular units
BP	blood pressure
BPH	benign prostatic hyperplasia
BTS	British Thoracic Society
CAP	community-acquired pneumonia
CDR	Clinical Dementia Rating
CFC	chlorofluorocarbon
CGIC	Clinician's Global Impressions of Change
CGIS	Clinician's Global Impressions of Severity
CHD	coronary heart disease
CHF	chronic heart failure
CIBIC	Clinician's Interview-Based Impression of Change
CIOP	corticosteroid-induced osteoporosis
CNS	central nervous system
COMT	catechol-O-methyltransferase
COPD	chronic obstructive pulmonary disease
COX-2	cyclo-oxygenase-2
CPMP	Committee for Proprietary Medicinal Products
CRCs	child-resistant containers

CRP	C-reactive protein
CSF	cerebrospinal fluid
CSM	Committee on Safety of Medicines
CTZ	chemoreceptor trigger zone
DCCT	Diabetes Control and Complications Trial
DG	Declaration of Geneva
DH	Declaration of Helsinki
DHEA	dehydroepiandrosterone
DMARDs	disease-modifying antirheumatic drugs
DPLD	diffuse parenchymal lung diseases
DPN	diabetic polyneuropathy
ECT	electroconvulsive therapy
EMEA	European Medicines Evaluation Agency
ESAS	Edmonton Symptom Assessment System
ESR	erythrocyte sedimentation rate
FEV	forced expiratory volume
FEV_1	forced expiratory volume in 1 s
FT_3	free tri-iodothyronine
FT_4	free thyroxine
FSH	follicle-stimulating hormone
FVC	forced vital capacity
GABA	γ-aminobutyric acid
GCP	Good (Research) Clinical Practice for Trials on Medicinal Products
GFR	glomerular filtration rate
GH	growth hormone
GnRH	gonadotrophin-releasing hormone
GORD	gastro-oesophageal reflux disease
HA	hyaluronic acid
HbA_{1c}	glycated haemoglobin
HDL	high-density lipoprotein
HimP	Health Improvement Programmes
HIV	human immunodeficiency virus
HLA	human lymphocyte antigen
HRCT	high-resolution computed tomography
HRT	hormone replacement therapy
5-HT	serotonin
IBD	inflammatory bowel disease
ICH	International Conference on Harmonisation
ICP	intracranial pressure
IGF-1	insulin-like growth factor 1

IHD	ischaemic heart disease
IL-1	interleukin-1
INR	international normalised ratio
IOP	intraocular pressure
ISH	isolated systolic hypertension
$[K^+]$	molar concentration of potassium ion
LAR	long-acting release
LFT	liver function test
LH	luteinising hormone
LTOT	long-term oxygen therapy
LVH	left ventricular hypertrophy
MAOI	monoamine oxidase inhibitor
MI	myocardial infarction
MMSE	mini-mental state examination
MND	motor neurone disease
MRSA	methicillin-resistant *Staphylococcus aureus*
$[Na^+]$	molar concentration of sodium ion
NG	nasogastric
NMDA	N-methyl-D-aspartate
NSAIDs	non-steroidal anti-inflammatory drugs
NSCLC	non-small-cell lung cancer
NSF	National Service Framework
OA	osteoarthritis
OC	oral contraceptives
OP	osteoporosis
Pa_{CO_2}	partial arterial pressure of carbon dioxide
Pa_{O_2}	partial arterial pressure of oxygen
PCG	Primary Care Group
pCO_2	partial pressure of carbon dioxide
PCT	Primary Care Trust
PILs	patient information leaflets
PL	product licence
pO_2	partial pressure of oxygen
PSA	prostatic-specific antigen
PTH	parathyroid hormone
RA	rheumatoid arthritis
RCP	Royal College of Physicians
RCT	randomised control trial
RECs	research ethics committees
RNI	reference nutrient intake
SCLC	small-cell lung cancer

SD	standard deviation
SERMs	selective oestrogen receptor modulators
SIADH	syndrome of inappropriate antidiuretic hormone secretion
SRVS	small round structured virus
SSRIs	selective serotonin reuptake inhibitors
T_3	tri-iodothyronine; liothyronine
T_4	levothryoxine; thyroxine; tetraiodothyronine
TB	tuberculosis
TBG	thyroid-binding globulin
TCA	tricyclic antidepressants
TDM	Therapeutic Drug Monitoring
TFR	total fertility rate
TGI	thyroid growth immunoglobulins
T_{max}	time taken for the blood level of a drug to achieve its maximum following an administered dose
TNF-α	tumour necrosis factor-α
TRH	thyrotrophin-releasing hormone
TSH	thyrotrophin-stimulating hormone
TSI	thyroid-stimulating immunoglobulins
TT_3	total tri-iodothyronine
TT_4	total thyroxine
TURP	transurethral resection of the prostate
UKPDS	United Kingdom Prospective Diabetes Study
UTI	urinary tract infection
UVB	ultraviolet B
V_d	volume of distribution
VTE	venous thromboembolism
WBPI	Wisconsin Brief Pain Inventory
WHO	World Health Organization

1

What is old age?

Peter H Millard and David Armour

All that lives must die, passing through nature to eternity.

Hamlet I.ii.72

Authors' note

In most later chapters of this book the chapter material is dealt with largely as reviews of available data. In Chapter 1, in contrast, the intention is to explore ideas about the nature of ageing and old age with the objective of stimulating the reader to explore the subject further. The opinions and theories presented are most certainly open to debate and no one should doubt that further illumination will be cast on this fascinating and vital subject in the course of time.

Introduction

There is a high level of awareness in developed countries that people of advanced years now constitute more of the population than hitherto and that the processes which have given rise to this state of affairs seem set to continue indefinitely. It is also widely perceived that older people become on the whole less capable of productive employment, as normal ageing processes give rise to progressive restriction of physical or mental abilities.

It is easy to create a subjective impression of a resultant 'top-heavy' population with an ever-decreasing proportion of working population supporting an ever-increasing elderly sector which consumes ever more health and social services resources.

Objectively, however, these daunting prospects may not be so threatening after all, certainly in the near future in the UK. There is some evidence that the proportion of elderly is indeed set to rise, but during the next decade this may amount to only about 3%, whereas the proportion of people aged between 45 and 59 (i.e. those of peak earning capacity) will increase by about 13%.[1] Not only are the latter high earners but they constitute a major source of informal caring. It is true that the proportion of elderly people in the UK population will go on rising for some time (until people born in the 'baby boom' years of the 1960s have begun to die off) but the main brunt of this demographic change has already been borne, certainly in the medium term (a different but related problem may arise in the long term as a consequence of the falling birth rate in the western world – see later).

Other populations may not be so lucky. In the UK the change from a high fertility/high infant-mortality scenario to one of low fertility/low infant-mortality has happened gradually over about a century. In developing countries such as Brazil and India, this process may take place much more rapidly, with the potential for consequent serious social upheaval. Figure 1.1 shows a diagrammatic population pyramid representing a population profile for the former case; Figure 1.2 shows for comparison the inverted pyramid of an ageing society.

However, whether or not the social structures of some countries are to be challenged by successively larger cohorts of old people, there is no doubt that people at the end of their lives, whatever their age, do consume more health resources than others and that a major part of this extra resource is medicine. Old age also offers a variable but general deterioration of various body systems giving decreased ability to cope

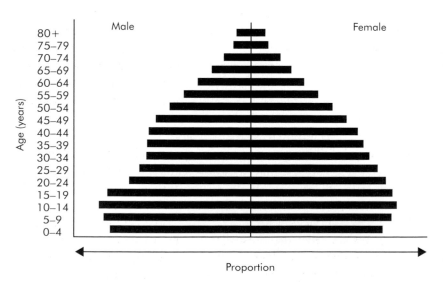

Figure 1.1 Theoretical population profile for high fertility/high mortality scenario.

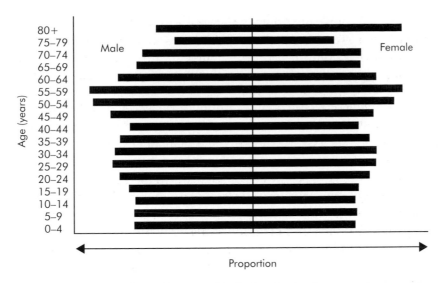

Figure 1.2 Theoretical population profile for low fertility/low mortality scenario.

with constraints. It follows that opportunities for experiencing complications of therapy such as adverse reactions and interactions are much
greater.

Characteristics of ageing

It is a universal experience that changes in our bodies make us less able
to function in physical capacities. One cannot envisage a person aged
over 60 winning major tennis tournaments or competing in Olympic
Games gymnastics events. Human life shows an unavoidable tendency
to physical (and possibly mental) deterioration, with death as an
inevitable end-point. Individual body organs start to function less effi-
ciently, tissues repair themselves more slowly and the individual must
alter lifestyle to accommodate these changes.

In some primitive organisms there appears to be no ageing or death
other than by violent external insult. When an amoeba reproduces it
divides into two – there is no death and no corpse. However, the evolu-
tion of sexual reproduction has given rise to a new entity – the parent –
who instead of staying around as one of the offspring remains a parent
who ultimately ages and dies. Mortality is the price of becoming a multicellular, multistructured organism with specialised organs like eyes
and limbs. The advantage of being able to pass on certain genetic material from two parents to their offspring gives the members of a species

long-term flexibility to combat external threats at the expense of supporting senescent individuals whose contribution to species survival may well be less than that of youth.

Ageing is a phenomenon which can be observed in cells, tissues, organs, individual creatures, populations and societies. In cell culture, cells can be studied as they first reproduce themselves then lose reproductive ability then decline to death. The only exception to this universal mortality is the cell which undergoes malignant transformation and becomes (in tissue culture and if ambient conditions permit) in practical terms immortal.

In a developing organism there comes a point at which some cells cease multiplying and start differentiating into masses of similar type, thereby losing (with some exceptions) the ability to multiply. A tissue is formed which can only function if its component cells and surrounding tissues can work together. The limiting factor of ageing tissue function is the cessation of ability of any of its component cells to contribute to the coordinated functions of the whole.

Tissues combined make up organs and the complexity of the ageing process multiplies accordingly. It becomes easier to observe symptoms rather than causes as changes in muscles, vision, lungs, etc. become more apparent because of their consequences in decreased function.

The degree of complexity involved in the ageing of an individual person is very great indeed but paradoxically it becomes very simple to predict that some of us will not be around after a certain time has passed. Despite differences between individuals which, as will be seen, become greater with the passing of time, actuarial tables predict with chilling accuracy the annual demise of so many people per thousand. This is because we are all put together in a broadly similar way, although exactly *who* will die at a given time is partly a reflection of the unique way in which the physical components of each individual are linked and integrated.

Old age tends to be characterised by such features as stooping posture, less confident gait, shrunken shanks, hair loss and wrinkled skin. All complex organisms grow old and die, because the biological processes that create them fail. From the moment of our conception, everything conspires to ensure that the genes survive; reproduction takes place, offspring are nurtured and ageing life forms die. This ageing process starts at the time of conception when two meiotic cells – one sperm, one ovum – unite. Thereafter, mitotic division transforms the cytoplasm of the ovum and the newly combined genes into a complex organism that can forage for food and reproduce.

Human ageing seems universal and inevitable. However, some creatures do not apparently age at all, for example, some sea anemones. Why is it that cells which have accomplished the great feat of differentiating during fetal growth are unable to maintain properly what is already formed? In theory, powerful repair mechanisms should be able to correct or repair defects in cells indefinitely. But in practice they don't. Is it possible that ageing serves some evolutionary purpose?

Natural selection permits successful strategies of living to persist while those which are detrimental die out. As ageing and death appear to be universal, possibly they confer biological success (for a species as a whole, perhaps). Maybe ageing accelerates the turnover of generations, allowing better adaptation to rapid or profound changes in the environment. Such effects cannot be demonstrated, however, because natural selection operates firstly at an individual level; any species effects follow after a time lag. Also, in the wild, such an effect would never be realised, as the near universality of predation or accident as causes of death makes old age very rare. It seems unlikely that death is an adaptive effect.

It may be that the prime component of ageing is not the run-down of individual cells or tissues but that of their ability to respond to one another, especially the cells of the nervous, immune and endocrine systems; the maintenance of receptors to enable this response is energy-intensive and ultimately the cell may not be able to maintain both its response capability and its internal homeostasis. The resulting chaos could lead to rapid senescence, even though most of the organism's cells may be perfectly healthy. In such a scenario, different organs could decay in different people of the same age, leading to differing causes of death, which accords nicely with reality. This possibility could also explain the 'immortality' of cells with malignant transformation – they no longer need to communicate with other cells and therefore need not expend energy on the synthesis and maintenance of receptor molecules.

Is it possible that ageing is merely a purposeless slow march towards death? If so, it might help if we explore what we mean by death before we can better understand ageing.

Cell death can occur either by necrosis (damage) or apoptosis (programmed cell death, e.g. the annual shedding of the leaves of deciduous trees). It can be observed as a cessation of metabolic activity, following which the material of the cell will start to decompose. However, the death of a person can be more difficult to define. Individuals have been fully resuscitated after prolonged immersion in ice-cold water following which no brain activity could be observed. People with 'flat' EEGs but functioning circulations (in persistent vegetative state, for example) may have fully functional organs which might be removed for transplantation. But is such a person dead? It seems that the moment of death may be difficult to define, even approximately in some cases.

Perhaps we have to be content with a pragmatic approach to death – we know it when we see it, especially after a lapse of time. As Shakespeare's Hamlet puts it, addressing Yorick's newly disinterred skull: 'Get thee to my lady's chamber and tell her, let her paint an inch thick, to this favour she shall come'. (Ironically, Yorick has achieved his own kind of immortality *because* his character is incontrovertibly dead.)

If we cannot know exactly what human death is, perhaps our understanding of ageing will not be as comprehensive as we would like; given this reservation, however, is it possible to arrive at a definition of ageing which will necessarily be deficient but will provide a pragmatic framework of understanding? Various theories have been advanced to explain ageing and perhaps elements of many of them should be taken into account to achieve a comprehensive and comprehensible standpoint.

Theories of ageing

There are almost as many theories about the cause of ageing as there are scientific viewpoints. Theories put forward in the past include body wear and tear, rate of living, free radical damage, random errors in DNA repair, mitochondrial damage, cross-linking in glucose and collagen and immune decline.[2] This is not the place to discuss each of these theories in detail. However closely some of them may accord with reality, they simply express, as all theories do, the opinions of the scientists who formulated them and none of them on its own appears to provide a comprehensive picture of what ageing is. In an attempt to reconcile some of these disparate ideas, Professor Tom Kirkwood, a biologist with an interest in mathematics, developed the *disposable soma theory*.[3]

The disposable soma theory considers complex biological organisms to be entities which are programmed to transform energy into progeny. Complex biological organisms have two significant parts, the germ cells and the soma, i.e. the rest of the body. Survival depends on energy expenditure being balanced between foraging, feeding, somatic maintenance and reproduction. As death in the wild is an inevitable consequence of biological hazard and predation, there is no point in investing large amounts of energy to maintain the soma after reproduction has ceased. So, other things being equal, organisms can gain a selective advantage by investing more energy in rapid and prolific reproduction, and less in somatic maintenance.

This balance will differ markedly between different species; hence the mouse has a short life span but rapid reproductive capacity and invests little energy in soma; the elephant has a long life span but slow reproduction and needs to invest large amounts of energy in soma. The relationship between optimum evolutionary fitness and optimum maintenance appears to be imprecise and this suggests considerable variability between individuals as they age – which again accords with reality, as will be seen later.

Too small an investment in the development and maintenance of the soma may therefore lead to death before reproduction and too great an investment in its maintenance may be wasteful and inefficient. The strength of the disposable soma theory is its recognition of the biological inevitability of death. Its weakness is that it does not explain how we age.

No theory provides a fully comprehensive account of ageing and to understand how we age we need to consider some elements of how we develop and grow.

Human growth, development and ageing

Intrinsic and extrinsic factors

Intrinsic factors determined by the intermingling of the somatic genes of our parents – the gender-determining chromosomes of our biological father and the mitochondrial genes and cell cytoplasm inherited from our biological mother – explain the processes that underpin human growth and development.[2] Biologically, we have to be transformed from a single fertilised cell (the zygote) into a fully formed adult that can think, plan, talk, change food into energy, breathe oxygen, excrete waste products and walk around.

The mitochondria in the cytoplasm of the fertilised ovum provide the powerhouse which drives the cell. Without these mitochondria we could not breathe oxygen or convert energy into power. Genetic abnormalities increase with the age of the mother. Although all oocytes are laid down in the first 3 months of an embryo's life, the second meiotic division only occurs at fertilisation. This may explain to some extent why the ageing process for each individual starts in earnest at conception, irrespective of the age of the parents. Abnormalities in mitochondrial genes can cause a syndrome that is like accelerated ageing, with weakness, wasting and difficulty in breathing.

To stand upright in a gravitational field a baby's bones and muscles have to be strong enough to support his or her weight. Alternative contraction and relaxation of antigravity muscles holds us upright; and blood pressure control in the upright posture ensures that sufficient oxygenated blood reaches the brain. Young bones break like green sticks. As we age, our bones first become stronger, then more brittle. When there is insufficient bone of normal quality, osteoporosis is evident and our bones, like chains, break at the weakest link.

Extrinsic factors, associated with diverse factors such as social class, income, habit and personal behaviour, interact with intrinsic factors to explain why some people live longer than others. Smoking is a good example of an extrinsic factor that accelerates ageing. Gaseous exchange in the alveoli is inhibited and microvascular changes adversely affect the functioning of the heart and circulation. Another less well-recognised factor is exposure to sunlight. The excessive use of sun beds or living in hot countries without adequate solar protection causes accelerated skin ageing in white people.[4]

Ageing changes and disease

The four characteristics of age changes are universality, intrinsicality, progressiveness and deleteriousness.[5] Cross-linking of collagen is a good example of an age change. It occurs in everyone (universal) whatever their race, social class or environment. It begins in the embryo (intrinsic) and continues until death (progressive), first strengthening then weakening tissues such as bone (deleterious).

At any age, total system failure can accompany serious infections. In old age, the total system often fails in association with seemingly minor infections. Such effects as falls, confusion or inability to cope are common presenting problems of simple illnesses in older people and that is why many such people need ready access to skilled medical help.

Population growth

The western world has an ageing population for three reasons. Firstly, at the end of the 19th century, public health measures led to a dramatic reduction in childhood mortality associated with substandard nutrition and susceptibility to infection. Consequently, children born during the first half of the 20th century had a better chance of living to be old. In the 1880s, 150 children per thousand born died in the UK in the first year of their lives. Now the UK death rate in the first year of life is 10 per thousand.[6]

Next, improved medical care, especially advances in drug treatment, anaesthetic and surgical techniques, provides the second reason why the western world has an ageing population. In the 19th century, people who survived childhood and childbirth had a reasonable chance of living to be old. Some experts consider that we are the first society to have an ageing population, yet the average expectancy in the Bible is recorded as three score years and ten, and Ecclesiastes comments that human life span is 100 years at most. From biblical times to well into the 20th century, individuals who survived into old age were probably very healthy. Now, because of medical advances, individuals who have had serious illnesses as well as fit people expect that they will live to be old.

Population control is the third, and probably the most important, cause of the western world's ageing population. Examination of the population pyramids derived from census data in all countries of Europe shows that the number of live births is below replacement rate. Population stability depends on 2.1 children being born for every female of child-bearing age, i.e. aged 15–49. Total fertility rates, for example in Russia (1995) of 1.34; Italy (1994) 1.22; United Kingdom (1996) 1.71; Spain (1994) 1.21 and Poland (1996) 1.60, indicate that the European nations are in danger of breeding themselves out of existence.[6]

In the UK the downward trend in fertility rates began in 1968. From 1960 to 1967 the average annual total fertility rate (TFR) was 2.82. Between 1968 and 1977 the UK TFR fell from 2.62 to 1.69. Since then the average annual TFR has been 1.77. Increasing numbers of older people, coupled with fewer children being born, explains why the UK has an ageing population. Between 1971 and 1997, the number of people aged 65 and over living in the UK increased by 1 800 000 to 9 246 000 individuals. During the same period the number of people aged less than 16 fell by over 2 000 000 to 12 103 000.[6] While the surge in numbers of elderly people has already largely happened for the UK, it is of concern that we appear to be heading for a time when there may be insufficient numbers of young people to support them.

Longevity, life expectation and life span

Longevity is species-specific.[7] Mice live for maybe 2 years; the average human life span is 75–80 years. Perhaps if everyone took regular exercise, ate a healthy diet and maintained a lifelong interest in current affairs many more of us could live to be 100 years old. However, whatever else we do, whatever advances are made in gerontological research, we are very unlikely to get a mouse to live for 10 years or a human being to live for 400 years.

In 1994 life expectancy at birth was 73.9 years for males and 79.2 years for females: why females live longer than males is not known. Perhaps the male phenotype brings with it inherent weakness or perhaps healthy men take more risks, including in recent times dying in large numbers on battlefields. Alternatively, as men die more frequently than they should (from all causes) in the first year after bereavement or retirement, it may be that men have a weaker hold on the life force than women do. Whatever the reason, women born at the end of the 20th century are expected to live almost 5 years longer than men do (it may be of interest that, for people reaching their late 80s, the life expectation gap *for that age* narrows greatly, although there is still a female advantage).

Are elderly people different?

There is considerable variation between individuals in the age at which a particular physiological function starts to decline and in the rate of that decline. It may be difficult to distinguish between functional decline in old people due to environmental influences or diseases and that of an intrinsic ageing process. With some measurable physiological functions youth and age can be compared quantitatively. For example, a group of 80-year-old subjects showed about 15% reduction in nerve conduction velocity, about 30% reduction in resting cardiac output and about 50% in respiratory vital capacity in comparison with a group of 30-year-old subjects.[8] Age-related impairment of autonomic function may present diversely as, for example, postural hypotension or defective temperature regulation.

Atypical presentation of illness is another consequence of ageing, largely because of impaired physiological response to stress factors (such as invading microorganisms) but there may also be sensory impairment with alteration of pain sensation – a heart attack may not produce any pain, perhaps only shortness of breath. Respiratory or urinary tract infections may show confusion as the main presenting sign.

The prevalence of many disorders rises with age and they tend to coexist with each other. Such conditions as arthritis, visual impairment and deafness become widespread (almost 'normal'). Because of the general decline in physiological functioning, disorder of one function may overwhelm the capacity of another (pneumonia may lead to cardiac failure, hypovolaemia due to gastric bleeding may lead to renal failure).

Because of the tendency to multiple pathology in old age (and inappropriate prescribing), old people tend to be taking more medicines than their younger counterparts. However, because of altered liver and kidney function, kinetics of drug disposal may alter profoundly. There may also be pharmacodynamic changes in receptors, making the elderly more susceptible to sedation, for example. Initiation of therapy may require reductions in dose amount and/or frequency. Drugs with a prolonged time course in the body, such as digoxin or phenobarbital, which may have been prescribed for many years may need a reduction in dose as the ageing kidney becomes less able to eliminate them or the ageing liver to inactivate them by metabolism (see Chapter 2).

Because of the loss of adaptive mechanisms to stress due to physiological ageing, the elderly person commonly needs a prolonged period of recovery from illness while a younger person does not, in general. The recognition of the need of people with chronic illnesses for rehabilitation was a major influence in the development of the medical discipline of geriatrics. The need to treat acutely ill elderly people in a specialist unit in general hospitals and then to provide rehabilitation in order to enable them to live independently again should become a standard feature of good elderly care provision in the UK.

What is old age?

The run-down of individual cells is a prime cause of the gradual ageing of each individual at the microscopic level. More immediately perceptible mechanisms of ageing affect people at the macroscopic level also. Clearly perceptible changes in the appearance of the face and the hair announce to the world that one is no longer young; loss of hearing may bring about false perceptions of stupidity and previous falls and arthritis may affect mobility and gait (and confidence).

What does it mean to be aged or old? Experience suggests that there is no absolute meaning for terms like these; they are purely relative. The parents of a child will always seem old to the child but young to their own parents. It would be unwise to use a particular value, such as the arbitrary pensionable age (currently 60 for females, 65 for males in the UK) as a scientifically valid dividing line between middle and old age, as many people live vigorous and healthy lives well into retirement, whereas others appear old well before this time, even in the absence of overt disease. This appears to be the prime characteristic of human old age: its heterogeneity. There is a problem therefore in making dose recommendations for many drugs solely on the basis of chronological age and perhaps individual dose recommendations should be based more on other factors such as physiological values derived from liver or kidney function. But if chronology is not a very useful guide to old age, is there a more meaningful definition?

Societies are made up of populations which differ in age, racial origin, economic status, intellectual abilities, education and a host of other ways. For a society to function properly these diverse groups must interact for mutual benefit (and if in the course of time they lose the ability to do so, the society may age and die out, in parallel with the ageing process in the body). If a group dominates, as well-off elderly may do in some towns, local resources will tend to be directed towards the needs of this group. Others will treat them with respect. One reason for this is economic; people with plenty of resources tend to be respected more than those who are more dependent. Another is that such people are not usually seen as being 'old' – senior citizens, possibly; elderly, maybe – but not 'old'. Perhaps 'old' carries inevitable connotations of inadequacy or uselessness and therefore possible dependence; ideas of physical or economic burden to other individuals or society as a whole may follow with a decrease in the respect in which others hold them.

There is thus a highly subjective element in our perceptions of old age. This is borne out by the historically changing perception of what old age is; only 100 years ago 60 was really old, whereas now 90 would be really old and perhaps in only 25 years' time you will have to be 100 to be really old.

Perhaps it is better to abandon chronological ideas and think in terms of physical decline. A possible approach would be to perceive ageing as a gradual deterioration in bodily structure and function resulting in increased vulnerability to external and internal constraints, which in turn leads to increased dependence and, ultimately, death.

Old age is a stage of life that will, with good fortune, come to us all, especially if we are lucky enough to be born in the western world. Living to see one's children's children is a blessing that now comes to many. In future years, that blessing may also be extended to include seeing your children's children's children. Yet, as one's life begins to pass into its 80th and 90th years, old age may be seen to bring with it burdens as well as pleasures.

The greatest burden may be the loss of agility. Incontinence may be a curse and frequent falls can paralyse the subject with fright. Some people – the lucky ones – maintain excellent bodily function, even up to 100 years of age; use it or lose it is a message that one needs to bear in mind. After retirement, mental function can decline, especially if one has no interest in current affairs or in intellectual spheres of activity and all too often, because of the differential survival rate, women outlive men.

Further burdens appear as one's children, now maybe grandparents in their own right, have to turn their attention on to you and your life. No one, least of all a parent, wants to depend on his or her children, neighbours or friends. However, this sharing, this communal gift of love, brings with it burdens as well as joys for the 'child'. There is great joy for an individual in knowing that one has been able to support one's mother, father, uncle or neighbour to live independently in his or her own home. Yet that joy comes at a price which the individual may ultimately find too great.

Other burdens may arise if hospital-based services, developed by pioneers of geriatric medicine to meet the needs of older people, have not been maintained or expanded to meet demand. When service to others is expected of you, such care can easily become overwhelming. The pressures of caring can crush the spirit even of (especially of) the most devoted daughter or son, husband or wife. For this reason, society should perhaps recognise that specially developed services, run by specially trained people, are essential and that access to them should not be limited by personal resources or the good offices of close relatives or friends. In this context the Royal Commission on Long Term Care[9] recommended that personal care for the elderly should be paid for according to need and out of general taxation; however, there is currently no sign of this actually happening. The risk of needing such care is about 1 in 3 for males and 1 in 5 for females[10] and is largely unpredictable for each individual.

Warning: the lottery of old age is the reality of *your* future existence.

Conclusion

Old age is difficult to define and for the concerned health professional chronological age is only a very rough guide at best to client needs. The characteristic of older people which distinguishes them most from younger people is heterogeneity; old age produces much more variation in physical and mental capabilities than is apparent within cohorts of younger people. In purely chronological terms there is no such thing as old age! When considering any intervention (especially involving drug treatment) for a person of advanced years the strategy should be don't treat the age, treat the person.

References

1. Raleigh V S. The demographic timebomb. *BMJ* 1997; 315: 442–443.
2. Timiras P S, Bittar E E, eds. *Advances in Cell Aging and Gerontology*, vol. 1: *Some Aspects of the Aging Process*. Greenwich, Connecticut: JAI Press, 1996: 248.
3. Kirkwood T B L. Biological aspects of ageing. In: Grimley Evans J, Franklyn Williams T, Beattie B *et al.*, eds. *Oxford Textbook of Geriatric Medicine*, 2nd edn. Oxford, England: Oxford University Press, 2000: 35–42.
4. Uitto J. Connective tissue biochemistry of the aging dermis. Age related alterations in collagen and elastin. *Dermatol Clin* 1986; 4: 433–446.
5. Strehler B L. *Time Cells and Ageing*, 2nd edn. London: Academic Press, 1962: 270.
6. Council of Europe. *Recent Demographic Developments in Europe 1997. United Kingdom Demography*. Strasbourg, France, Council of Europe, 1997: 363–372.
7. Comfort A. *The Biology of Senescence*, 3rd edn. New York: Elsevier, 1979: 414.
8. Briggs R S J. Historical overview: definitions and aims. In: *Principles and Practice of Geriatric Medicine*, 3rd edn. Chichester: John Wiley, 1999: 2.
9. Royal Commission on Long Term Care. *With Respect to Old Age*. London: Stationery Office, 1999.
10. Heath I. Dereliction of duty in an ageist society. *BMJ* 2000; 320: 1422.

Further reading

Carter N D, ed. *Development, Growth and Ageing*. London: Croom Helm, 1980.
Pathy M S J, ed. *Principles and Practice of Geriatric Medicine*, 3rd edn. Chichester: John Wiley, 1999.
Ross I K. *Aging of Cells, Humans and Societies*. Dubuque, IA: Wm C Brown: 1995.

2

Altered drug response in the elderly

Alison B Ewing

As people grow older significant changes in average body composition tend to happen. This is an inevitable part of the continuing ageing process. The extent to which drug response is dependent on time course of drug concentration in the body (pharmacokinetics) and events at the intracellular site (pharmacodynamics) inevitably alter as a result of these changes. All aspects – absorption, distribution, metabolism, excretion and target organ sensitivity – may be affected.

These changes will result in more problems with drug handling in the elderly population. This has been proved by research showing that as many as 28% of hospital admissions in the USA of older people are as a result of drug-related problems, with 70% of those being attributed to adverse drug reactions (ADRs).[1] The changes mean that the use of medicines in the elderly requires careful management to give optimum care.

There is little that can be done to modify the ageing process itself but an understanding of what is happening will allow drugs to be used appropriately with minimum complications.

Understanding of the nature of the physiological changes has increased greatly, and now it is possible to predict drug effects in the elderly. However, as well as predictable physiological changes, the extent of the influence of lifestyle, concomitant medication, environment, underlying disease and genetics must be considered carefully when using drugs.

Inappropriate prescribing is not only the cause of many ADRs, but it is also expensive and preventable. The total annual cost is impossible to measure but must be considerable. Careful management of medication will undoubtedly be cost-effective.

Pharmacokinetic changes

Liberation and absorption

To reach the blood stream, a solid oral dosage form must first disintegrate, dissolve and cross the gut wall into the blood stream. The gastrointestinal environment influences both the dissolution rate and the rate of absorption.

Due to a reduction in the amount of saliva produced in old age, oral doses that are absorbed through the buccal mucosa, such as glyceryl trinitrate, may show a reduced rate of absorption (increased T_{max}) which will increase the time to maximum drug effect. This will not decrease the overall amount of drug absorbed.

In older people, we see a decrease in the volume of gastric secretion, and gastric fluid is less acidic. Additionally, peristalsis is weakened and gastric emptying delayed.[2] This may potentially delay the dissolution of orally administered drugs. The delay in gastric emptying time together with reduced peristalsis will result in decreased intensity of the mixing of the gastrointestinal contents.

As ageing progresses, there is increasing atrophy of the intestinal epithelium (age-related reduction in jejunal mucosal surface area) which results in a decreased surface area for drug absorption.[3] Most drugs are absorbed by passive diffusion, which is dependent on a concentration gradient. In the elderly, there is diminished blood flow in the splanchnic area and decreased mesenteric blood flow, both of which will reduce the concentration gradient. This often results in a slower rate of absorption, which in turn causes an increased time to reach peak drug levels. The extent of absorption is seldom affected by increasing age. In reality, there would appear to be few effects on kinetics of drugs as a result of changes in their absorption.[3,4]

One important exception to the 'no effect of ageing on absorption' is levodopa. This drug is widely used in the elderly population to treat Parkinson's disease. There is a substantial increase in the absorption of this drug in old age, presumably due to a reduced amount of dopa-decarboxylase in the gastric mucosa.[5]

The absorption of vitamin B_{12}, iron and calcium through active transport mechanisms is reduced,[2] although many other drugs transported actively are not affected. Even poorly absorbed drugs such as ampicillin are equally absorbed in the elderly and the younger population.[4]

Gastric pH increases with age, which could theoretically affect absorption, but so far this is not proven.[2]

Table 2.1   Summary of absorption changes

Reduced amount of saliva
Increasing gastric pH
Reduced gastric acid secretion
Increased gastric emptying time
Decreased gastric surface area
Decreased gastrointestinal motility
Decreased active transport mechanisms

The decrease in regional blood flow in older people may alter the rate of absorption after intramuscular or subcutaneous injections. Few clinically significant effects occur as a result of this effect. The decrease in blood flow is often caused by replacement of well-perfused tissue by connective tissue and fat.[6]

The changes in absorption are summarised in Table 2.1.

In conclusion, there is little evidence that changes in liberation and absorption in older people will influence their handling of drugs, hence the dose of most drugs need not be altered in old age because of altered gastrointestinal function.

Distribution

Changes in drug distribution in old age are generally related to either changes in body fat and water or changes in protein binding. In addition, cardiac output is reduced and peripheral vascular resistance increases, resulting in a reduction in the total systemic perfusion of organs. The kidneys and liver receive reduced amounts of blood that will in turn reduce the capability for metabolism and excretion (see below).[7]

The ageing body changes significantly in composition, which will influence drug distribution. In the older person, lean body mass declines by as much as 12–19%.[8] This will cause higher blood levels for drugs distributed in muscle such as digoxin.[9] Adipose tissue mass increases by 14–35% in relation to total body weight even in the absence of overt obesity. There is a decrease in total body water. The effect of these changes on drug distribution depends largely on a drug's lipid- or water-solubility.

These changes will result in an alteration to the volume of distribution (V_d) of drugs. The V_d is a proportionality constant, defined as the amount of drug in the body (A) divided by the concentration (Cp) in the plasma (i.e. as the amount in the body increases or decreases –

depending on when the last dose was taken – the plasma concentration also increases or decreases).

$$V_d = \frac{A}{Cp}$$

The lower the V_d, the less well distributed the drug is in body tissue (e.g. warfarin) and the higher the V_d, the more extensively it is distributed (e.g. nortriptyline, amiodarone).

Clearly, altered V_d will produce changes in drug half life and the duration of drug effect. If a drug is lipid-soluble, then it is expected that there would be a rise in the V_d because of the increase in body fat in elderly people. This holds true for drugs such as diazepam,[10] thiopental, lidocaine (lignocaine)[11] and clomethiazole, where increased V_d and $t_{1/2}$ have been shown. For these drugs there will be increased tissue levels and prolonged duration of effect.

The converse is true for water-soluble drugs, where it is expected that there would be a decrease in V_d with the decrease in total body water, resulting in increased plasma levels. Gentamicin, digoxin,[9] ethanol, theophylline and cimetidine fall into this category. Loading doses of digoxin need to be reduced to accommodate these changes.

As well as alterations in V_d, protein binding is affected. This accounts for many adverse drug effects. There are two principal changes – a decrease in plasma albumin and an increase in α_1-acid glycoprotein.[12] The influences of altered protein binding are complex and become especially significant in those with chronic hepatic or renal disease and people who are undernourished and debilitated.

For the elderly, the plasma albumin decrease is between 10 and 20%.[13] Acidic drugs, such as cimetidine and furosemide (frusemide), tend to bind extensively to albumin, hence there is a increased free fraction of these drugs. There are obvious implications for other highly protein-bound drugs such as non-steroidal anti-inflammatory drugs (NSAIDs),[14] oral anticoagulants, phenytoin and sulphonylureas. Dosage reductions should be considered. Lidocaine, a basic drug, binds to α_1-acid glycoprotein. The free fraction may be reduced due to higher levels of the protein.[15]

Phenytoin is significantly bound to plasma albumin, hence there is an increase in the unbound fraction in elderly people. However, as a result of the increased free fraction, there is an increased proportion of drug available for elimination, resulting in increased clearance.[16] This means that dosage need not be altered (however, measured drug serum levels will tend to be reduced as they may not reflect any changes in free

Table 2.2   Summary of distribution changes

Reduced cardiac output
Increased peripheral vascular resistance
Decreased renal blood flow
Decreased hepatic blood flow
Reduced body water
Increased body fat tissue
Altered V_d (increased for lipid-soluble and decreased for water-soluble drugs)
Reduced serum albumin levels

fraction and allowance for this effect should be made in their interpretation). This is a good example of the complexity of the implications of pharmacokinetic changes in the elderly.

It is in the acute phase of drug administration that these changes are most significant; when a new dose regimen has settled down to a steady state, homeostatic mechanisms will tend to counteract and negate any kinetic changes.

Changes in distribution are summarised in Table 2.2.

Metabolism

Drug metabolism is mainly carried out in the liver but occurs to a limited extent in other organs such as the kidney and lungs. The reduced hepatic blood flow of up to 40% in the elderly severely reduces the amount of drug delivered to the liver.[17]

Many lipid-soluble drugs undergo first-pass metabolism after oral administration, as they are transported via the portal circulation to the liver. This causes a significant reduction in systemic bioavailability. Even small decreases in the first-pass effect will result in major alterations in bioavailability as often 90–95% first-pass metabolism occurs. Drugs such as nifedipine, labetalol, nitrates and verapamil will be affected. For nifedipine, there will be a clinically significant reduction in blood pressure, due to an increased amount of drug being available.[18]

For those drugs eliminated by hepatic metabolism, the metabolic capacity of the liver is reduced significantly, by up to 60%, resulting in increased plasma concentrations and longer half-lives. Examples include NSAIDs, antiepileptics and analgesics.[14, 16]

The rate of drug delivery to the liver is an important factor in metabolic capacity. In the elderly, liver perfusion is reduced and this significantly affects the metabolism of hypnotics and antipsychotic drugs such as clomethiazole and chlorpromazine. There is a delicate

Table 2.3   Summary of metabolic changes

Reduced microsomal hepatic oxidation
Reduced clearance
Increased steady-state levels
Increased half-lives
Increased levels of active metabolites
Reduced first-pass metabolism due to reduced hepatic blood flow

balance between the reduced perfusion, increased free fractions (from the plasma protein changes) and clearance. Drugs can be divided into three groups – those of high, medium and low clearance.[18]

High-clearance drugs have a high hepatic extraction ratio. This means that there is a high proportion of the drug removed from the circulation on one pass through the liver. This means that their rate of metabolism is highly dependent on hepatic blood flow.[19] Included in this category are morphine, propranolol and many of the calcium antagonists. Their clearance will be decreased as a result of reduced first-pass metabolism and reduced blood flow, which may cause clinically significant problems. Levels of the calcium channel blockers may be 1.5–2 times higher in an elderly population compared to the population at large.

For drugs with lower clearance and a lower hepatic extraction ratio, the intrinsic metabolic capacity of the liver will be the major rate-determining factor.[19] There are few conclusive studies about the absolute effect of ageing on the liver enzymes, but it is generally felt that there is a tendency for drugs subject to oxidative phase I metabolism to show decreased elimination with a lesser tendency for an age-associated reduction in phase II conjugative function.

Changes in metabolism are summarised in Table 2.3.

Elimination

Many drugs are eliminated solely or mainly by renal excretion of the unchanged drug – digoxin and gentamicin are two examples. It can be clearly shown for these drugs that elimination rate is related to glomerular filtration rate (GFR). Between the ages of 20 and 80 years, there is a 20% decrease in kidney size with a 30% loss of functioning glomeruli. This may result in up to 50% loss of normal renal function.[20] As well as a reduced number of nephrons, there is also a reduction in active tubular secretion and reabsorption. The clinical significance of this is yet to be established.

If renal disease results in impairment, it will exaggerate the age-reduced clearance. Elderly people may have normal plasma creatinine levels but still have a reduced creatinine clearance, because serum creatinine concentrations are a result of a balance between production of creatinine by muscle tissue and clearance of creatinine by the kidney. Creatinine production is less as there is a decrease in muscle mass, so the decreased renal clearance is compensated, thus giving 'normal' serum levels.[21]

Since GFR and tubular secretion decrease at a constant rate with increasing age, renal elimination can be correlated with creatinine clearance. This allows dosing to be adjusted downwards if creatinine clearance can be calculated.

It is essential that the declining renal function be taken into account when doses of highly toxic drugs with a narrow therapeutic range are used. Digoxin and gentamicin are two examples of critical importance. Detailed nomograms have been developed to help calculate both loading and continuing doses in the elderly, taking into account the declining renal function. The most commonly used is the Cockcroft and Gault equation:

$$\text{Cr clearance}_{(males)} = (140 - age) \times (weight\ in\ kg)/72 \times serum\ Cr\ (mg/dl)$$

For females, the result is multiplied by 0.85.

Acute illness can lead to a rapid decrease in renal clearance. Hence an elderly patient already established and stable on a drug with a narrow therapeutic index – such as digoxin – may rapidly develop toxicity and adverse effects when he or she contracts a severe chest infection or has a myocardial infarction.

Pharmacodynamic changes

As well as kinetic changes, the natural loss of function of body tissues at the cellular level must be taken into account when considering drug use in the elderly.

Central nervous system (CNS) changes may be significant. Movement disorders and forgetfulness may be due to faulty neurotransmitter metabolism rather than loss of neurons. Increased confusion may be related to reduced cerebral blood flow. Changes in autonomic function may cause bradycardia and a significant incidence of thermoregulatory disorders. Failure of vasoconstriction in cold weather can produce hypothermia. Alcohol can worsen the situation as it also decreases awareness of temperature.[22]

In the very old (over 85 years), manifestations of normal ageing may be mistaken for disease and lead to inappropriate prescribing. The most common example of this is the long-term use of prochlorperazine for giddiness due to age-related loss of postural stability. Not only is such treatment ineffective, but the patient may experience serious side-effects such as drug-induced parkinsonism, postural hypotension and mental confusion.

As well as having reduced function, older people appear to exhibit altered responses to drugs. This is a very difficult aspect to study or quantify because of the many other factors in elderly people, which may confuse the results, such as coexisting disease and poor nutritional state.

The possible mechanisms underlying altered responses include bio-mechanical responses, receptor mechanisms, homeostatic changes and altered CNS function in old age (Table 2.4).

A great many drugs exhibit their primary action at specific receptor sites. These include receptors in the adrenergic, cholinergic and dopaminergic systems; calcium antagonist action at the calcium channel sites; digoxin actions at sodium/potassium ATPase; and receptors for benzodiazepines, opioids, anticonvulsants and some antidepressants.

Changes in receptors may result in changes in drug responses in several ways. There may be an alteration in receptor density (numbers of receptors), affinity (receptor–ligand interaction), receptor membrane environment or mechanism of binding. Any or all of these may alter the physiological response to a drug.

Drugs affecting the β-adrenergic system are the most widely studied group in this category. Both salbutamol (agonist) and propranolol (antagonist) show decreased responses in the elderly. These effects are caused by decreased β-receptor function due to reduced production of cyclic AMP following receptor stimulation. The total number of receptors seems to be the same but the postreceptor events are changed because of the altered intracellular environment.[23,24]

Homeostasis – the body's ability to maintain a constant biochemical and physiological environment by a complex integrated set of peripheral

Table 2.4 Possible sources of pharmacodynamic effects in the elderly

- Drug–receptor interactions
- Receptor–cell membrane interactions
- Postreceptor events
- Structural changes in organs or tissues
- Homeostatic functions

Table 2.5 Drugs that are particularly affected by changes in the older population

Analgesics	Opioids show an increased level of side-effects such as nausea, hypotension and central nervous system effects due to higher blood levels. Pentazocine, pethidine and dextropropoxyphene (ingredient of co-proxamol) are to be used with extreme care
	Non-steroidal anti-inflammatory drugs (NSAIDS) with long half-lives such as piroxicam should be avoided altogether. All NSAIDs cause fluid retention that may negate treatments for heart failure and hypertension. There is also an increased risk of both renal failure and gastrointestinal toxicity
Digoxin	In long-term use, the dose should be reduced to reflect reduced renal excretion
Diuretics	Predictable side-effects such as hyponatraemia, postural hypotension and incontinence are more common. Loop diuretic doses may need to be higher because their effect is reduced. Thiazides should be used in the lowest possible dose to minimise side-effects
H_2-antagonists	Excretion is reduced, giving rise to higher blood levels, resulting in increased risk of confusional states. Lower doses should be used
Warfarin	The anticoagulant effect is increased so smaller starting doses should be used
Angiotensin-converting enzyme (ACE) inhibitors	Small initial doses will minimise the risk of hypotension. Increased risk of renal impairment
β-Blockers	Small initial doses should be used. Bradycardia and precipitation of heart failure are more likely. Atenolol and sotalol have a renal excretion pathway that may be impaired, resulting in higher blood levels. Propranolol has reduced first-pass metabolism that will also increase levels
Benzodiazepines	Smaller doses should be used and for the minimum possible period. Those with short half-lives are best, e.g. lormetazepam
Phenothiazines	There is an increased risk of tardive dyskinesia, extrapyramidal effects and anticholinergic effects such as urinary retention and constipation. Hypothermia, especially in winter, is more common. Small doses with regular reviews are essential
Antiparkinsonian drugs	For levodopa, all predictable side-effects – confusion, postural hypotension and psychosis – are more common. Selegiline causes more agitation and confusion in elderly people and the anticholinergic drugs have their effects enhanced (constipation, dry mouth and urine retention)

and central feedback mechanisms – is essential to maintain life. This system becomes compromised in old age.[25] Postural hypotension is common. There is a blunting of the reflex tachycardia that occurs in younger people on standing or in response to vasodilation. One theory for this is that there is decreased baroreceptor response and reduced sodium conservation.[26] Many drugs will cause exaggerated postural hypotension as a result of these changes.

Phenothiazines have α-adrenergic blocking effects and will reduce blood pressure. Diuretics will reduce plasma volume, augmenting the poor homeostatic response.

There is increased susceptibility to many commonly used CNS drugs.[27] The brain shows particularly increased sensitivity and patients may become confused and disoriented at doses of drugs which are well tolerated in normal younger people where confusion is not a usual side-effect. These include benzodiazepines, antidepressants, neuroleptics and even NSAIDs. It is well documented that older people are more sensitive to the effects of the benzodiazepines even if there are no demonstrable kinetic changes. This may be due to increased penetration of the drug into the brain or an altered benzodiazepine receptor response.[27]

CNS effects are also seen with other drugs. In particular, the H_2-receptor antagonists, especially cimetidine, can cause confusion. Others that have been implicated include antiparkinsonian drugs, barbiturates, diuretics, hypoglycaemic agents, steroids and tricyclic antidepressants. (See Table 2.5 for drugs that are particularly affected by changes in the older population.)

Conclusion

It is essential that, as well as considering pharmacokinetic and pharmacodynamic changes in elderly people, the other influences on drug handling are also taken into account. While changes in kinetics with age may be significant, their predictive value and clinical significance may often be outweighed by the other variables such as disease, concomitant medication and environmental factors.

Dealing with elderly people's medication is complex, with many variables – altered handling and sensitivity; underlying disease; polypharmacy; social circumstances and environmental factors. The natural ageing process will impair communication with defects in hearing and eyesight as well as mobility. It is essential to consider each elderly person individually and tailor-make each treatment as there are so many variables.

One important aspect to be aware of is the 'prescribing cascade'[28] effect – where medication is prescribed when an ADR is mistaken for a change in medical condition. The greater the number of drugs an old person is taking, the greater the chance of drug interactions and ADRs.

One example of the prescribing cascade is the use of NSAIDs that cause fluid retention and possibly oedema. If a thiazide diuretic is then prescribed to treat the oedema, hyperuricaemia may result, which may lead to treatment for gout being started.

To ensure that there is minimal risk in using medication for this already vulnerable group of people, a few simple rules should be followed:

1. Medication should be kept to a minimum and only used where there is established benefit. One should always consider carefully whether or not a drug is actually needed before it is given. Could non-drug alternatives such as dietary advice be used instead? This could be of particular importance for laxatives. Hypnotics cause multiple problems and should be avoided if at all possible.
2. Drugs which have the potential to interact or oppose each other should be avoided. Equally, drugs should be prescribed bearing in mind the other diseases present in an individual. A patient with bladder instability is unlikely to be happy with a diuretic used to treat mild hypertension. Suitable alternatives should be considered.
3. Regular reviews of prescribing should take place. Symptoms should be investigated and not just treated with medication. Body ageing is a constant process and vigilance is essential to stay aware of the dynamic situation, such as the possible development of reduced cardiac function.
4. Kinetic changes must always be borne in mind. Highly metabolised drugs require low starting doses with careful upward titration against response, for example, clomethiazole. Creatinine clearance should be used as a measure of renal function to help choose doses for renally cleared drugs such as gentamicin.
5. Drugs that are known to affect homeostatic feedback should be used with caution.
6. Therapeutic drug monitoring should be employed where appropriate, to ensure optimal dosing.
7. Concordance must always be considered and suitable dosage forms used to maximise the potential for full concordance with a prescribed regimen.

As pharmacists, we have a major role in monitoring the use of medication in older people. We can help reduce hospital admissions and unnecessary suffering by optimising drug therapy.

References

1. Col N, Fanale J E, Kronholm P. The role of medication in non-compliance and adverse drug reactions in hospitalisations of the elderly. *Arch Intern Med* 1990; 150: 841–845.
2. Bhanthumnavin K, Schuster M M. Ageing and gastrointestinal function. In: Finch C E, Hayflick L, eds. *Handbook of the Biology of Ageing*. New York: Van Nostrand Reinhold, 1977: 709–723.
3. Castleden C M, Volans C N, Raymond K. The effect of ageing on drug absorption from the gut. *Age Ageing* 1977; 6: 138–143.
4. Iber F L, Murphy P, Connor E S. Age-related changes in the gastrointestinal system. Effects on drug therapy. *Drugs Aging* 1994; 5: 34–38.
5. Klawans H L. Emerging strategies in Parkinson's disease. *Neurology* 1990; 40 (suppl 3): 1–76.
6. Editorial. Drug use in the elderly: a review of problems and special considerations. *Drugs* 1978; 16: 358–382.
7. Woodhouse K W, Ewynne H A. Age-related changes in liver size and hepatic blood flow: the influence of drug metabolism in the elderly. *Clin Pharmacokinet* 1988; 15: 328–344.
8. Main A. Elderly patients and their drugs. *Pharm J* 1988; 240: 537–539.
9. Cusack B, Horgan J, Kelly J G *et al.* Digoxin in the elderly: pharmacokinetic consequences of old age. *Clin Pharmacol Ther* 1979; 25: 772–776.
10. Klotz U, Avant G R, Hoyumpa A *et al.* The effects of age and liver disease in the distribution and elimination of diazepam in adult man. *J Clin Invest* 1975; 55: 347–359.
11. Nation R L, Triggs E J, Selig M. Lidocaine kinetics in cardiac patients and elderly subjects. *Br J Clin Pharmacol* 1977; 4: 439–448.
12. Reidenberg M M, Erill S, eds. *Drug–Protein Binding*. New York: Praeger, 1986: 163–171.
13. Wallace S M, Verbeeck R V. Plasma protein binding of drugs in the elderly. *Clin Pharmacokinet* 1987; 12: 41–72.
14. Solomon D H, Gurwitz J H. Toxicity of nonsteroidal anti-inflammatory drugs in the elderly: is advanced age a risk factor? *Am J Med* 1997; 102: 208–215.
15. Cusack B, O'Malley K, Lavan J *et al.* Protein binding and disposition of lidocaine in the elderly. *Eur J Clin Pharmacol* 1985; 29: 323–329.
16. Bach B, Molholm-Hansen J, Kamomann J P *et al.* Disposition of antipyrine and phenytoin correlated with age and liver volume in man. *Clin Pharmacokinet* 1981; 6: 389–396.
17. Tregaskis B F, Stevenson I H. Pharmacokinetics in old age. *Br Med Bull* 1990; 46: 9–21.
18. Durnas C, Loi C, Cusack B. Hepatic drug metabolism and ageing. *Clin Pharmacokinet* 1990; 19: 359–389.
19. Wilkinson G R, Shand D G. A physiological approach to hepatic drug metabolism. *Clin Pharmacol Ther* 1975; 18: 377–390.
20. Davies D F, Shock N W. Age changes in glomerular filtration rate, effective renal plasma flow and tubular excretory capacity in adult males. *J Clin Invest* 1950; 29: 496–501.

21. Rowe J W, Andres R, Tobin J D *et al*. The effect of age on creatinine clearance in man: a cross sectional and longitudinal study. *J Gerontol* 1976; 31: 155–163.
22. Feeley J, Coakley D. Altered pharmacodynamics in the elderly. *Clin Geriatr Med* 1990; 6: 269–283.
23. Vestal R E, Wood A J J, Shand D G. Adrenoreceptor status and cardiovascular function in ageing. *J Hypertens* 1988; **6** (suppl 1): S59–S62.
24. Vestal R E, Wood A J J, Shand D G. Reduced beta-adrenoreceptor sensitivity in the elderly. *Clin Pharmacol Ther* 1979; 26: 181–186.
25. Swift C G. Pharmacodynamics: changes in homeostatic mechanisms, receptor and target organ sensitivity in the elderly. *BMJ* 1977; 1: 10–12.
26. McGarry K, Laher M, Fitzgerald D *et al*. Baroreflex function in elderly hypertensives. *Hypertension* 1983; 5: 763–766.
27. Gordon M, Preiksaitis H G. Drugs and the ageing brain. *Geriatrics* 1988; 43: 69–78.
28. Rochon P A, Gurwitz J H. Optimising drug treatment for elderly people: the prescribing cascade. *BMJ* 1997; 315: 1096–1099.

Further reading

Beeley L. *Safer Prescribing*, 5th edn. London: Blackwell Scientific Publications, 1992.
Grimley Evans J, Franklyn Williams T, eds. *Oxford Textbook of Geriatric Medicine*. Oxford: Oxford Medical Publications, 1992.
Shetty H, Woodhouse K. Geriatrics. In: Walker R, Edwards C, eds. *Clinical Pharmacy and Therapeutics*. Edinburgh: Churchill Livingstone, 1994: Chapter 8.

3

Gastrointestinal medicines in the elderly

Anne E Kinnear and Moira Kinnear

The gastrointestinal tract shown in Figure 3.1 is subject to age-related pathophysiological changes placing the elderly at an increased risk of gastrointestinal diseases and associated increased morbidity. Diseases of the elderly, such as stroke, Parkinson's disease and hypothyroidism, are often associated with decreased gastrointestinal motility resulting in disorders of the gastrointestinal tract from the oesophagus to the colon, the most common of which will be covered in this chapter.

Constipation is probably the most common chronic digestive complaint among the elderly population. The prevalence increases with age and is more common in women than men. However, defining constipation is complicated by differences in understanding of normal bowel function. Many older patients are under the impression that a daily bowel movement is required for good health. The prevalence therefore depends on the definition used.

Decreased gastric acid secretion is another physiological change associated with ageing and predisposes the elderly to bacterial overgrowth and associated complications of malabsorption.

Increases in plasma and biliary cholesterol concentrations predispose the elderly to coronary heart disease and gallstones. Gallstones can lead to acute pancreatitis which may also rarely be caused by drugs such as azathioprine and diuretics. Pancreatitis is not discussed in this chapter.

Approximately 10% of admissions to hospital are caused by drug-induced disorders and it is estimated that 40% of adverse drug reactions affect the gastrointestinal tract. Adverse drug effects on the gastrointestinal tract can be grouped into: pharmacological mode of action, impairment of gastrointestinal defences, direct injury and alteration in colonic bacterial flora. Polypharmacy in elderly patients increases the risk of drug-related adverse effects compared with younger individuals and increased morbidity associated with these reactions. Non-steroidal anti-inflammatory drugs (NSAIDs) are responsible for more toxicity in

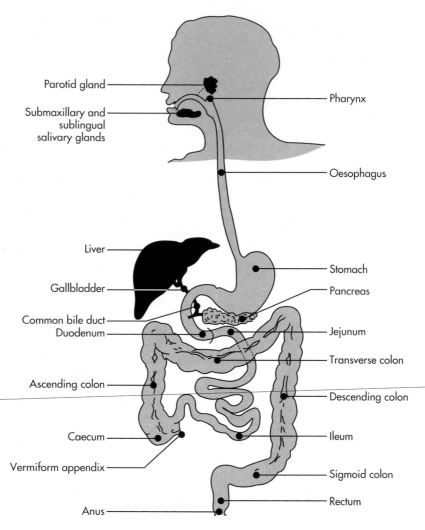

Figure 3.1 A schematic diagram of the gastrointestinal system.

elderly patients than any other single group of drugs: gastrointestinal toxicity plays a major role.

Altered bioavailability because of reduced liver blood flow and liver capacity are risk factors for adverse drug reactions in the liver, as is impaired hepatic metabolism.[1]

Drug-induced hepatotoxicity and the management of liver disease in the elderly will not be further discussed.

This chapter describes the therapeutic management and pharmaceutical care issues associated with gastrointestinal disorders, focusing on specific problems which occur commonly in the elderly population. The journey will commence at the oesophagus and will descend through the gastrointestinal tract, omitting the liver, pancreas and malignant diseases.

Dysphagia

Dysphagia can result from a variety of defects affecting the oral, pharyngeal or oesophageal phases of swallowing. In elderly patients with recent-onset dysphagia, cancer is a primary initial consideration. Such patients present with rapidly progressive dysphagia and weight loss.

Conditions particularly associated with dysphagia in the elderly include stroke, Parkinson's disease and, rarely, hypothyroidism. Pharmaceutical care issues often arise in patients who have difficulty swallowing and patients who receive enteral tube feeding, in particular, drug administration issues.[2] Case study 3.1 illustrates some of these issues.

Case study 3.1 JT, a 75-year-old man, presented with left-sided hemiparesis, slurred speech, hemianopia and dysphagia. Computer tomography revealed an infarct in the right cerebral hemisphere. Assessment confirmed he was unable to receive any oral intake and subsequently a nasogastric (NG) tube was passed. On admission he was taking nifedipine LA 30 mg in the morning for control of hypertension and phenytoin 300 mg at night for control of epileptic seizures

Drug administration issues	
Verify formulations are suitable for administration via NG tube	Long-acting preparation of nifedipine unsuitable for crushing Phenytoin liquid available
Verify bioequivalence of alternative formulations	Dosage calculation required for phenytoin liquid
Verify interactions with feeding solutions	Appropriate timing of doses
Verify appropriate process of administration	Flushing of tube

Xerostomia (dry mouth)

Drug-associated xerostomia is a problem in elderly patients, particularly since salivary production is known to decrease in this population. This may affect the ability to swallow solid dosage forms and absorption of sublingual or buccal preparations. Examples of drugs which commonly cause dry mouth are listed in Table 3.1.

Table 3.1 Drug-induced xerostomia

Drugs with antimuscarinic effects	
Drug class	Examples
Tricyclic antidepressants	Amitriptyline
Antiparkinsonian drugs	Benzatropine
Antiemetics	Prochlorperazine
Drugs for urinary frequency	Oxybutynin
Antispasmodics	Hyoscine
Antipsychotics	Phenothiazines
Antiarrhythmics	Disopyramide
Antidiarrhoeals	Co-phenotrope

Gastro-oesophageal reflux disease (GORD)

Diseases of the oesophageal mucosa are common in the elderly population and may present with symptoms of heartburn, dysphagia and chest pain. Although heartburn is the characteristic symptom of GORD, dysphagia, chest pain, acid reflux and a variety of respiratory symptoms such as coughing and wheezing may also occur. GORD may also be a contributing factor in elderly patients with chronic respiratory symptoms, even when they have no typical symptoms of GORD.[3] Prevalence, patterns and features of symptomatic GORD appear to be generally similar regardless of age. Symptoms in Barrett's oesophagus (replacement of squamous epithelium with metaplastic columnar epithelium and associated with increased risk of adenocarcinoma) appear to be less severe in elderly patients compared to their younger counterparts, although there appears to be an increased frequency of erosive oesophagitis, strictures and Barrett's oesophagus in elderly patients.[4] Endoscopy is the best diagnostic test and can establish a diagnosis of Barrett's oesophagus which can be found in up to 25% of older patients who receive endoscopic investigation of GORD symptoms.[5]

Symptomatic stricturing of the oesophagus complicates the course of about 10–15% of patients with GORD, particularly if elderly or if Barrett's oesophagus is making treatment more difficult and complex.[6]

Causes of GORD include abnormal oesophageal clearance, abnormalities in the lower oesophageal sphincter, delayed gastric emptying and oesophageal injury. Decreased salivary volume and bicarbonate production in elderly patients together with a higher incidence of hiatus hernia in elderly patients may contribute to an increased frequency of oesophagitis in this patient group. However, one study suggested that only 9% of patients with a hernia actually have typical reflux symptoms, suggesting that hiatus hernia alone has little importance as a cause of GORD.[7] Hiatus hernia is therefore not synonymous with GORD but can be considered a cofactor in patients who also have reduced lower oesophageal sphincter pressure.

Drug-induced oesophagitis occurs in all age groups and usually presents with difficulty and pain on swallowing and retrosternal chest pain. Difficulty in swallowing is often the only presenting symptom in the elderly. Medications either cause direct mucosal injury or pharmacologically they increase the risk of gastro-oesophageal reflux and/or mucosal injury from gastric acid. Examples of drug-induced oesophagitis are listed in Table 3.2.

Elderly patients are especially at risk of drug-induced oesophagitis because they have multiple factors which delay oesophageal transit time of medications, such as decreased salivation, multiple medications and bed rest and they are more likely to have anatomical or motility abnormalities. The symptoms associated with damage to the oesophageal mucosa usually occur several hours after ingestion of medication, particularly if taken at bedtime with minimal fluid.[4] Medications associated with complications and severe oesophageal injury include alendronate, potassium chloride and NSAIDs.[8] NSAIDs inhibit the mucosal cytoprotective mechanisms, increasing the risk for injury from gastric acid and other substances, whereas bisphosphonates such as alendronate or potassium chloride are caustic agents themselves. Patients should be advised to discontinue these drugs if symptoms such as retrosternal pain or dysphagia occur.

Table 3.2 Drug-induced oesophagitis

Drugs affecting lower oesophageal sphincter tone
Drugs with antimuscarinic effects
Calcium channel blockers
Nitrates
Theophylline
Alcohol, nicotine, caffeine

Drugs causing oesophageal mucosal injury
Non-steroidal anti-inflammatory drugs
Potassium chloride
Alendronate and other bisphosphonates
Iron
Tetracycline, doxycycline

Treatment of GORD

Treatment of drug-induced oesophagitis involves removal of the causative agent and treatment of the associated oesophagitis. Many cases of drug-induced oesophagitis can be prevented by educating patients about medication administration. If the oesophagus is partially obstructed it may be necessary for all oral drug therapy to be given as liquid formulations where possible.

Infectious oesophagitis caused by *Candida* or viruses such as herpes simplex or cytomegalovirus occasionally occurs in immuno-compromised elderly patients. Antifungal and antiviral treatments are required to treat such oesophagitis.[3]

The management of patients with GORD is similar in all age groups. GORD includes patients with oesophagitis in addition to endoscopy-negative patients who describe heartburn as the dominant symptom. The goals of treatment are to provide and maintain symptom relief and heal oesophagitis if present. A combination of pharmacological treatment and lifestyle modification are the principal treatments. Reflux surgery is an option in young patients but may be considered in otherwise fit elderly patients who do not respond to medical treatment. Eradication of *Helicobacter pylori* has no known role in the healing or maintenance of reflux disease.

Patients with erosive oesophagitis usually require therapy with proton pump inhibitors for complete symptom relief and healing. Proton pump inhibitor therapy heals a significantly higher proportion of patients with oesophagitis than H_2-receptor antagonists and healing occurs after a shorter duration of therapy.[9] Recurrence of erosive oesophagitis is observed in up to 80% of patients within 3–6 months if therapy is stopped. These patients usually require long-term therapy.[10]

The increased risk of adenocarcinoma in patients with Barrett's oesophagus has led to the practice of regular endoscopic surveillance and, if necessary, oesophageal resection. This practice is controversial and is only undertaken in patients who would benefit from oesophageal resection. Many centres repeat endoscopy every 12–24 months, more frequently if dysplastic changes are seen. Patients with Barrett's oesophagus require long-term proton pump inhibitor therapy to eliminate the acid-induced injury.

Recent evidence is now challenging the established stepped approach to the management of patients with heartburn symptoms or mild oesophagitis. Most practitioners continue to support changes in lifestyle and use of antacids as initial management of heartburn symptoms. If symptoms continue some patients respond to H_2-receptor antagonists, prokinetic agents or a combination of both.[11] The next step is proton pump inhibitor therapy. It has been suggested that early use of proton pump inhibitors may mask early gastric cancer and patients should be investigated endoscopically prior to initiating this therapy.[12] A more accurate diagnosis is obtained from endoscopy prior to management with proton pump inhibitors and, since elderly patients are at increased risk of gastric cancer and Barrett's oesophagus, they should be investigated endoscopically if there is no good response to initial antacid therapy.

Successful intermittent treatment with either omeprazole or ranitidine has recently been reported in patients with either normal endoscopy findings or mild oesophagitis.[13] In this study, symptom control was better at 2 weeks in those patients who received omeprazole 20 mg daily, but after 12 months approximately half the patients in both groups required maintenance therapy. Those who responded quickly to therapy were less likely to require maintenance treatment. The outcome was poorer in patients who smoked but age, unexpectedly, did not influence outcome. Proton pump inhibitor therapy is currently suggested as the initial medical treatment of choice in GORD and maintenance therapy should be chosen by step down to the least costly but effective regimen.[14]

Changes in lifestyle can help to provide symptom relief but do not allow healing of oesophagitis.[14] Although objective evidence to support lifestyle modification is lacking, advice includes: elevate the head of the bed, reduce fat in the diet, avoid eating within 2 h of retiring to bed, consume less coffee, chocolate and alcohol, and decrease or stop

---

Case study 3.1 (continued). JT experienced severe nausea and hiccups. He was prescribed metoclopramide 10 mg three times daily as required with no improvement. Hyoscine 20 mg was then prescribed four times daily, with little effect. Endoscopy confirmed a diagnosis of severe erosive oesophagitis and a proton pump inhibitor was prescribed

---

Pharmaceutical care issues

Verify appropriate symptomatic treatment	Symptoms not specific to gastro-oesophageal reflux disease
	Risk of antimuscarinic effects of hyoscine
Verify appropriate choice and duration of acid suppressant in severe oesophagitis	Proton pump inhibitor appropriate
	Appropriate formulation choice for NG administration

smoking. A review of patients' medication and the discontinuation of medicines which may contribute to oesophageal injury is advisable.

The major side-effects associated with proton pump inhibitors are headache and diarrhoea. Side-effects are rarely reported with H_2-receptor antagonists, although confusion in the elderly has been reported with cimetidine. Pharmaceutical care issues are discussed in the case study given on the previous page (continued).

Drug interactions

Other pharmaceutical care issues commonly associated with drugs used to treat upper gastrointestinal disorders include drug interactions which result in either decreased efficacy or increased toxicity. Very few of these drug interactions are clinically significant or an important cause of morbidity. Interactions between antacids and tetracyclines can be avoided by adjusting the timing of drug administration. The absorption of keto-conazole is reduced with concomitant administration of H_2-receptor antagonists and proton pump inhibitors. Most other clinically important interactions involve the effect of one drug on the metabolism of another. Interactions can be predicted if the specific isoenzyme of the cytochrome P450 system responsible for drug metabolism is known. For example, cis-apride is metabolised by CYP 3A4. Antifungals, macrolide antibiotics and protease inhibitors reduce the metabolism of cisapride resulting in QT interval prolongation and ventricular arrhythmias. Fatal interactions have led to the withdrawal and review of the licence for cisapride. Omeprazole inhibits CYPs 2C9 and 2C19, the isoenzymes involved in the metabolism of, for example, phenytoin (2C9), S-warfarin (2C9), diazepam (2C19), R-warfarin (2C19). Omeprazole 40 mg daily has been shown to decrease the clearance of phenytoin,[15, 16] but phenytoin levels were unchanged after a dose of 20 mg omeprazole daily. Monitoring of phenytoin plasma concentrations is recommended. Omeprazole may increase the coagulation time in patients receiving warfarin therapy, especially if doses higher than 20 mg daily are given. Changes in the plasma concentration of the less potent (R) enantiomer of warfarin have been observed, therefore monitoring of the international normalised ratio (INR) is recommended during concomitant therapy. The less potent enantiomer, R-warfarin, also interacts with cimetidine[17] which is also known to reduce the clearance of theophylline and phenytoin. Food and antacids can reduce the bioavailability of lansoprazole,[18, 19] although all proton pump inhibitors are most effective if taken about 30 min before a meal as they inhibit only actively secreting proton pumps.

Peptic ulcer disease

NSAIDs

The principal causes of peptic ulcer disease are use of aspirin or NSAIDs and the presence of *H. pylori* infection. These are more common in elderly patients and therefore place elderly patients at higher risk than younger patients for developing peptic ulcer disease and its complications of major bleeding and perforation. There is also a greater prevalence of comorbid diseases such as cardiovascular disease. The average mortality from complicated peptic ulcer disease in the elderly is about 30%; the complication rate is approximately 50%.[20] The use of NSAIDs is associated with approximately 50% of complicated ulcers. The incidence of ulceration is on average three times higher in NSAID users than in non-users; the relative risk in patients greater than 60 years is 5.5.[21] Age-related reduction in the synthesis of prostaglandins and bicarbonate by the gastrointestinal mucosa provides a rationale for the increased risk of NSAID-induced damage to the gastric mucosa in elderly patients who often present without the warning symptoms of dyspepsia and abdominal pain. 'Silent' ulcers are usually detected at endoscopy.

Another rationale for increased incidence of toxicity in the elderly population is the increased frequency of prescriptions. Long-term aspirin therapy is used for thromboprophylaxis in elderly patients who have coronary artery disease, unstable angina and in those at risk for myocardial infarction or stroke. A meta-analysis to assess the incidence of gastrointestinal haemorrhage found that about 1 in 100 patients taking aspirin over 28 months will experience a gastrointestinal haemorrhage.[22] There was no evidence that reduction of dose lowered the risk and another study has confirmed that enteric coating does not reduce risk.[23] The risk of long-term aspirin in the elderly needs to be weighed against the potential benefits in thromboprophylaxis. NSAIDs are routinely prescribed for elderly patients with musculoskeletal conditions such as rheumatoid arthritis and osteoarthritis. Ibuprofen is recommended as the initial drug of choice as it has the lowest incidence of reported adverse drug reactions.[24, 25] Azapropazone is associated with the highest risk of gastrointestinal toxicity followed by piroxicam then indometacin and ketoprofen followed by diclofenac and naproxen.[24]

Although there is scepticism surrounding the use of topical NSAIDs, a systematic review has concluded that these agents are more effective than placebo in pain control.[26] Gastrointestinal toxicity has not been reported with topical administration of NSAIDs. Contrary to common belief, corticosteroids alone are an insignificant ulcer risk but potentiate the risk when taken concomitantly with NSAIDs.[27] Concomitant warfarin therapy increases the risk of gastrointestinal bleeding associated with peptic ulcer disease.

Enteric coating of NSAIDs does not reduce ulcer risk, as the major mechanism of NSAID-induced toxicity is the reduction of mucosal prostaglandin synthesis,[28] as illustrated in Figure 3.2.

Newer NSAIDs such as the cyclo-oxygenase-2 (COX-2) inhibitors have been designed to be gastro-protective through selectively inhibiting COX-2 enzyme, and sparing COX-1, the enzyme responsible for the synthesis of prostaglandins which protect the gastrointestinal mucosa. Celecoxib and rofecoxib have greater selectivity for COX-2 than meloxicam and etodolac. Large prospective, blinded, randomised trials have been completed looking at the toxicity and risk factors associated with COX-2 inhibitors compared with NSAIDs over a 6-month exposure period. The results showed that celecoxib, at dosages greater than those indicated clinically, was associated with a lower incidence of symptomatic ulcers and ulcer complications, compared with ibuprofen and diclofenac at standard dosages. The decrease in upper gastrointestinal toxicity was strongest among patients not taking aspirin concomitantly.[29]

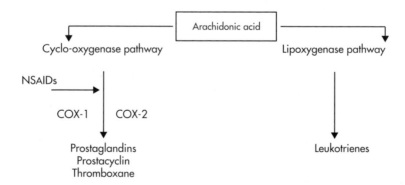

NSAIDs inhibit the synthesis of prostaglandins through inhibition of the enzyme cyclo-oxygenase (COX)
       COX-1 yields protective prostaglandins in the stomach
       COX-2 is induced in inflammation, producing pain, swelling and stiffness
Theory: selective COX-2 inhibitors may reduce inflammation without damage to the stomach

Figure 3.2 Mechanism of non-steroidal anti-inflammatory drug (NSAID)-induced gastrointestinal toxicity.

The other study in rheumatoid arthritis patients, none of whom took aspirin, shows that rofecoxib at a dose greater than recommended was also associated with a lower incidence of symptomatic ulcers and ulcer complications compared with naproxen at normal doses.[30] However, there was a higher rate of cardiovascular events in the rofecoxib group, a finding that requires further investigation. Caution should be exercised in patients with a history of cardiac failure or hypertension. Further data are needed to establish the long-term safety of these agents.

For further discussion of these issues, see Chapter 11.

H. pylori

The prevalence of *H. pylori* infection increases with age, with approximately 60% of those over 60 years of age being infected. The organism is thought to be acquired in childhood and infection rates are falling as living standards improve. High prevalence rates in elderly patients reflect the infection rate when they were children.

Over 95% of duodenal ulcers and over 80% of gastric ulcers are *H. pylori*-positive. Successful eradication alters the otherwise chronic relapsing nature of peptic ulcer disease by reducing ulcer recurrence rate and complications from peptic ulcer disease.

The particular method selected to determine the presence of *H. pylori* depends on whether an ulcer has already been diagnosed. In elderly patients receiving maintenance therapy for proven peptic ulcer disease, a urea breath test can be used. It is important to remember that both breath tests and endoscopic tests for *H. pylori* may produce false-negative results when performed within 4 weeks of eradication therapy, other antibiotic therapy or treatment with proton pump inhibitors. Serological tests for *H. pylori* are less accurate and false-positive rates of 30% have been reported in the elderly.[31] This method is unsuitable for assessing successful eradication as it takes several months for antibody levels to fall.

Endoscopy is the preferred means of diagnosis. It is well tolerated in elderly patients and it allows biopsies to be taken in order to exclude malignancy and test for the presence of *H. pylori*. Repeat endoscopy is necessary to confirm healing of gastric ulcers but is not necessary for uncomplicated duodenal ulcers.

Treatment of peptic ulcer disease

The management of patients with peptic ulcer disease is similar in all age groups. *H. pylori* eradication rates above 90% can be achieved by triple therapy, consisting of a proton pump inhibitor plus two of the following anti-infectives: amoxicillin, metronidazole, clarithromycin. Combinations which include clarithromycin are effective when metronidazole-resistant strains of *H. pylori* are present. Bismuth-containing quadruple therapy achieves eradication in some patients who repeatedly fail triple therapy.[32] Compliance is an important factor in successful eradication. Effective 7-day, twice-daily regimens cause fewer adverse effects than previously recommended therapies of longer duration. The most common adverse effect associated with recommended regimens is diarrhoea. Some patients find this intolerable and in some elderly patients when eradication has failed or when eradication therapy is contraindicated because of adverse effects or drug interactions, it may remain appropriate to continue maintenance therapy with H_2-receptor antagonists.

Patient management of NSAID-associated ulcers should include discontinuation of the NSAID, substituting simple analgesics and other non-drug means of management when possible. Ulcer healing is slower in patients who must continue NSAID therapy. Both H_2-receptor antagonists and proton pump inhibitors heal ulcers effectively, with similar healing rates after discontinuation of the NSAID. If the NSAID is continued, omeprazole 20 mg daily has better healing rates than ranitidine 150 mg twice daily and misoprostol 200 μg four times daily after 8 weeks' treatment.[33, 34] Once healed, omeprazole 20 mg daily has been shown to be more effective than misoprostol 200 μg twice daily or ranitidine 150 mg twice daily in preventing ulcer recurrence in those who continue NSAID therapy.[33, 34] Studies are required to compare the relative risk reduction associated with the use of gastro-protection and/or COX-2 inhibitors.

H. pylori and NSAIDs have been described as 'independent, though possibly additive, risk factors for the development of ulcer disease'.[32] One study has suggested that successful eradication before NSAIDs are started could lessen the incidence of ulceration.[35] Another study has demonstrated that *H. pylori* eradication impairs ulcer healing in NSAID users.[36] Long-term studies are needed to clarify these findings.

Endoscopic injection therapy arrests bleeding in most complicated ulcers. Surgery is required for those with continuing or recurrent bleeding or those with perforation.

Non-ulcer dyspepsia

Elderly patients with symptoms of dyspepsia should be investigated, preferably by endoscopy, in view of the higher proportion of patients in whom a diagnosis of peptic ulcer or GORD is made and also the higher risk of malignancy.[37] Non-ulcer dyspepsia or functional dyspepsia is the term used to describe dyspepsia symptoms when no lesion is observed on endoscopic investigation. It is common in both sexes of all age groups and accounts for approximately 50% of all cases of dyspepsia. Approach to management in patients with predominant symptoms of heartburn should be similar to that for patients with GORD.

Even though *H. pylori* is prevalent in approximately 60% of the elderly population, eradication of the organism in non-ulcer dyspepsia is controversial. Randomised controlled trials have given conflicting results but a meta-analysis has demonstrated a small but significant benefit associated with eradication.[38] Elderly patients are more likely to suffer adverse effects associated with eradication therapy and therefore the benefit must be weighed against this risk.

Drugs associated with peptic ulcer disease and with oesophagitis, as previously listed, may cause dyspepsia symptoms without causing mucosal damage. It is important to take a drug history and, if required, review the need for and choice of drugs which are associated with dyspepsia.

Some patients experience pain which resembles myocardial ischaemia but no cardiac or oesophageal abnormalities are identified. This type of pain is often not responsive to acid-suppressing agents which should not be continued beyond a trial period of a few weeks if symptoms do not respond.

Malabsorption

The only age-related defect in intestinal absorption that has been demonstrated is the absorption of calcium, a risk factor for osteoporosis. However, dietary vitamin D deficiency and impaired renal function are considered to be more important factors than a decline in gastrointestinal function. Malabsorption in elderly patients is generally considered, as in younger individuals, to be caused by disease processes affecting the gastrointestinal tract and not to the ageing process *per se*. Calcium deficiency in elderly patients responds to oral calcium supplementation.

Diseases associated with malabsorption include chronic pancreatitis, coeliac disease and Crohn's disease. Deficiency of iron, vitamin B_{12} and folic acid may occur and require replacement.

Bacterial overgrowth can occur in the presence of anatomical changes secondary to gastrointestinal surgery, changes in intestinal motility and also in the presence of achlorhydria.[39] It usually presents with painless diarrhoea and is best confirmed using the breath hydrogen test. Treatment with broad-spectrum antibiotics aims to remove the causative organisms.

Constipation

A number of definitions of constipation exist, including a functional inability to produce stool at regular intervals. The *British National Formulary* (No 41, 2001) definition is 'the passage of hard stools less frequently than the patient's own normal pattern'.

Constipation is more common in the elderly population, affecting 20% of people aged over 65. In long-stay elderly patients, the prevalence of chronic constipation has been reported to be as high as 40%. Most elderly people have a normal bowel habit but use a greater number of laxatives. This may be because elderly people are under the impression that a daily bowel movement is required. In this case laxative use is inappropriate as there is no organic cause.[40, 41]

Contributory factors

Physiological changes that contribute to constipation include deficient colonic propulsion, pain on defecating, ignoring the urge to stool and impaired rectal sensation.

Constipation in the elderly develops in association with immobility and is therefore more common in institutions. Although whole gut transit time is unchanged with healthy old age, it has been found to be significantly prolonged in immobile constipated patients. Regular exercise reduces whole gut transit times. The sigmoid colon and rectum

Table 3.3 Disease-induced constipation

Anorectal abnormalities	Neurological
	Stroke
Gut lesions	Parkinson's disease
Colorectal carcinoma	Multiple sclerosis
Intestinal obstruction	Paraplegia
Idiopathic megacolon	
Aganglionosis	**Metabolic and endocrine**
	Hypercalcaemia
Psychiatric	Hypokalaemia
Depression	Hypothyroidism
Dementia	

Table 3.4 Drug-induced constipation

Drugs with antimuscarinic effects
Opioid analgesics
Diuretics
Aluminium antacids
Iron
Calcium channel blockers
Prolonged use of laxatives
Digoxin toxicity

appear to be the sites of delay. This, in turn, may have an effect on drug transit time and absorption.

Dehydration and low-fibre diets also contribute to constipation. A fluid intake of 2000 ml/day and an increase in dietary fibre may be all that is required in such cases.[42]

Disease may lead to constipation. Diseases causing constipation are listed in Table 3.3.

Drugs may also cause constipation. Common causative agents are listed in Table 3.4.

Constipation is often associated with faecal impaction in the elderly. Faecal impaction is often considered to represent rectal loading with hard faeces. However, many elderly patients have faecal loading with soft or liquid faeces, which may lead to faecal soiling.

Treatment of constipation

A review of the effectiveness of laxatives in the elderly by the NHS Centre for Reviews and Dissemination at York in 1997 concluded that information on the effectiveness of laxatives in the elderly is limited. Trials carried out have been small and not representative of the elderly population in the community. There is little evidence to suggest major differences in effectiveness between the different laxatives.[43]

Initial treatment of faecal impaction is to empty the rectum and colon using enemas or suppositories on a daily basis until the mass is cleared. Laxatives or stool softeners are inappropriate if impaction is with soft stools, as further softening may increase incontinence. Manual evacuation may be required with hard faeces impaction, especially in patients with spinal cord lesions. The goal is to maintain an empty rectum to prevent recurrence. High dietary fibre intake should be avoided as it has been shown to add to existing constipation in immobile elderly patients.

For soft stools, a stimulant laxative should be used, for example, senna. For hard stools, an osmotic laxative is an appropriate choice.

Table 3.5 Indications for laxative use

- When patients cannot achieve a regular pattern of bowel movement, despite dietary changes, increased exercise and fluid intake
- Where it is desirable to avoid straining at stool, for example, bleeding piles, ischaemic heart disease, lumbar disc prolapse
- In order to re-educate the bowel, for example in elderly patients who are chronically laxative-dependent with overflow diarrhoea or urinary incontinence due to faecal impaction
- To overcome side-effects of necessary drug therapy
- Treatment of irritable bowel syndrome or diverticular disease

A combination laxative, such as co-danthrusate, may occasionally be required.[40] Once the diagnosis has been made and any underlying cause corrected, laxative treatment may be necessary (Table 3.5).

Laxatives can be divided into bulking agents, osmotic agents, stimulant agents and faecal softeners.[44–47]

There are four main types of bulking agents: wheat bran, methyl-cellulose, mucilaginous gums such as sterculia and mucilaginous seed coats and husks such as ispaghula. These act by increasing both water retention and microbial growth, thereby increasing faecal weight, water and gas content and so stimulating peristalsis. The onset of action may take days. All agents require to be taken with plenty of fluid to lubricate the colon in order to reduce the risk of obstruction. Patients with very slow gut transit time may not fully respond and may require the addition of a stimulant. Some patients may suffer from abdominal discomfort, flatulence and bloating and some may find preparations unpalatable. Bulk-forming agents should be avoided in patients with stenosis, intestinal ulceration or adhesions as there is a risk of impaction.

The main osmotic laxative in use is lactulose, which is a synthetic disaccharide, broken down by bacteria in the colon to short-chain organic acids. These promote bacterial growth which increase faecal mass and osmotic pressure, thus producing an increase in stool water content and volume. The short-chain acids are absorbed in the colon so the effect does not continue throughout the whole colon. The onset of action may take 2 or 3 days. Abdominal discomfort and flatulence may be problematic at higher doses and tolerance may develop with long-term use.

A number of clinical trials have shown lactulose to be effective in elderly constipated patients. Studies have demonstrated that lactulose is superior to bulk laxatives and to stimulant laxatives but less effective than both used in combination.[41]

Other osmotic agents include the saline laxatives, for example, the phosphate and citrate salts which are administered rectally for relief of acute constipation and bowel evacuation prior to investigation and surgery. Their regular use should be avoided due to their sodium- and water-retaining properties. Magnesium salts may also be employed where rapid evacuation is required. Care must be taken in patients with renal impairment as accumulation may occur, leading to hypotension and central nervous system depression. Magnesium also reduces iron absorption.

Stimulant laxatives such as senna, bisacodyl and dantron act by direct stimulation of the colon and act within 12 h of ingestion, although rectal preparations act within 20–60 min where rapid relief of symptoms is required. Dose-related abdominal cramping is the most troublesome side-effect. Stimulants should be avoided in intestinal obstruction. Prolonged use may precipitate hypokalaemia. Large doses taken over many years have been reported to lead to atonic colon.

Dantron was withdrawn from use in 1987 following links with tumour formation in rodents. It is currently licensed only for the terminally ill and patients who must avoid straining at stool. The licence was changed in 1999 to exclude the elderly, a group which had previously been specifically mentioned. The report from the NHS Centre for Reviews and Dissemination at York indicates that costly dantron laxatives should not be routinely used, as evidence indicates that they are no more effective than cheaper alternatives.[43]

Docusate is the main faecal softener in use. It is an anionic surfactant which lowers the intestinal content surface tension, leading to fluid and fat penetration. It may also have a stimulant effect. An effect will take 1–3 days and may be an option for patients in whom straining must be avoided.

Movicol, a polyethylene glycol/electrolyte solution is a non-absorbed laxative which speeds up transit time and induces a dose-related increase in stool volume and water. The solution, formed by dissolving the sachet contents in 125 ml of water, is iso-osmolar and therefore does not upset overall fluid balance. There is no bacterial action required and therefore no excess wind production. It has been shown to be effective in the elderly and to be superior to lactulose.[48]

Diarrhoea

Common causes of diarrhoea in elderly patients include infection, faecal impaction, inflammatory bowel disease (IBD), irritable bowel syndrome, small-bowel bacterial overgrowth and drugs.

Drug-induced diarrhoea

Drug-induced diarrhoea can result from altered defences, mucosal damage and disruption of normal physiological fluid and electrolyte balance. Examples of drugs which induce diarrhoea are listed in Table 3.6.

Proton pump inhibitors and H_2-receptor antagonists reduce acid secretion and allow proliferation of gastric microflora. Diarrhoea is a reported adverse effect of these drugs and bacterial overgrowth as a result of achlorhydria is considered to be an underlying factor. Bacterial overgrowth is also associated with hypomotility. Anticholinergic drugs are frequently associated with constipation but rarely may be associated with diarrhoea secondary to hypomotility. Tacrine, the cholinesterase inhibitor used in Alzheimer's disease, causes diarrhoea due to its cholinergic activity.

Broad-spectrum antibiotics are probably the most common drugs which cause diarrhoea in the elderly. Disruption of normal colonic flora allows organisms such as *Clostridium difficile* to proliferate. The organism produces toxin which in severe cases can cause pseudomembranous colitis. Clindamycin, ampicillin, amoxicillin and the cephalosporins have been associated with this condition. Elderly patients in hospital or long-term care are at particular risk, especially if incontinent or if they have multiple pathology. Oral vancomycin or metronidazole are equally efficacious in the treatment of pseudomembranous colitis.[49]

Erythromycin produces diarrhoea as a result of its motilin-like prokinetic activity. Misoprostol, olsalazine, digoxin, auranofin and colchicine all cause secretory diarrhoea through different mechanisms. Magnesium-containing antacids cause osmotic diarrhoea. Other drugs such as NSAIDs cause diarrhoea through direct mucosal damage.

Inflammatory bowel disease

IBD shows a bimodal peak age of onset – 15–25 years and 50–80 years. The presentation of ulcerative colitis and Crohn's disease is similar in

Table 3.6 Drug-induced diarrhoea

Acid suppressants	Antibiotics
Tacrine	Digoxin
Theophylline	Auranofin
Magnesium	Olsalazine
Non-steroidal anti-inflammatory drugs	Colchicine
Amantadine	Misoprostol
Statins	

elderly and younger patients, although rectal bleeding appears less frequently in Crohn's disease of the elderly. Both diseases can have extensive colonic involvement but distal colonic disease is reported more frequently in older patients.[50] Elderly patients may present with non-specific symptoms which can be confused with infectious or ischaemic colitis, diverticulitis, carcinoma of the colon or pseudomembranous colitis.[51] In younger patients, irritable bowel syndrome is the main differential diagnosis. The most common symptoms are diarrhoea and abdominal pain. Anorexia and weight loss often feature but can occur in elderly patients with comorbid conditions. Diagnosis is usually confirmed by colonoscopy and biopsy in patients with signs of inflammation, such as raised C-reactive protein and erythrocyte sedimentation rate.

Medical treatment in IBD is similar for all age groups. Prolonged use of prednisolone in elderly patients may exacerbate diabetes mellitus, hypertension, congestive heart failure, osteoporosis or mental disturbances. Oral budesonide has been shown to be as effective as prednisolone in active Crohn's disease after 8 weeks' treatment and was associated with fewer adverse effects.[52] Budesonide has not however been shown to be effective in maintaining remission in Crohn's disease. Corticosteroids alone are not associated with peptic ulcer disease but add to the risk associated with NSAIDs in elderly patients.[27] Enteric-coated preparations of prednisolone are not recommended in IBD as there is a risk of reduced drug absorption. There is no difference in efficacy between the corticosteroid foam enema preparations and patient preference should be taken into consideration. This is particularly important in elderly patients who may have difficulty manipulating the device during the administration process.

The 5-aminosalicylate preparations sulfasalazine, mesalazine, olsalazine and balsalazide appear to be equally efficacious in ulcerative colitis and only sulfasalazine is licensed in active Crohn's disease. Haematological monitoring should be undertaken in patients receiving these agents which have been associated with blood disorders. Renal function should be monitored regularly in elderly patients and these agents should not be used in patients with moderate or severe renal impairment. Sulfasalazine is associated with a greater proportion of reported hypersensitivity reactions and olsalazine is known to cause watery diarrhoea.

Adverse effects associated with azathioprine treatment do not appear to be any different in the elderly population than in younger patients. Azathioprine-induced diarrhoea or pancreatitis are rare adverse effects. Regular haematological monitoring should be undertaken no matter the age of the patient.

NSAIDs are known to activate quiescent IBD and should be avoided whenever possible. Many patients with IBD present with systemic complications such as arthropathy or ankylosing spondylitis, for which NSAIDs may be of benefit, but their use must be balanced with the associated risks.

Faecal incontinence

Faecal incontinence, which is nearly always accompanied by urinary incontinence, can be due to a number of factors, including anorectal incontinence, dementia, immobility, unconsciousness and faecal impaction.

Anal and perianal disorders

Haemorrhoids

Common symptoms are bleeding, prolapse and discomfort. More serious pathology associated with these symptoms needs to be excluded. Topical preparations have no proven value. If necessary, surgical treatment is preferred.

Anal fissure

Most anal fissures heal spontaneously. Bulking laxatives, non-constipating analgesics and local anaesthetic gels may provide symptom relief. Glyceryl trinitrate ointment 0.2% has successfully reduced anal canal pressure and healed approximately 50% of patients with fissures.[53] Headaches associated with this treatment have occasionally curtailed its use.

Acknowledgements

We would like to thank Dr M Ford and Dr S Ghosh, Consultant Physicians at the Western General Hospital, Edinburgh and Dr C Stewart, Consultant Physician at the Royal Infirmary of Edinburgh, for their valuable comments.

References

1. Schmuker D L. Aging and the liver: an update. *J Gerontol* 1998; 53A: B315–B320.
2. Thomson F C, Naysmith M R, Lindsay A. Managing drug therapy in patients receiving enteral and parenteral nutrition. *Hosp Pharm* 2000; 7: 155–164.
3. Ouatu-Lascar R, Triadafilopoulos G. Oesophageal mucosal diseases in the elderly. *Drugs Aging* 1998; 12: 261–276.
4. Triadafilopoulos G, Sharma R. Features of symptomatic gastro-esophageal reflux disease in elderly patients. *Am J Gastroenterol* 1997; 92: 2007–2011.
5. Collen M J, Abdulian J D, Chen Y K. Gastroesophageal reflux disease in the elderly: more severe disease that requires aggressive therapy. *Am J Gastroenterol* 1995; 90: 1053–1057.
6. Barkun A N, Mayrand S. The treatment of peptic oesophageal strictures. *Can J Gastroenterol* 1997; 11 (suppl B): 94B–97B.
7. Palmer E D. The hiatus hernia–esophagitis–esophageal stricture complex. *Am J Med* 1968; 44: 566–572.
8. Kikendall J W. Pill-induced esophageal injury. *Gastroenterol Clin North Am* 1991; 20: 835–846.
9. Chiba N, De Gara C J, Wilkinson J M *et al.* Speed of healing and symptom relief in grade II to IV gastroesophageal reflux disease: a meta-analysis. *Gastroenterology* 1997; 112: 1798–1810.
10. Hetzel D J, Dent J, Reed W D *et al.* Healing and relapse of severe peptic esophagitis after treatment with omeprazole. *Gastroenterology* 1988; 95: 903–912.
11. Vigneri S, Termini R, Leandro G *et al.* A comparison of five maintenance therapies for reflux esophagitis. *N Engl J Med* 1995; 333: 1106–1110.
12. Griffen S M, Raimes S A. Proton pump inhibitors may mask early gastric cancer. *BMJ* 1998; 317: 1606–1607.
13. Bardhan K D, Muller-Lissner S, Bigard M A *et al.* Symptomatic gastro-oesophageal reflux disease: double blind controlled study of intermittent treatment with omeprazole or ranitidine. *BMJ* 1999; 318: 502–507.
14. Dent J, Brun J, Fendrick A M *et al.* An evidence-based appraisal of reflux disease management – the Genval workshop report. *Gut* 1999; 44 (suppl 2): S1–S16.
15. Gugler R, Jensen J C. Omeprazole inhibits oxidative drug metabolism: studies with diazepam and phenytoin *in vivo* and 7-ethoxycoumarin *in vitro*. *Gastroenterology* 1985; 89: 1235–1241.
16. Pritchard P J, Walt R P, Kitchingman G K *et al.* Oral phenytoin pharmacokinetics during omeprazole therapy. *Br J Clin Pharmacol* 1987; 24: 543–545.
17. Niopas I, Toon S, Aarons L, Rowland M. The effect of cimetidine on the steady-state pharmacokinetics and pharmacodynamics of warfarin in humans. *Eur J Clin Pharmacol* 1999; 55: 399–404.
18. Delhotal-Landes B, Cournot A, Vermerie N *et al.* The effect of food and antacids on lansoprazole absorption and disposition. *Eur J Drug Metab Disposition* 1991; 111: 315–320.

19. Bergstrand R, Grind M, Nyberg G, Olofsson B. Decreased oral bioavailability of lansoprazole in healthy volunteers when given a standardised breakfast. *Clin Drug Invest* 1995; 9: 67–71.

20. Peterson W L. Bleeding peptic ulcer: epidemiology and nonsurgical management. *Gastroenterol Clin North Am* 1990; 19: 155–170.

21. Gabriel S E, Jaakkimainen L, Bombardier C. Risk for serious gastrointestinal complications related to use of nonsteroidal anti-inflammatory drugs; a meta-analysis. *Ann Intern Med* 1991; 115: 787–796.

22. Derry S, Loke Y K. Risk of gastrointestinal haemorrhage with long term aspirin: meta-analysis. *BMJ* 2000; 321: 1183–1187.

23. Sorensen H T, Mellemkjaer L, Blot W J *et al.* Risk of upper gastrointestinal bleeding associated with use of low dose aspirin. *Am J Gastroenterol* 2000; 95: 2218–2224.

24. Rodriguez L A G, Jick H. Risk of upper gastrointestinal bleeding and perforation associated with individual non-steroidal anti-inflammatory drugs. *Lancet* 1994; 343: 769–772.

25. Langman M J S, Weil J, Wainwright P *et al.* Risks of bleeding peptic ulcer associated with individual non-steroidal anti-inflammatory drugs. *Lancet* 1994; 343: 1075–1078.

26. Moore R A, Tramer M, Carroll D *et al.* Quantitative systematic review of topically applied non-steroidal anti-inflammatory drugs. *BMJ* 1998; 316: 333–338.

27. Conn H O, Poynard T. Corticosteroids and peptic ulcer: meta-analysis of adverse events during steroid therapy. *J Intern Med* 1994; 236: 619–632.

28. Wolfe M M, Lichtenstein D R, Singh G. Gastrointestinal toxicity of non-steroidal antiinflammtory drugs. *N Engl J Med* 1999; 340: 1888–1899.

29. Silverstein F E, Faich G, Goldstein J L *et al.* Gastrointestinal toxicity with celecoxib vs nonsteroidal anti-inflammatory drugs for osteoarthritis and rheumatoid arthritis. The CLASS study. *JAMA* 2000; 284: 1247–1255.

30. Bombardier C, Laine L, Reicin A *et al.* Comparison of upper gastrointestinal toxicity of rofecoxib and naproxen in patients with rheumatoid arthritis. VIGOR study group. *N Engl J Med* 2000; 343: 1520–1528.

31. Liston R, Pitt M A, Banerjee A K. IgG ELISA antibodies and detection of *Helicobacter pylori* in elderly patients. *Lancet* 1996; 347: 269.

32. Lam S K, Talley N J. *Helicobacter pylori* consensus. Report of the 1997 Asia Pacific Consensus Conference on the management of *Helicobacter pylori* infection. *J Gastroenterol Hepatol* 1998; 13: 1–12.

33. Yeomans N D, Tulassay Z, Juhasz L *et al.* A comparison of omeprazole with ranitidine for ulcers associated with nonsteroidal antiinflammatory drugs. *N Engl J Med* 1998; 338: 719–726.

34. Hawkey C J, Karrasch J A, Szczepanski L *et al.* Omeprazole compared with misoprostol for ulcers associated with nonsteroidal antiinflammatory drugs. *N Engl J Med* 1998; 338: 727–734.

35. Chan F K, Sung J J, Chung S C *et al.* Randomised trial of eradication of *Helicobacter pylori* before non-steroidal anti-inflammatory drug therapy to prevent peptic ulcers. *Lancet* 1997; 350: 975–979.

36. Hawkey C J, Tulassay Z, Szczepanski L *et al.* Randomised controlled trial of *Helicobacter pylori* eradication in patients on non-steroidal anti-inflammatory drugs: HELP NSAIDs study. *Lancet* 1998; 352: 1016–1021.

37. British Society of Gastroenterology. *Dyspepsia Management Guidelines.* London: British Society of Gastroenterology, 1996.
38. Moayyedi P, Shelly S, Deeks J *et al.* Systematic review and economic evaluation of *Helicobacter pylori* eradication treatment for non-ulcer dyspepsia. *BMJ* 2000; 321: 659–664.
39. Salzman J R, Russell R M. The aging gut. *Gastroenterol Clin North Am* 1998; 27: 309–324.
40. Barrett J A. Colorectal disorders in elderly people. *BMJ* 1992; 305: 764–766.
41. Lederle F A. Epidemiology of constipation in elderly patients. *Drugs Aging* 1995; 6: 465–469.
42. The National Prescribing Centre. The management of constipation. *MeRec Bull* 1999; 10: 33–36.
43. Petticrew M, Watt I, Sheldon T. Systematic review of the effectiveness of laxatives in the elderly. *Health Technol Assessment* 1997; 1, 7–13.
44. O'Donoghue N, Moriarty K. GP guide to laxative choice in constipation. *Prescriber* 1996; 7: 29–41.
45. Black D. Constipation in the elderly: causes and treatments. *Prescriber* 1998; 9: 105–108.
46. Gerbino P P, Gans J A. Antacids and laxatives for symptomatic relief in the elderly. *J Am Geriatr Soc* 1982; 30 (suppl 11): S81–S87.
47. Nathan A. Laxatives. *Pharm J* 1996; 257: 52–55.
48. Attar A, Lemann M, Ferguson A *et al.* Comparison of a low dose polyethylene glycol electrolyte solution with lactulose for treatment of chronic constipation. *Gut* 1999; 44: 226–230.
49. Teasley D G, Gerding D N, Olson M M *et al.* Prospective randomised trial of metronidazole versus vancomycin for *Clostridium difficile*-associated diarrhoea and colitis. *Lancet* 1983; 2: 1043–1046.
50. Grimm I S, Friedman L S. Inflammatory bowel disease in the elderly. *Gastroenterol Clin North Am* 1990; 19: 361–389.
51. Akerkar G A, Peppercorn M A. IBD in the elderly. Practical treatment guidelines. *Drugs Aging* 1997; 10: 199–208.
52. Campieri M, Ferguson A, Doe W *et al.* Oral budesonide is as effective as oral prednisolone in active Crohn's disease. *Gut* 1997; 41: 209–214.
53. Carapeti E A, Kamm M A, McDonald P J *et al.* Randomised controlled trial shows that glyceryl trinitrate heals anal fissures, higher doses are not more effective, and there is a high recurrence rate. *Gut* 1999; 44: 727–730.

4

Cardiovascular medicines in the elderly

Andrzej Kostrzewski

With advancing age, disorders of cardiovascular functioning become more prevalent. Available longitudinal data suggest that individuals vary greatly in the rate and degree of functional decline, even in full health. This variability of rate of ageing when added to the differential effects of any superimposed disease states means that there is very considerable heterogeneity in old age. The elderly are much less like one another than younger people are to each other, particularly in their susceptibility to disease.

Generalisations about old people should reflect such factors, therefore, but in those afflicted with cardiovascular problems some differences between younger and older people are recognisable.

Some conditions may present atypically, especially in the very old. For example, myocardial infarction (MI) is more likely to present as dyspnoea without pain or other discomfort. There is a tendency for a higher incidence of comorbidity; pneumonia may precipitate heart failure because compensating mechanisms may be easily overwhelmed in old age. Such effects mean that the outlook for the sick old person is more uncertain than for the young – hospital stays may be prolonged and rehabilitation lengthy. Because of these effects prevention is extremely important and risk factor control imperative.

Risk factors for cardiovascular disease

Death rates from cardiovascular diseases have fallen recently in developed countries, largely because of reductions in cigarette smoking, better blood pressure (BP) control and lifestyle changes.[1]

Hypertension is common, asyptomatic, dangerous and controllable. It is the dominant risk factor for cardiovascular disease. Systolic hypertension (systolic BP 140 mmHg or more) is said to be a more consistent predictor than the diastolic variety (diastolic BP > 90 mmHg), possibly because of the tendency of the former to rise with age and of the latter to reach a peak, then fall.[2] One possible consequence of raised BP in the elderly is left ventricular hypertrophy (LVH) which is itself a risk factor for cardiovascular mortality and MI.

Cigarette smoking is associated with increases in platelet aggregation, hypoxia, fibrinogen levels and ischaemic heart disease (IHD); it also affects factors such as glucose tolerance and indirect factors such as ability to exercise.

The blood lipid profile shows raised total cholesterol in old age but, for the over-70s, this effect may be less important than in the young.

Dietary factors are important; western populations are eating healthier diets but are becoming more obese,[3] the exact balance of risk being obscure.

Physical fitness protects against cardiovascular disease and a high level of fitness gives a better chance that illness will be survived. Some of this protection may be due to decreased body weight.

Diabetes mellitus tends to be associated with more severe heart disease and the occurrence of MI carries a greater risk of death.[4]

Oestrogen levels are important protective factors against cardiovascular disease in women; hormone replacement therapy (HRT) is protective in immediately postmenopausal women but data are lacking about any protective effect in the very old.

Dysrhythmias are common in the elderly, especially atrial fibrillation (AF), which is a potent predictor of stroke and heart failure.

Changes in cardiac function with age

Advancing age is associated with various changes to the cardiovascular system. The inherent rhythmicity of the sinoatrial node declines with greater possibility of arrhythmias. There is relative resistance to sympathetic stimulation because of a decline in the numbers and sensitivity of β-receptors. α_1-Receptors show little change, whereas α_2 presynaptic and postsynaptic responses show attenuation during ageing. Pulse rate declines but cardiac output is maintained by an increase in left ventricular stroke volume. There is reduced left ventricular wall compliance, thereby reducing ventricular relaxation during diastole, which can lead to heart failure. For reasons which are unclear, severe cardiac pain, for example from MI, may not be experienced at all.

The human aorta becomes progressively less able to dilate with increasing age, becoming almost completely rigid by the age of 85 years.[5] The rest of the arterial system shows a progressive rigidity with increasing age. This leads to a progressive increase in peripheral vascular resistance to blood flow.

Apparent increased susceptibility to calcium antagonists and angiotensin-converting enzyme (ACE) inhibitors are probably due to reduced baroreceptor function. Studies of atrial and brain levels of natriuretic peptide have shown increases with age and may be used in the future as markers of heart failure.

Cardiovascular drugs comprise the most frequently used class of agents since cardiovascular disease represents the greatest cause of morbidity, mortality and hospitalisation. It has been estimated that 40% of the drugs prescribed to the elderly, including diuretics, exhibit specific cardiovascular actions.

Hypertension

Aetiology

The elderly have a higher prevalence of hypertension than younger adults. The Health Survey for England 1996[6] showed the prevalence of hypertension to be 50% between the ages of 65 and 74 years and it is higher above this age. Isolated systolic hypertension (ISH) is defined as a systolic BP of $\geqslant 160$ mmHg with diastolic BP $\leqslant 90$ mmHg. The prevalence of ISH rises from about 12% at 70 years to about 23% at 80 years. Systolic hypertension appears to be more closely related to cardiovascular risk in the elderly than the diastolic variety. In addition, cardiovascular risk factors such as obesity, LVH, hyperlipidaemia, sedentary lifestyle and diabetes are more common in the elderly with hypertension. Two most widely discussed mechanisms for BP elevation with ageing are increased peripheral vascular resistance in diastolic hypertension and increased artery rigidity in ISH; even in the latter, increased peripheral vascular resistance appears to have an important role.

It has been postulated that a high salt intake combined with decreased elimination causes a rise in peripheral vascular resistance. Decreased β-activity in association with unaltered α-adrenergic activity is thought to be an important contributor to the vasoconstriction. An important age-related physiological change is the decrease in efficiency of BP homeostasis and this results in an increased likelihood of precipitating drug-related hypotensive events, such as postural hypotension or syncope.

Understanding the derangement in volume regulation and baroreflex activity is a useful way of explaining some of the problems of BP control. The elderly are highly vulnerable to volume depletion from almost any stress. Renin levels decline with ageing and are thought to be a major factor in impaired sodium conservation.

Water homeostasis is also impaired because maximal urinary concentration after water deprivation decreases with age.

The elderly also have impaired heart rate increase and vaso-constriction in response to low BP due to posture. This is thought to be due to decreased sensitivity of the baroreceptors. The high-pressure sinoaortic baroreceptor sensitivity is also impaired and possibly contributes to elderly hypertension. Others have suggested a resetting of the reflex mechanism in response to chronic high arterial pressures.

Risk factors – evidence base

Inadequately treated hypertension gives rise to two major causes of morbidity and mortality: stroke and MI. In the Veterans Administration Co-operative Study 1972[7] people over 60 years comprised 20% of the hypertensive study population, yet suffered 63% of all morbid outcomes during the 5-year follow-up. In the Framingham study the average annual incidence of cardiovascular events for older hypertensives (65–74 years) was twice that of age-matched normotensives.

The Cochrane Collaboration 1998 reported on 15 drug trials including 21 908 elderly subjects.[8] Most were 60–80 years old and most were conducted in western, industrialised countries and evaluated diuretic therapy and β-blockers. Cardiovascular morbidity and mortality were reduced from 177 to 126 events and total mortality was reduced from 129 to 111 deaths.

Three trials restricted to ISH indicated significant benefits in respect of coronary heart disease mortality and morbidity,[9] or cerebro-vascular mortality and morbidity.[9–11] The incidence of ISH increases with advancing age because, in contrast to diastolic BP which shows a plateau in the 60s, systolic BP continues to increase into the 80s.[2] The increase in systolic pressure is attributed to arteriosclerotic changes of the media of the aorta and its larger branches. As the less elastic aorta becomes rigid, higher systolic pressures are required to force blood into the resultant confined and narrow aortic area. In studies of ISH there has been no definite conclusion as to whether age-associated arterio-sclerosis or the systolic pressure itself was responsible for the increased adverse outcomes. A recent meta-analysis of eight trials with 15 693 patients with ISH aged 60 years or more found that the absolute benefit of drug treatment is larger in men aged 70 or more and in those with previous cardiovascular complications or wider pulse pressure. Treatment prevented stoke more effectively than coronary events.[12]

It is possible that the distinction between systolic and diastolic hypertension may be less important than supposed hitherto, and treatment should be aimed at optimising both systolic and diastolic BPs rather than distinguishing between the patterns of hypertension.[13] The British Hypertension Society had advised that BP be reduced to 160/90 mmHg up to the age of 80 years.[14] The new British Hypertensive Society recommend that the minimum acceptable level of control is < 150/ < 90 mmHg in uncomplicated patients.[15] Recently, the World Health Organization–International Society of Hypertension produced new guideline limits for the elderly: 140/90 mmHg.[16]

The EWPHE[11] study had no upper age limit and recruited patients up to the age of 97 years, with 155 patients over 80 years, and in the STOP study[10] patients were recruited up to the age of 84 years, with 269 patients aged over 80 years; these two studies did not show any benefit from treatment over the age of 80 years, but the numbers were too small to exclude a possible advantage. In the SHEP study 649 patients over 80 years with ISH showed a 45% reduction in stroke incidence.[9]

In the Syst-Eur study a total of 4695 study participants (who were at least 60 years old with diagnosis of ISH (systolic pressure 160–219 mmHg) were treated with nitrendipine (10–40 mg/day) and enalapril, hydrochlorothiazide or both. There was a 42% difference in stroke incidence in favour of treatment. The authors concluded that treatment of 1000 patients for 5 years should prevent 29 strokes or 53 major cardiovascular incidents.[17]

A recent meta-analysis collected data from subgroups of randomised controlled trials to assess the evidence for and against antihypertensive treatment in people over 80 years of age.[18] It covered seven trials which included 1670 participants. Stroke was the main outcome measure and results suggested a 34% prevention of strokes and that treatment benefit was restricted to non-fatal stroke. Rates of major cardiovascular events and heart failure were significantly decreased, by 22% and 39% respectively; however, there was no treatment benefit for cardiovascular death, and a non-significant relative excess of death from all causes. The conclusion was that an age threshold beyond which hypertension should not be treated cannot be justified. However, the positive results from this meta-analysis were not considered robust. The HYVET study has recruited 1284 patients but the results are not expected to be available until 2004. The researchers say that the benefits in reducing morbidity and mortality are well established in the young elderly (65–74) but unknown for the over 80s.[19]

Treatment options

Dietary alterations should be considered before the use of drugs. Salt restriction[20] and calorie restriction, whether separately or combined, suggested a limit of 2–3 g of sodium per day. Independent effects of salt reduction, exercise, weight reduction and alcohol reduction on BP have been reported, although changes over a lifetime are not easily managed.

The preferred first-line drugs are thiazide diuretics and β-blockers. Atenolol is the most widely used β-blocker, usually used as a second-line agent; thiazides are usually better tolerated than atenolol in the elderly. Low-dose thiazide diuretic therapy has been endorsed by the Joint National Committee on prevention, detection, evaluation and treatment of high blood pressure[21] as first-line monotherapy. A recent review of 12 trials[22] concluded that first-line diuretics reduced cerebrovascular events, coronary heart disease, stroke, cardiovascular and all-cause mortality. First-line β-blockers reduced only cerebrovascular events. Concerns on the use of diuretics include symptomatic hyponatraemia, postural hypotension because of impaired baroreceptors, hyperuricaemia and glucose intolerance.

β-Blockers may be particularly suited to patients with coronary artery disease but peripheral vasoconstriction is a potential problem, especially in elderly people who may thereby experience cold hands and feet; however, evidence suggests no worsening of intermittent claudication. Calcium channel blockers decrease peripheral resistance and, in the Syst-Eur study, nitrendipine in ISH demonstrated a relative reduction in stroke of 42% and total cardiac end-points of 26%.[17] Nitrendipine is not currently licensed in the UK. Orthostatic hypotension, fluid retention and constipation may limit the use of this group of drugs in the elderly.

ACE inhibitors as single agents in the elderly vary in effectiveness from 15 to 50%. They do decrease cardiac preload and afterload and are therefore useful in elderly people with heart failure. ACE inhibitors in combination with diuretics lessen the diuretic-induced metabolic problems.[23] Additional indications include diabetic nephropathy and LVH (excluding renal artery stenosis). ACE inhibitors are acceptable as first-line agents but combination with diuretics may be necessary for optimum control.

Peripheral α_1-adrenergic receptor antagonists like doxazosin may be useful in elderly male hypertensives who also have bladder-emptying problems due to prostatic hypertrophy, although first-dose syncope and orthostatic hypotension can be particular problems.

Heart failure

Aetiology

Chronic heart failure (CHF) is found in over 80% of people aged 65 years. The Framingham study data showed that both the incidence and prevalence of CHF increase with age, approximately doubling with each decade. Approximately 5% of all geriatric admissions are due to congestive heart failure.[24] Mortality from CHF at 5 years from onset is about 50% and annually can be as high as 60%.

The diagnosis of congestive heart failure may be difficult in the elderly because concurrent symptoms and physical signs can be misleading. Heart failure is often due to coronary artery disease and in 10% of cases it is associated with AF,[25] but in the elderly it may develop insidiously without obvious cause.

Risk factors – evidence base

The two principal risk factors for heart failure are hypertension and MI.[26] Although MI carries the greatest relative risk, hypertension contributes substantially in the elderly. The Hillingdon Heart Failure Study in West London identified heart failure within a population of 151 000 served by 81 general practitioners. In a 20-month period 220 patients met the criteria for study admission, the median age of presentation being 76 years. Coronary artery disease accounted for 40% of cases, hypertension 13% and valve disease 7%. In developing countries it is likely that heart disease associated with valvular and nutritional deficiencies are more common.[26]

Hypertension is a main risk factor for LVH and carries three adverse consequences for left ventricular function. Firstly, LVH is a potent risk factor for MI; secondly, it predisposes to ventricular and atrial diastolic dysfunction, leading to increased risk for AF and, thirdly, there is an association with ventricular systolic dysfunction without the occurrence of an MI. Diastolic ventricular dysfunction has an incidence of 40% of older heart failure patients.[26] The pathophysiology is varied but usually involves impaired left ventricular relaxation and/or increased ventricular stiffness, partially related to the normal ageing process, as well as underlying cardiovascular diseases. There is no specific therapy to treat diastolic dysfunction but diuretics, calcium channel blockers, β-blockers and ACE inhibitors offer symptomatic relief and may prevent progression of the disorder.[27]

Treatment options

Diuretics

There are few comparisons of loop and thiazide diuretics in cardiac failure, but thiazides may be as effective as loops in relatively mild failure with preserved cardiac function, although thiazides have a tendency to cause more hyponatraemia than loop diuretics.

Although diuretics alleviate symptoms of oedema and dyspnoea, they do not improve left ventricular function and are best used with an ACE inhibitor, where possible. The elderly in particular have mobility problems and in patients with predominantly diastolic dysfunction, diuretics can cause large reductions in intravascular volume and reduce cardiac output, causing hypotension and dizziness.[24]

In the Randomised Aldactone Evaluation Study of 1600 patients with NYHA class III–IV heart failure (i.e. more severe) and systolic dysfunction, spironolactone 25 mg daily increased to 50 mg once daily after 8 weeks in addition to standard treatment (including ACE inhibitors) reduced total mortality by 27% and decreased the combined end-point of nonfatal hospitalisations and total mortality by 22%.[28] The study was terminated 18 months early as the results were so significantly favourable to treatment that it would have been unethical to continue. Spironolactone and other potassium-sparing diuretics must only be used with an ACE inhibitor with extreme caution, as life-threatening hyperkalaemia may occur.

Angiotensin-converting enzyme inhibitors

Despite the benefits with ACE inhibitors in heart failure, trials have generally excluded subjects who are aged 75 years or more. However, the benefits for older patients have been illustrated by a 6-month mortality reduction of up to 40%.[29] In a review of 1016 elderly patients, the 1-year survival was significantly higher among patients who did, compared with those who did not, receive ACE inhibitor therapy.[30] The benefits of doses in the higher ranges of these drugs are well established but many patients discharged from hospital on ACE inhibitors remain on their treatment inception doses, which may be insufficient in the long term.[26] The older person, often frail or living alone, presents the greatest practical difficulties in establishing optimal ACE inhibition.

Patients with left ventricular systolic dysfunction should be given a trial of ACE inhibitors unless contraindicated, and may be considered as sole therapy in patients without volume overload. There have been concerns of severe hypotension and renal dysfunction but a survey suggested that ACE inhibitors are used without serious side-effects in the elderly; the problems are avoided if treatment is commenced with proper hydration and monitoring of electrolytes.

Morbidity may be a more clinically relevant measure in the elderly with established heart failure. A few trials have used end-points such as 25-m walking times. In a study evaluating patients over 60 years with congestive heart failure using generic health status measures, ACE inhibitors were found to have had little impact on the quality of life.[24]

After starting with a low dose, the ACE inhibitor should be titrated over the next few days or weeks to the target dose which is based on the larger trials in heart failure and post-MI and left ventricular dysfunction. Hypotension itself should not prevent dose titration and some renal dysfunction is common and usually acceptable (creatinine < 120 μmol/l, urea < 12 mmol/l). A recent study of 20 902 patients aged 65 years and older, after a confirmed MI found that ACE inhibitors safely reduce mortality with moderate renal insufficiency.[31] If hypoperfusion is a problem, this is usually reversed by reducing the patient's diuretic dose, or withdrawing other hypotensive agents that are of no value in heart failure, e.g. nitrates, calcium channel blockers, α-blockers.

Angiotensin II receptor antagonists (ACE II inhibitors)

These agents inhibit angiotensin II without increasing levels of bradykinin, which is thought to be responsible for many of the side-effects of ACE inhibitors. In the ELITE trial, in which two-thirds of the patients were over 70 years, an ACE II inhibitor, losartan, in a dose of 50 mg once daily, was compared with an ACE inhibitor, captopril, in a dose of 50 mg three times a day (other drug therapy was permitted except for other open-label ACE inhibitors). This study reported a significantly lower all-causes mortality in the losartan group, but this was not a primary end-point and needs confirmation.[32] ELITE II, in 3152 patients aged 60 years, showed that there was no significant difference between losartan and captopril seen in the earlier ELITE study, but better tolerability.[33] In the RESOLVD study[34] 769 patients with mild heart failure were assigned to enalapril alone (ACE), candesartan (ACE II) or a combination of both. A non-significant trend toward increased mortality was observed with candesartan alone or in combination, but this was not an end-point for which the study was empowered. A recent study of 71 patients examined the use of candesartan plus captopril in elderly patients (65 years or more) who were not thrombolised. The drugs were given within 3 days of admission and followed up at 90 days. The data suggest that the combination has more effect than captopril alone.[35] The role of angiotensin II receptor antagonists will have to await the results of further studies.

Digoxin

Digoxin is one of the most commonly prescribed medications in patients over 65 years.[36] When added to diuretic therapy, digoxin reduces the symptoms and signs of heart failure and improves exercise capacity. The evidence for this comes from a number of randomised controlled trials and a meta-analysis; most were digoxin withdrawal trials. None of these identified a negative influence of digoxin. The PROVED[37] and RADIANCE[38] trials were designed specifically to demonstrate the efficacy and safety of digoxin alone or in combination with ACE inhibition in patients with normal sinus rhythm and mild to moderate congestive heart failure. Both were randomised double-blinded, placebo-controlled trials of digoxin withdrawal. Withdrawn patients in both studies exhibited clinical deterioration, a reduction in exercise tolerance and worsening cardiac function.[36] The Digitalis Investigators Group[39] has been the only randomised, placebo-controlled trial of digoxin reporting morbidity and mortality in 6800 patients in sinus rhythm. The mean age was 64 years and 27% of all patients were more than 70 years old. Digoxin added to background diuretic therapy and ACE inhibitor therapy did not change overall mortality.

However, a study on the use of digoxin in the elderly who did not have congestive heart failure or AF during a 12-year follow-up found the mortality rate was significantly higher in digoxin recipients compared with untreated individuals. In contrast, proper use of digoxin was not associated with an increase in mortality.[40] In addition, there was a substantial reduction in all-cause hospitalisation. The administration of digoxin in combination with ACE inhibitors and diuretics can be considered in all patients, including the elderly, who have significant heart failure and AF. The role of digoxin in patients with relatively preserved systolic function remains controversial. This syndrome of diastolic heart failure with relatively preserved systolic function is common in the older age and may be one of the factors underlying inappropriate digoxin administration.[40]

Digoxin toxicity in the elderly may be due to multiple predisposing factors,[36] including a reduction in lean body mass, decreased glomerular filtration rate, decreased skeletal muscle, diuretic-induced potassium loss, drug interactions and concomitant diseases. Often the elderly patient presents with digoxin toxicity manifested as anorexia, cognitive changes, hazy vision or arrhythmia compared to that of younger patients, who usually develop anorexia and vomiting.[36]

Hydralazine with isosorbide dinitrate

The combination of hydralazine 25 mg four times daily and isosorbide dinitrate 10 mg four times daily, with diuretics and digoxin, with or without enalapril, has been shown to increase left ventricular ejection fraction and exercise capacity more than enalapril but survival was significantly greater in the enalapril-treated patients.[26]

β-Adrenoceptor blocking drugs (β-blockers)

There is evidence that a small dose of a β-blocker started cautiously and titrated upwards over weeks or months provides long-term benefit. In 1999 two studies, CIBIS-II[41] and MERIT-HF,[42] were consistent with each other and superimposed the findings of a previous meta-analysis.[43] The effect of β-blockade seems additive to ACE inhibition. Both trials showed that sudden death was significantly reduced and deaths from progressive heart failure were significantly reduced. The patients were relatively young, predominantly male and had left ventricular systolic dysfunction. However, the elderly may have coexisting disorders and relatively preserved left ventricular systolic function and any benefit for this group is currently not known.[43] Recently, a Canadian study of 13 623 survivors of an MI who were 66 years or older investigated the relation between the use of β-blockers, the dose used, hospital admission for heart failure and 1-year survival. Compared with high-dose β-blocker therapy, low-dose treatment was associated with a lower rate of hospital admission for heart failure and a similar 1-year survival benefit. The need for a randomised controlled trial comparing doses of β-blockers in the elderly was recommended.[44]

Cardiac arrhythmias

Atrial fibrillation

AF is the most common arrhythmia in patients with structural heart disease and those with normal hearts. The prevalence increases with age from 0.5% in the 50–59-year group to 8.8% in the 80–89-year bracket.[45] AF is more common in more severe congestive heart failure and is associated with embolic stroke. In addition elderly patients may have 'sick sinus syndrome'; this may result in patients having heart failure as a result of uncontrolled AF and/or prolonged periods of bradycardia, so the use of digoxin to treat the tachycardia is a problem as it may exacerbate the bradycardia. The ideal management of AF is cardioversion, failing this, long-term anticoagulation should be considered in all patients regardless of age.[46]

Despite the use of antiarrhythmic drugs, recurrence can be up to 50% of patients within 1 year during a particular regimen.[45]

Paroxysmal AF is associated with significant risk for thromboembolism and is often a precursor to chronic AF. The elderly may have increased vagal tone and so respond best to antiarrhythmic drugs with anticholinergic properties.[47] Paroxysmal AF with a rapid ventricular rate should be slowed initially with intravenous verapamil or β-blockers, although the preferred treatment is cardioversion with success rates of 75–91% in patients of all ages. Increased age itself is not an independent risk factor for the success of cardioversion. More research is needed in the very elderly as cardioversion has little evidence for its use in this group.

The ventricular rate can be slowed by using three classes of drugs: digitalis compounds, β-blockers and calcium channel blockers.[48] Digoxin is no more effective than placebo in terminating new-onset AF[44] nor is it effective in maintaining sinus rhythm once cardioversion has occurred. However, the DIGAF study[49] indicated that high doses of digoxin can convert AF to sinus rhythm within 18 h in most cases (maximum total dose 1.8 mg). It may be necessary to add another drug, and amiodarone is the first choice. Amiodarone interacts with digoxin, resulting in an increase in the serum digoxin level so the maintenance dose of the latter needs to be reduced by half.

β-Blockers are effective in controlling ventricular response during AF. If the patient has borderline left ventricular function small doses should be tried first. Calcium channel blockers such as verapamil or diltiazem are effective, although verapamil has greater atrioventricular nodal blocking and negative inotropic effects. Verapamil increases serum digoxin levels and may precipitate ventricular fibrillation in patients with AF and pre-excitation syndrome.[49] Restoration to sinus rhythm is more likely if the AF has been present for less than 12 months and if the left atrium is not enlarged. For other patients, Vaughan-Williams classes IA, IC and III antiarrhythmic agents can be used. These increase the chance of maintaining sinus rhythm from 30–50% to 50–70% of patients per year after cardioversion.

Newer alternatives include new class III agents such as dofetilide (in view of the DIAMOND trial[50]) or ibutilide.

The class IC agent flecainide is reserved for patients without structural heart disease with documented life-threatening arrhythmias in whom it is considered that benefits outweigh risks. The CAST trial[51] found excessive mortality and non-fatal cardiac arrest in patients treated with flecainide and encainide, compared with placebo. Therefore, before antiarrhythmic drugs are used, precipitating or aggravating factors should be excluded, including digoxin toxicity, hypokalaemia, hypomagnesaemia, hyperkalaemia or exacerbation of pump dysfunction with calcium channel blockers. Many antiarrhythmics exacerbate heart failure (see CAST study[51]) but amiodarone has a neutral effect on mortality and is effective in symptomatic control of arrhythmias. Amiodarone may be well tolerated in the elderly, as most of its side-effects are due to slow tissue accumulation and the elderly may not need to take it for prolonged periods.

Digoxin and verapamil must be avoided in patients with Wolff–Parkinson–White syndrome with AF as these drugs can cause ventricular tachycardia by speeding up AV conduction.

Paroxysmal and sustained AF are associated with a high incidence of thromboembolism and many of the patients recruited into trials had heart failure. Warfarin reduces the risk of stroke by about 70% but many physicians do not use anticoagulation in elderly people because the risk-to-benefit ratio is perceived to be too high.[52] In addition, most of the evidence for anticoagulation is based on patients younger than 80 years of age. In patients with AF, current evidence suggests that the best ratio of benefit to risk is achieved when the target international normalised ratio (INR) is 2.0–3.0. The benefits of aspirin are likely to be less than those of warfarin and there is no evidence of the efficacy of aspirin in doses of less than 325 mg daily.[46]

Adenosine

Adenosine blocks the atrioventricular node transiently and can terminate atrioventricular nodal re-entry arrhythmias. Its use is mainly as a diagnostic agent and treatment of narrow QRS complex tachycardias acutely. It has to be given as a rapid injection over 2 s and has a half-life of 2–10 s. It is of note that theophylline and other xanthines are potent antagonists of adenosine and therefore larger doses of adenosine may be required in patients on those drugs. In contrast dipyridamole inhibits adenosine uptake, causing toxicity.

Ischaemic heart disease (IHD)

Angina affects 15–17% of people aged 65 years, and the prevalence does not seem to increase further in older people.[52] In addition, 50% of elderly patients with unstable angina have asymptomatic ischaemic episodes which are associated with an increased risk of MI and cardiac death.

Statins are effective in reducing mortality and morbidity from coronary heart disease, in particular in secondary prevention, although no trial has demonstrated beneficial effects in patients over 75 years of age. The CARE study showed a greater risk reduction for major coronary events in 60–75-year-old patients than in younger patients.[53] A follow-up analysis of 1283 patients aged 65–75 years demonstrated a risk reduction of fatal coronary heart disease and non-fatal MI from 17.3 to 10.8%.[54] In the 4S (Scandinavian Simvastatin Survival Study) follow-up, simvastatin reduced the risk of fatal coronary heart disease and non-fatal MI from 33.4 to 23.6% in 1021 patients aged 65–80 years.[55] The benefits of statin therapy may be observed within 2 years of starting.[56] Treating hyperlipidaemia may also reduce the risk of stroke, dementia and hip fracture. Older patients should be assessed with an emphasis more on biological than chronological age.[57] The results of FAME (Fluvastatin Assessment of Morbidity-Mortality in the Elderly) and PROSPER (Prospective Study of Pravastatin in the Elderly at Risk) will help the situation in the over-75 years group. The Antihypertensive, Lipid Lowering after Heart Attack Trial (ALLHAT) should also clarify the role of statins[58] in the near future. From a recent review of over 72 000 patients 65 years or older with a diagnosis of coronary heart disease, β-blockers were least likely to be administered compared to calcium channel blockers and nitrates. This is of concern as β-blockade is well documented to reduce the risk of mortality and non-fatal reinfarction.[59,60]

Myocardial infarction

The prevalence of MI increases from 11% at age 65–69 years to 18% at age 80–84 years.[52] In 1995, 74.4% of deaths from acute MI (AMI) in

England and Wales occurred in people aged 70 years or more.[61] Reduction of infarct size with thrombolysis improves survival in patients older than 70 and the net benefit seems to increase incrementally with age up to 75 years.[62]

In a prospective cohort study 1225 patients aged 70 years were less likely to receive standard therapy with β-blockers and thrombolysis than younger patients and take longer to get to hospital.[62] However, patients aged 70 or older without left ventricular failure had significantly better survival at 1 year after AMI than patients under 60 years of age with left ventricular failure. Older patients with MI have a higher risk of complications with thrombolytic therapy but this should not preclude its use.

Intracranial haemorrhage occurs in 0.3–0.5% of younger treated patients, but this increases progressively with advancing age. Tissue plasminogen activator has been associated with a 60% greater risk of intracranial haemorrhage than streptokinase, and this risk is most pronounced in patients older than 75 years of age.[63]

Subcutaneous heparin reduces the risk of venous thrombo-embolism in patients hospitalised with AMI but the role of full-dose intravenous heparin in AMI remains controversial, although enoxaparin has been shown to be more effective than heparin in patients older than 65 years.[64] Ongoing studies should clarify the role of low-molecular-weight heparin in older AMI patients.

Glycoprotein IIb/IIIa inhibitors are more potent antiplatelet agents than aspirin. Tirofiban with heparin and aspirin was shown to reduce the risk of death and AMI compared with heparin and aspirin alone in patients with non-Q-wave AMI or unstable angina. This was more pronounced in patients greater than 65 years of age.[65] More trials will define the role of these agents in the future.

As older AMI patients do not receive a thrombolytic agent, the results of the earlier β-blocker trials remain applicable. Pooled data from three large trials of 23 200 patients indicate that early treatment with intravenous β-blockers reduces mortality by 23% in older patients, but has no significant effect in younger patients. The agents used were atenolol 5 mg intravenously administered twice at 10-min intervals followed by oral atenolol and metoprolol 5 mg intravenously at 5-min intervals for three doses followed by oral metoprolol 50 mg every 6 h and progressing to 100 mg twice daily after 24–48 h. Lower doses would be appropriate in older patients.[66]

Oral ACE inhibitors initiated within the first 24 h of an acute infarct have demonstrated small but statistically significant reductions in mortality.[66]

A patient with a large anterior infarct who is haemodynamically stable and has complications of heart failure or ejection fraction less than 40% should be considered for early ACE inhibitor therapy starting with a low dose.[66]

Aspirin reduces mortality and recurrent ischaemic events in patients with AMI or unstable angina. In a study among 3411 patients more than 70 years of age, aspirin reduced vascular deaths by 21% and the absolute benefit was greatest in this age group,[66] the daily dose used being 162.5 mg. In order to achieve prompt antiplatelet effect, the first dose should be 300 mg, chewed rather than swallowed and the daily maintenance dose 75–150 mg.[67]

References

1. Sytkowski P A, Karmel W B, D'Agostina R. Changes in risk factors and the decline in mortality from cardiovascular disease: the Framingham study. *N Engl J Med* 1990; 332: 1635–1641.

2. Volkonas P S, Kannel W B, Cupples L A. Epidemiology and risk of hypertension in the elderly. *J Hypertens* 1998; 6: S3–S9.

3. Posner B M, Fraz M M, Quatrononi P A *et al*. Secular trends in diet and risk factors for cardiovascular disease: the Framingham study. *J Am Diet Assoc* 1995; 95: 171–179.

4. Jenkins J S, Flaker G C, Nolte B *et al*. Causes of higher in-hospital mortality in women than in men after acute myocardial infarction. *Am J Cardiol* 1994; 73: 319–322.

5. Swift CG, ed. *Clinical Pharmacology in the Elderly*. New York: Marcel Dekker, 1987: 17.

6. Prescot-Clarke P, Primatesta P. *Health Survey for England 1996: A Survey Carried out on Behalf of the Department of Health*. London: Stationery Office, 1998: 3.

7. Veterans Administration Cooperative Study Group on Antihypertensive Agents. Effects of treatment on morbidity in hypertension. III. Influence of age, diastolic pressure and prior cardiovascular disease: further analysis of side effects. *Circulation* 1972; 45: 991–1004.

8. Mulrow C, Lau J, Cornell J, Brand M. *Pharmacotherapy for Hypertension in the Elderly*. The Cochrane Library issue 4. Oxford: Update Software, 1999.

9. SHEP cooperative research group. Prevention of stroke by antihypertensive drug treatment in older persons with isolated systolic hypertension: final results of the Systolic Hypertension in the Elderly Program (SHEP). *JAMA* 1991; 265: 3255–3264.

10. Dahlof B, Lindholm L H, Hansson L *et al*. Morbidity and mortality in the Swedish Trial in Old Patients with Hypertension (STOP-Hypertension). *Lancet* 1991; 338: 1281–1285.

11. Amery A, Bixko P, Clement D *et al*. Mortality and morbidity results from the European working party on high blood pressure in the elderly trial. *Lancet* 1985; 1: 1349–1354.

12. Staessen J A, Gasowski J, Wang J G *et al*. Risks of untreated and treated isolated systolic hypertension in the elderly: meta-analysis of outcome trials. *Lancet* 2000; 355: 865–872.

13. Walker H, Jackson G. Hypertension: broadening the approach. *Update* 1999; 28 Jan: 96–104.

14. Sever P, Beevers G, Bulpitt C *et al*. Management guidelines in essential hypertension: report of the second working party of the British Hypertension Society. *BMJ* 1993; 306: 983–987.

15. Ramsey L E, Williams B, Johnston G D *et al*. British Hypertensive Society guidelines for hypertension management 1999: summary. *BMJ* 1999; 319: 630–635.

16. World Health Organization–International Society of Hypertension guidelines for the management of hypertension: guidelines subcommittee. *J Hypertens* 1999; 17: 151–183.

17. Staessen J A, Fagard R, Thijs L *et al*. Randomised double-blind comparison of placebo and active treatment for older patients with isolated systolic hypertension. *Lancet* 1997; 350: 757–764.

18. Gueyffier F, Bulpitt C, Boissel J-P *et al*. Antihypertensive drugs in very old people: a subgroup meta-analysis of randomised controlled trials. *Lancet* 1999; 353: 793–796.

19. Bulpitt C J, Fletcher A E, Amery A *et al*. The Hypertension in the Very Elderly Trial (HYVET): rationale, methodology and comparison with previous trials. *Drugs Aging* 1994; 5: 171–183.

20. Weinberger M H, Fineberg N S. Sodium and volume sensitivity of blood pressure: age and pressure change over time. *Hypertension* 1991; 18: 67–71.

21. The sixth report of the Joint National Committee on prevention, detection, evaluation, and treatment of high blood pressure. *Arch Intern Med* 1997; 157: 2413–2446.

22. Messerli F H, Grossman E, Goldbourt U. Are beta-blockers efficacious as first-line therapy for hypertension in the elderly? A systematic review. *JAMA* 1998; 279: 1903–1907.

23. Todd P A, Fitton A. Perindopril: a review of its pharmacological properties and therapeutic use in cardiovascular disorders. *Drugs* 1991; 42: 90–114.

24. Gillespie N D, Darbar D, Struthers A D, McMurdo M E T. Heart failure: a diagnostic and therapeutic dilemma in elderly patients. *Age Ageing* 1998; 27: 539–543.

25. McAnaw J, Hudson S, McGlynn S, Watson A. Chronic heart failure. *Pharm J* 1999; 262: 502–509.

26. Coats A, Cleland J G F. *Controversies in the Management of Heart Failure*. London: Churchill Livingstone, 1997.

27. Tresch D D, McGough M F. Heart failure with normal systolic function: a common disorder in older people. *J Am Geriatr Soc* 1995; 43: 1035–1042.

28. Pitt B, Zannad F, Remne W J *et al*. The effect of spironolactone on morbidity and mortality in patients with severe heart failure. Randomised aldactone evaluation study investigators. *N Engl J Med* 1999; 34: 709–717.

29. Farnsworth A. Angiotensin-converting enzyme inhibitors in heart failure: target dose prescription in elderly patients. *Age Ageing* 1998; 27: 653–654.

30.   Havranek E P, Abrams F, Stevens E, Parker K. Determinants of mortality in elderly patients with heart failure: the role of angiotensin-converting enzyme inhibitors. *Arch Intern Med* 1998; 158: 2024–2028.

31.   Frances C D, Noguchi H, Massie B M *et al*. Are we inhibited? Renal sufficiency should not preclude the use of ACE inhibitors for patients with myocardial infarction and depressed left ventricular function. *Arch Intern Med* 2000; 160: 2645–2650.

32.   Pitt B, Segal R, Martinez F A *et al*. Randomised trial of losartan versus captopril in patients over 65 with heart failure (evaluation of losartan in the elderly study, ELITE). *Lancet* 1997; 349: 747–752.

33.   Pitt B, Poole-Wilson P A, Segal R *et al*. Effect of losartan compared with captopril on mortality in patients with symptomatic heart failure: randomised trial – the Losartan Heart Failure Survival Study ELITE II. *Lancet* 2000; 355: 1568–1569.

34.   Tsuyuki R T, Yusuf S, Rouleau J L *et al*. Combination neurohormonal blockade with ACE inhibitors, angiotensin II inhibitors and beta-blockers in patients with congestive heart failure: design of the Randomised Evaluation of Strategies for Left Ventricular Dysfunction (RESOLVD) pilot study. *Can J Cardiol* 1997; 13: 1166–1174.

35.   di Pasuale P, Cannizzaro S, Giubilato A *et al*. Effects of the combination of candesartan plus captopril in elderly patients with anterior myocardial infarction – a pilot study. *Clin Drug Invest* 2000; 19: 173–182.

36.   Haas J G, Young J B. Inappropriate use of digoxin in the elderly. How widespread is the problem and how can it be solved? *Drug Safety* 1999; 20: 223–230.

37.   Uretsky B F, Young J B, Shahidi F E *et al*. Randomised study assessing the effect of digoxin withdrawal in patients with mild to moderate chronic congestive heart failure: results of the PROVED trial. PROVED investigative group. *J Am Coll Cardiol* 1993; 22: 955–962.

38.   Packer M, Gheorghiade M, Young J B *et al*. Withdrawal of digoxin from patients with chronic heart failure treated with angiotensin-converting enzyme inhibitors. RADIANCE study. *N Engl J Med* 1993; 329: 51–53.

39.   The Digitalis Investigators Group. The effect of digoxin on mortality and morbidity in patients with heart failure. *N Engl J Med* 1997; 336: 525–533.

40.   Casiglia E, Tikhonoff V, Pizziol A *et al*. Should digoxin be prescribed in elderly subjects in sinus rhythm free from heart failure? A population-based study. *Jpn Heart J* 1998; 39: 639–651.

41.   CIBIS-II investigators. The Cardiac Insufficiency Bisoprolol Study II (CIBIS-II): a randomised trial. *Lancet* 1999; 353: 9–13.

42.   MERIT-HF study group. Effect of metoprolol CR/XL in chronic heart failure: Metoprolol CR/XL Randomised Intervention Trial in congestive cardiac failure (MERIT-HF). *Lancet* 1999; 353: 2001–2007.

43.   Sharpe N. Benefit of beta-blockers for heart failure: proven in 1999. *Lancet* 1999; 353: 1988–1989.

44.   Rochon P A, Tu J V, Anderson G M *et al*. Rate of heart failure and 1-year survival for older people receiving low-dose beta-blocker therapy after myocardial infarction. *Lancet* 2000; 356: 639–644.

45.   Chandramouli B V, Kotler M N. Atrial fibrillation: drug therapies for ventricular rate control and restoration of sinus rhythm. *Geriatrics* 1998; 53: 46–60.

46. English K M, Channer K S. Managing atrial fibrillation in elderly people. *BMJ* 1999; 318: 1088–1089.

47. Reardon M, Camm A J. Cardiac arrhythmias. In: Pathy M S J, ed. *Principles and Practice of Geriatric Medicine*, 3rd edn. Chichester: John Wiley, 1998: 543.

48. Aronow W S. Management of the older person with atrial fibrillation. *J Am Geriatr Soc* 1999; 47: 740–748.

49. Stuhlinger H G, Domanovits H, Gamper G *et al*. The DIGAF study. Reversion of AF with high dose digoxin (preliminary results). *J Am Coll Cardiol* 1997; 29 (suppl 2): 177A.

50. Norgaard B L, Watchtell K, Christensen P D *et al*. Efficacy and safety of intravenously administered dofetilide in acute termination of atrial fibrillation and flutter: a multicenter, randomised, double-blind, placebo-controlled trial. *Am Heart J* 1999; 137: 1062–1069.

51. The Cardiac Arrhythmia Suppression Trial (CAST) investigators. Increased mortality due to encainide or flecainide in a randomised trial of arrhythmia suppression after myocardial infarction. *N Engl J Med* 1989; 321: 406–412.

52. Mittelmark M B, Psaty B M, Rautaharzu P M *et al*. Prevalence of cardiovascular diseases among older adults: the Cardiovascular Health Study. *Am J Epidemiol* 1993; 137: 311–317.

53. Phehn J F, Davis B R, Sacks F M *et al*. Reduction of stroke incidence after myocardial infarction with pravastatin: the Cholesterol and Recurrent Events (CARE) study. *Circulation* 1999; 99: 216–223.

54. Lewis S J, Moye L A, Sacks F M *et al*. Effect of pravastatin on cardiovascular events in older patients with myocardial infarction and cholesterol levels in the average range. *Ann Intern Med* 1998; 129: 681–689.

55. Miettinen T A, Pyorala K, Olsson A G *et al*. Cholesterol lowering therapy in women and elderly patients with myocardial infarction or angina pectoris: findings from the Scandinavian Simvastatin Survival Study (4S). *Circulation* 1997; 96: 4211–4218.

56. Carlsson C M, Carnes M, McBride P E *et al*. Managing dyslipidemia in older patients. *J Am Geriatr Soc* 1999; 47: 1458–1465.

57. Kelly J, Rudd A. Statins for stroke should be considered in biologically fit people over 75. *BMJ* 2000; 320: 1278.

58. Machado F. An age limit for statin therapy. *Update* 1999; 10 Jun: 1050.

59. Lapane K L, Barbour M M, Van Haaren A B, Gambassi G. Antiischaemic therapy in patients with coronary heart disease living in long-term care. *Pharmacotherapy* 1999; 19: 627–634.

60. Gollub S B. Is intensive drug therapy appropriate for older patients? *Lancet* 1999; 353: 940–941.

61. Office for National Statistics. *Mortality Statistics*. Cause series DH2 no. 22. London: Stationery Office, 1997.

62. Barakat K, Wilkinson P, Deaner A *et al*. How should age affect management of acute myocardial infarction? A prospective cohort study. *Lancet* 1999; 353: 955–959.

63. Fibrinolytic Therapy Trialists' (FTT) collaborative group. Indications for fibrinolytic therapy in suspected acute myocardial infarction: collaborative overview of early mortality results from all randomised trials of more than 1000 patients. *Lancet* 1994; 343: 311–322.

64. Cohen M, Demers C, Gurfinkel E P *et al*. A comparison of low molecular weight heparin with unfractionated heparin for unstable coronary artery disease. *N Engl J Med* 1997; 337: 447–452.
65. The Platelet Receptor Inhibition in Ischemic Syndrome Management in Patients Limited by Unstable Signs and Symptoms (PRISM-PLUS) study investigators. Inhibition of the platelet glycoprotein IIb/IIIa receptor with itrofiban in unstable angina and non-Q-wave myocardial infarction. *N Engl J Med* 1998; 338: 1488–1497.
66. Rich M W. Therapy for acute myocardial infarction in older persons. *J Am Geriatr Soc* 1998; 46: 1302–1307.
67. Hardman S M C, Cowie M R. Anticoagulation in heart disease. *BMJ* 1999; 318: 238–244.

Further reading

Pathy M S J, ed. *Principles and Practice of Geriatric Medicine*, 3rd edn. Chichester: John Wiley, 1998.

5

Respiratory medicine in the elderly

Anne C Boyter and Kenneth Dagg

The main function of the respiratory system is gas exchange. Efficient gas exchange depends on: delivery of air to the alveoli; a concentration gradient across the alveolar capillary membrane; matching of ventilation and perfusion within the lung and adequate blood supply to the tissues. During inspiration the respiratory muscles contract, creating a negative intrapleural pressure which draws air into the thoracic cavity. At the end of inspiration intrinsic elastic recoil within the lungs and chest wall and to a lesser extent active expiratory muscle contraction results in waste gases being expelled. This process remains under the control of the respiratory centre sited in the medulla and pons via a series of afferent and efferent nerves. Respiratory illnesses in the elderly are common and result in significant morbidity and mortality.[1] Considerable resources within hospital and community trusts are allocated to the management of these illnesses. Despite these resources there is considerable evidence to suggest that elderly patients are less likely to receive appropriate investigation and management of respiratory illnesses.[2, 3]

This chapter describes the ageing respiratory system; and discusses some of the more common respiratory illnesses which affect the elderly.

Changes to the ageing respiratory system

Structural changes

A number of functionally important changes occur in the respiratory system with ageing.[4] The costochondral articulations of the ribs, sternum and vertebrae become ossified, reducing chest wall expansion.[4] The vertebral bodies become osteopenic and collapse, resulting in loss of vertebral height and predisposing elderly patients to kyphoscoliosis and impaired ventilation.[4] The muscle fibres of the chest wall and diaphragm have been classified into type I (slow fatigue-resistant), type

IIa (fast fatigue-resistant) and type IIb (fast fatigable) according to myosin ATPase activity.[5] There is evidence to suggest that inspiratory and expiratory muscle strength diminishes with age and that this is probably due to atrophy of type II muscle fibres.[4] Within the lung itself the major histological change is a loss of elastin and collagen fibres. This loss at the junction of the terminal bronchiole and alveolus results in destruction of the normal architecture and the formation of air spaces, not unlike emphysema. This process leads to a reduction in lung compliance and premature airway closure with resultant air trapping and loss of elastic recoil.[4] It has been estimated that the alveolar surface area falls from 75 m^2 at the age of 30 years to 60 m^2 at 70 years.[6] In larger airways there is a loss of glandular epithelial cells with reduced mucus secretion and impairment of mucociliary clearance which may predispose older patients to lower respiratory tract infections.[4]

Physiological changes

The reduction in respiratory muscle strength, chest wall compliance and elastic recoil leads to a number of important physiological changes. The major change observed is an increase in residual volume due to premature airway closure. This occurs due to a loss of elastin which disrupts the normal lung architecture. Despite this, total lung capacity is preserved.[5] Maximum inspiratory and expiratory mouth pressures fall, reflecting respiratory muscle weakness. There is an increased tendency towards airflow obstruction as the forced expiratory volume in 1 s (FEV_1) falls at a greater rate than the forced vital capacity (FVC).[4] Arterial PaO_2 also falls due to ventilation–perfusion mismatch from early airway closure during tidal breathing. Arterial $PaCO_2$ is essentially unchanged.

Changes in ventilatory drive

Ventilation remains under the control of the respiratory centre. In studies the elderly exhibit reduced ventilatory drive to arterial hypoxia and hypercapnia when compared to younger subjects.[4] This may be explained by failure of the peripheral and central chemoreceptors to detect changes in blood gas tensions. During exercise, however, elderly subjects increase their minute ventilation at a greater rate than younger subjects for similar exercise loads. There is evidence to suggest that older subjects' perceptions of the change in mechanical loads during exercise are blunted, leading to this inappropriate ventilatory response.[4,7] While sleeping, older patients have more prolonged and frequent apnoeas and increased arousals. This results in significant sleep fragmentation, reduced quality of sleep, increased daytime somnolence and poor daytime functioning.[4]

While there are measurable physiological changes in the ageing respiratory system it is unlikely that they result in clinically significant symptoms in healthy subjects. In patients with acute respiratory illnesses, however, these changes reduce respiratory reserve and the ability to cope with acute illness.[4]

Airways disease

It has been estimated that 40% of elderly patients have reversible or partially reversible airways obstruction. Patients with airways disease typically present with breathlessness which may be effort-related or paroxysmal, wheeze, cough and sputum production. The most common causes of airway obstruction are chronic obstructive pulmonary disease (COPD) and asthma. Differentiation between these conditions in the elderly is difficult because of their similar clinical presentation and the inability of elderly patients to cooperate with pulmonary function testing.[4] The presence of troublesome nocturnal symptoms, atopy or a family history may suggest underlying asthma but the clinical symptoms show considerable overlap with COPD.

Stable chronic obstructive airways disease

Diagnosis and incidence

COPD is defined as a chronic, slowly progressive disorder characterised by airflow obstruction that does not vary markedly with time. Although in the majority of cases airflow obstruction is fixed, some patients exhibit minor degrees of reversibility to inhaled bronchodilator therapy. Diagnosis is based on demonstrable airways obstruction on spirometry (Table 5.1).

Other diagnostic labels encompassed by COPD include chronic bronchitis, emphysema, chronic airflow limitation and some cases of chronic asthma which have become irreversible. Risk factors which have been identified for the development of COPD include smoking, increasing age, gender (male > female), environmental pollution and occupational exposure to a number of factors. Occupational groups

Table 5.1 Severity of chronic obstructive pulmonary disease

Category	FEV_1	Signs/symptoms	Treatment
Healthy	80–100% predicted/best	No symptoms	Smoking cessation
Mild	60–79% predicted/best	Smoker's cough Little/no breathlessness	Inhaled short-acting β_2-agonist or anticholinergic as required
Moderate	40–59% predicted/best	Shortness of breath ± wheeze Cough ± sputum Lung hyperinflation	Inhaled short-acting β_2-agonist or anticholinergic as required Long-acting β_2-agonist Steroid trial Pulmonary rehabilitation
Severe	< 40% predicted/best	Shortness of breath on exertion and at rest Wheeze and cough Lung hyperinflation Cyanosis Peripheral oedema	Inhaled short-acting β_2-agonist or anticholinergic as required Long-acting β_2-agonist Steroid trial Home nebuliser Theophylline Long-term oxygen therapy Pulmonary rehabilitation

which may develop airflow obstruction include coal miners, farm workers, cement workers and cotton workers.[8] It is recognised, however, that tobacco use is the single most important aetiological factor.[3]

In the age group 65–74, COPD accounts for 7.3% of male and 3.2% of female hospital admissions[3] with an average hospital stay of 8 days.[9] This age group also accounts for 9% of general practitioner consultations related to COPD.[3] Community studies based on questionnaires and simple spirometry have estimated that between 10 and 30% of the elderly population will have evidence of obstructive airways disease. Approximately half of these patients do not have a formal diagnosis of airways obstruction and less than 40% are receiving treatment with inhaled bronchodilators or steroids.[10] As a result of these figures some physicians have advocated screening programmes in an attempt to reduce undertreatment of this condition.

Management

The British Thoracic Society (BTS) guidelines for the management of COPD[3] describe the treatment for patients (Table 5.1). The mainstay of management of COPD is inhaled therapy with β_2-adrenoceptor stimulants (β_2-agonists) and anticholinergics. These drugs provide symptomatic relief, although their mechanism of action remains unclear. Their useful-ness in individual patients should not be based solely on reversibility testing. Short-acting β_2-agonists may be taken either as required or regularly. The long-acting β_2-agonist, salmeterol, has been shown to improve quality of life in patients with COPD.[11] There is little or no evidence to suggest that oral β_2-agonists are superior to low-dose inhaled bronchodilators and their routine use is not recommended. In elderly patients who have difficulty using inhaler devices, however, oral agents can provide a useful alternative strategy.

The role of inhaled corticosteroids in the management of stable COPD remains controversial despite several large studies.[12,13] Patients who demonstrate an objective response to a formal steroid trial (oral prednisolone 30 mg daily for 14 days) may benefit from the addition of regular inhaled corticosteroids. Patients who fail to respond should not be routinely prescribed corticosteroids.

Oral methylxanthines (theophylline and aminophylline) act as bronchodilators and may increase exercise tolerance and reduce symptoms in COPD.[3] Their narrow therapeutic index and multiple drug interactions suggest they should be prescribed with caution in the elderly.[4] Drugs such as nedocromil sodium, sodium cromoglicate, anti-histamines and mucolytic agents have not been shown to be effective in the treatment of COPD.[3]

Hypoxaemia complicating COPD is common. Long-term oxygen therapy (LTOT) has been shown to improve survival in patients with an FEV_1 less than 1 l and a PaO_2 less than 7.3 kPa when used for more than 15 h/day. LTOT in these patients may prevent the progression of pulmonary hypertension. It is recommended that patients who are to be considered for LTOT should be assessed by a respiratory physician prior to commencement of therapy (Table 5.2).[14, 15]

Pulmonary rehabilitation programmes are currently being evalu-ated as an adjunct to drug treatment for patients with moderate to severe COPD. Following optimisation of drug management a rehabilita-tion programme will provide education, psychosocial support and an individually tailored exercise programme to improve physical decondi-tioning. Other modalities which may improve the well-being of patients with COPD include dietary advice and vaccination against influenza.

Smoking cessation may be the single most important factor in the improvement in the patient's health. Smoking cessation programmes are however effective in less than one-third of patients with COPD. Sudden rather than gradual cessation combined with nicotine replacement and

Table 5.2 Prescription of long-term oxygen therapy (LTOT) in chronic obstructive pulmonary disease

Criteria	Measurements
Arterial blood gas measurements	Taken when the patient is stable on two occasions at least 3 weeks apart
Arterial blood gases	• PaO_2 < 7.3 kPa ± hypercapnia and FEV_1 < 1.5 l • PaO_2 7.3–8.0 kPa and pulmonary hypertension, peripheral oedema or nocturnal hypoxaemia
Smoking	Patients should have stopped smoking
Prescription of oxygen concentrator	Scotland: only via a respiratory consultant England/Wales: general practitioner may prescribe but referral to respiratory specialist is recommended
Settings	Flow rate should be 2–4 l/min via nasal prongs Therapy must be for at least 15 h/day
Monitoring	Blood gases should be repeated to ensure that a PaO_2 > 8 kPa is achieved without an increase in $PaCO_2$
Reassessment	Patients on LTOT should be reassessed every 6 months at home

attendance at a smoking cessation clinic has been shown to be the most effective method.[16] The current smoking cessation guidelines do not recommend the use of other drug therapies, including anxiolytics or antidepressants, as an aid to cessation because of insufficient evidence for their effectiveness.[17]

Acute exacerbations of COPD

Diagnosis and incidence

Acute exacerbations of COPD are common and often linked to infection, either bacterial or viral. An average health district of 250 000 people can expect 700 hospital admissions per annum, accounting for approximately 10 000 inpatient bed days.[3] The presenting features of an exacerbation of COPD include worsening of a stable condition, increased wheeze, increased dyspnoea, increased sputum volume and purulence, chest tightness and fluid retention. Baseline investigations, including chest X-ray, ECG, pulse oximetry and/or arterial blood gases and simple spirometry should confirm the diagnosis and exclude other conditions such as pulmonary oedema, pneumonia and lung cancer which may mimic acute exacerbations of COPD.[3]

Management

The mainstay of management during acute exacerbations is the addition of, or increase in, bronchodilator therapy[3] (Table 5.3).

Bronchodilator therapy includes β_2-agonists and/or anticholinergic drugs given regularly. In patients already receiving these drugs attention should be given to ensuring that the most appropriate device is used to optimise drug delivery.

Antibiotic therapy should be considered if the patient exhibits two of the following three signs: increased breathlessness; increased sputum volume and purulent sputum. First-line antibiotic therapy varies

Table 5.3 Treatment for acute exacerbations of chronic obstructive pulmonary disease

Home	*Hospital*
Add or increase bronchodilator: the inhaled route is preferred but the inhaler device and technique should be checked for suitability. Nebulised salbutamol or terbutaline is not usually required	Add or increase bronchodilator: nebulised bronchodilators, salbutamol 5 mg or terbutaline 10 mg is preferred initially. Ipratropium 500 μg may be added in severe cases
Add antibiotic if the patient has two or more of the following: increased breathlessness, increased sputum volume, development of purulent sputum	Add antibiotic if the patient has two or more of the following: increased breathlessness, increased sputum volume, development of purulent sputum
Steroid: if first exacerbation, evidence of reversibility, patient is already receiving steroid therapy or airflow obstruction fails to respond to increased bronchodilator dose	Steroid: if first exacerbation, evidence of reversibility, patient is already receiving steroid therapy or airflow obstruction fails to respond to increased bronchodilator dose
	Controlled oxygen therapy: maximum for patients over 50 years of 28% via a Venturi mask
	Intermittent positive pressure ventilation: decision should be made by a senior physician based on knowledge of the patient's previous history

according to local antibiotic policy and organism resistance.[3] The treatment of respiratory infections in the elderly is dealt with in Chapter 8.

Oral corticosteroids are routinely used in the treatment of exacerbations of COPD, although the evidence that their use is beneficial is controversial.[3] A dose of 30 mg of prednisolone for 7–14 days will adequately treat the reversible component of any airflow obstruction. It is recognised, however, that there is considerable variation in the dose and duration of oral corticosteroids used by individual clinicians. Adverse effects of short-term corticosteroids in the elderly include weight gain, fluid retention, hyperglycaemia and psychosis and are similar to those experienced by younger patients.[3]

Controlled oxygen therapy should be administered to the patient to maintain the PaO_2 above 7.5 kPa without a significant increase in the serum hydrogen ion concentration. A hydrogen ion concentration of more than 55 mmol/l, despite the above, should prompt consideration of additional treatment strategies such as intravenous doxapram or theophylline, nasal or mechanical ventilation. Loop diuretics should be considered in patients with peripheral oedema.

Not all patients with acute exacerbations of COPD require to be treated in hospital. In selected patients, treatment at home is as effective as hospital management.[18] The decision to treat at home following hospital assessment is based mainly on the patient's ability to cope; arterial blood gas analysis, level of consciousness and social factors are also important[18] (Table 5.4). Patients admitted to hospital who are discharged early with an appropriate domiciliary treatment package do as well as patients who remain in hospital.[9]

Table 5.4 Indications for admission to hospital for treatment of chronic obstructive pulmonary disease

Inability to cope at home
Severe breathlessness
Poor or deteriorating general condition
Inactivity or confined to bed
Worsening of peripheral oedema
Impaired consciousness
Acute confusion
Changes on the chest X-ray
Arterial pH < 7.35

Asthma

Diagnosis and incidence

Asthma is characterised by variable airflow obstruction, airway inflammation and airway hyperresponsiveness to a variety of stimuli.[2] Asthma
in the elderly is underdiagnosed and patients often receive suboptimal
treatment.[2,4,5] This may be due, in part, to a reluctance of physicians to
investigate older patients, underreporting of symptoms and difficulty in
the assessment of asthma-like symptoms. Patients may also be misdiagnosed. Conditions which may mimic the symptoms of asthma
include smoking-related COPD, cardiac failure and ischaemic heart
disease. Routine chest X-ray and ECG will help to exclude other diagnoses. Simple spirometry may be used to demonstrate variable airflow
obstruction. This may occur spontaneously, following a single dose of
inhaled bronchodilator (salbutamol 400 μg or terbutaline 500 μg) or oral
corticosteroids (prednisolone 40 mg daily for 10–14 days). An increase in
FEV_1 of 15% and 200 ml from baseline is suggestive of reversible airflow
obstruction. Patients with asthma may also demonstrate increased
airways responsiveness to inhaled histamine or methacholine. It is well
recognised that older patients may be unable to comply with pulmonary
function testing and that in some cases a symptom diary may be a more
useful diagnostic tool.[2] Asthma accounts for 0.34% of all hospital admissions in patients over 65 in the USA.[19] The reported prevalence of asthma
in patients over 65 in the UK is between 6.5% and 17%. It is more
common in women than men.[4] The prevalence of associated atopy is
lower in older patients with asthma. The significance of this observation
in terms of response to treatment and outcome is unknown.[20]

Management

Acute Acute exacerbations of asthma in the elderly are common and
associated with increased mortality. A recent Scottish confidential
inquiry into asthma deaths has suggested that there are avoidable
factors in approximately 60% of deaths.[21] Increased mortality may
reflect blunted perception of bronchoconstriction in older patients,
resulting in later presentation.[4] The emergency treatment of asthma is
based on severity criteria (Table 5.5).[2] Mild-to-moderate asthma can be
treated by doubling the dose of inhaled corticosteroids and more
frequent use of bronchodilator therapy. In some circumstances a course
of oral corticosteroids should be considered. Such mild or moderate

Table 5.5   Management of acute asthma

Assessment	Features	Treatment
Mild to moderate	Peak expiratory flow rate > 50% of predicted/best Speech normal Pulse < 110 beats/min Respiratory rate < 25 breaths/min	Double dose of inhaled corticosteroid Increase frequency of inhaled bronchodilator Add oral corticosteroid if peak expiratory flow rate 50–75% of predicted/best on maximum dose of inhaled corticosteroid
Acute severe	Fall in peak expiratory flow rate to less than 50% of predicted/best Inability to complete sentences Respiratory rate ⩾ 25 breaths/min Pulse ⩾ 110 beats/min	Oxygen 40–60% Nebulised β_2-agonist (salbutamol 5 mg or terbutaline 10 mg). Nebuliser should be oxygen-driven Oral (prednisolone 50 mg) or intravenous steroid (hydrocortisone 200 mg)
Life-threatening	As above plus: Peak expiratory flow rate ⩽ 33% of predicted Silent chest Decreased pulse Hypotension Exhaustion	As above plus: Nebulised ipratropium 500 μg Intravenous β_2-agonist (salbutamol or terbutaline 250 μg over 10 min) Intravenous aminophylline (avoid loading dose if maintained on oral)
Additional management	Oxygen saturation monitoring If < 92% then arterial blood gases: PaO$_2$ < 8.0 kPa PaCO$_2$ normal or high Deteriorating peak expiratory flow rate, PaO$_2$ or rising PaCO$_2$ Exhaustion, confusion, drowsiness or coma	Consider transfer to intensive care unit

The above assessments should be repeated every 15–30 min until the patient is improving.

exacerbations can be safely treated at home. In severe exacerbations, high-dose bronchodilators (either via a nebuliser or a large-volume spacer device), high-dose systemic corticosteroids and high-flow oxygen should be commenced. The oral and intravenous routes for cortico-steroids are equally effective. Patients should normally be admitted to hospital for monitoring. Patients who do not respond to this therapy may benefit from intravenous aminophylline or a β_2-agonist.

Aminophylline should be used with caution and a loading dose avoided in patients on maintenance theophylline. Indications for referral to intensive care are the same for patients of all ages.[4] Antibiotics in the treatment of exacerbations of asthma are not routinely recommended.

Chronic The BTS guidelines for the management of chronic asthma in adults contain few specific recommendations for the elderly and are essentially the same for all age groups (Table 5.6).[2] It is now recognised that the anti-inflammatory actions of inhaled corticosteroids provide the basis for the treatment of asthma. The choice of delivery device is more important than the individual corticosteroid used. In older patients some physicians recommend the early introduction of inhaled steroids coupled with regular inhaled bronchodilators as an alternative to step 1.[2]

Table 5.6 Asthma guidelines: the management of chronic asthma

Step	Treatment
1	Inhaled short-acting β_2-agonist as required
2	Inhaled short-acting β_2-agonist as required *plus* Low-dose inhaled steroid (beclometasone or budesonide 100–400 micrograms twice daily *or* fluticasone 50–200 micrograms twice daily)
3	Inhaled short-acting β_2-agonist as required *plus* High dose of inhaled steroid (beclometasone or budesonide 800–2000 micrograms/day or fluticasone 400–1000 micrograms/day via a large-volume spacer) *or* Low-dose inhaled steroid (as step 2 above) *plus* long-acting β_2-agonist (salmeterol 50 micrograms twice daily *or* formoterol (eformoterol) 6–12 micrograms once or twice daily) *or* Consider use of leukotriene receptor antagonists
4	Inhaled short-acting β_2-agonist regularly *plus* High-dose inhaled steroid (as step 3 above) then sequential therapeutic trial of: Long-acting β_2-agonist (as step 3 above) Leukotriene receptor antagonist *or* Oral theophylline *or* Inhaled anticholinergic *or* Oral β_2-agonist
5	Addition of oral steroids to current therapy
Stepping-down treatment	Treatment should be reviewed every 3–6 months and stepping down should be considered if control has been achieved Stepping down should be based on the least symptom, least need for bronchodilators, least limitation of activity, least variation in peak flow, least adverse effects from medicine and best peak flow

Table 5.7 Some inhaler devices

Type	Device	Drugs available	Comments
Aerosols	Pressurised metered-dose inhaler	β_2-Agonists: short- and long-acting Steroids Anticholinergics: short- and long-acting Combination preparations	Spacer devices may be useful Haleraid may improve use Difficult for the elderly to coordinate Inefficient drug delivery to the lungs Local side-effects due to drug deposition in the mouth Inexpensive
	Breath-actuated metered-dose inhaler	Salbutamol, budesonide, ipratropium	Click on actuation with breath-actuated devices may be offputting
Dry powder	Turbohaler	Terbutaline, budesonide, formoterol (eformoterol)	Low inspiratory pressure required Counting device Attachment available for the Turbohaler More expensive
	Accuhaler	Salbutamol, salmeterol, fluticasone, Seretide	
	Diskhaler	Salbutamol, salmeterol, beclometasone	Some easier to use, but Diskhaler difficult to load and prime
Nebuliser		Salbutamol, terbutaline, budesonide, fluticasone, ipratropium	Easy to use Steroids require the use of a mouthpiece rather than mask Inefficient Costly

Sodium cromoglicate and nedocromil sodium have limited value in the treatment of elderly asthmatics and are not routinely recommended.[4] Anticholinergic drugs may be more effective in older patients.[22] Leukotriene receptor antagonists have recently been licensed in the UK for use in patients with asthma, although their role in elderly patients has not been defined. These drugs have both bronchodilator and anti-inflammatory actions. As an oral preparation they may have advantages in the elderly and can currently be used as add-on therapy at step 3. Their use as a first-line agent is not recommended.[23] It is crucial that elderly patients are capable of administering and monitoring their treatment. As with elderly patients with COPD, the elderly patient with asthma should be offered vaccination against influenza.

Devices

Inhaler devices are important in the management of asthma and COPD but there are many problems associated with the use of inhaled drugs (Table 5.7). These include significant differences in the pattern of drug deposition in the airways and the number and type of manipulations required for correct actuation of aerosol and dry powder devices. It has been shown that metered-dose inhalers and Diskhaler are used incorrectly in over 40% of patients despite repeated instruction.[24] Newer devices, such as the Turbohaler and Accuhaler, may be preferred by patients in terms of ease of use. The use of large-volume spacers should be encouraged in all patients on inhaled corticosteroids administered via a metered-dose inhaler.[25] Patient choice or ability to use a device overrides the choice of drug in some cases. Combination inhalers may improve compliance in the elderly. Chlorofluorocarbon (CFC)-free inhalers are currently being introduced. Due to differences in drug deposition with non-CFC inhalers, the dose of inhaled steroids should be reduced according to manufacturers' recommendations.

Lung cancer

Incidence

Lung cancer is now the most common malignancy in the western world and in the West of Scotland has overtaken breast cancer as the most common cause of death in women with malignancy.[8] It accounts for approximately 40 000 deaths per annum in the UK with the highest mortality in patients over 65 years of age. In the UK mortality from lung cancer in males of all ages is now declining but continues to rise in women. This observation reflects changes in tobacco use since the 1970s.[8] The development of lung cancer is almost exclusively linked to tobacco use.[25] Lesser associations occur with passive smoking, air pollution and occupations involving exposure to substances including asbestos, arsenic, beryllium and soot.[8] The mean age at presentation of patients with lung cancer is rising and it is estimated that by the year 2000 more than 40% will be over 75 years of age and an increasing proportion of them will be women.[27] Despite being an illness of the elderly, it is recognised that older patients are less likely to have a histological diagnosis or be referred for active treatment.[28] This observation may be explained in part by a perception among physicians of the poor prognosis in lung cancer, particularly in the elderly. The estimated 6-month survival in a patient over 70 years old presenting with lung cancer is 20% compared to 50% in those under 40. The poorer prognosis in older patients may be accounted for by their presentation with more advanced disease. Later presentation may occur for a number of reasons, including reduced expectations of quality of life, the masking of early symptoms of cancer by comorbid conditions and reluctance on the part of physicians to investigate symptoms in the elderly. Despite the poor prognosis of lung cancer in the elderly there is good evidence to show that, with appropriate staging and careful patient selection, benefits in survival and quality of life observed with active treatment are the same for patients of all ages.[27]

Presentation

The clinical presentation of lung cancer includes a change in pre-existing respiratory symptoms or the development of new symptoms including cough, wheeze, breathlessness, haemoptysis, hoarseness and thoracic discomfort or pain. Extrathoracic manifestations of lung cancer include musculoskeletal pain, neurological deficit, lymphadenopathy and a variety of neuroendocrine effects.[8] Systemic symptoms such as weight loss and anorexia are common and associated with more advanced disease. Lung cancer as an incidental finding is more common in the elderly due to investigation of comorbid conditions.[4]

Investigations

The recommended minimum investigations in patients with suspected lung cancer include routine haematology and biochemistry (serum calcium, alkaline phosphatase and liver function), chest X-ray, flexible

Table 5.8 WHO/ECOG performance status in patients with lung cancer

0	Fully active
	Able to carry out all activities as before disease
1	Restricted in physically strenuous activities but ambulatory and able to carry out work of a light nature
2	Ambulatory and capable of all self-care but unable to carry out many work activities. Up and about for more than 50% of waking hours
3	Capable of only limited self-care. Confined to a bed or chair for more than 50% of waking hours
4	Completely disabled, unable to carry out any self-care, totally confined to a bed or chair

fibreoptic bronchoscopy or sputum cytology and an assessment of performance status (Table 5.8).[29] In patients being considered for surgical resection or radical radiotherapy additional computed tomography of the chest, pulmonary function tests and organ-specific scans according to symptoms, signs and biochemical abnormalities are required to exclude disseminated disease.

Histological types

The management of lung cancer depends on the histological type and stage of disease (Table 5.9a and 5.9b). Lung cancer can be subdivided

Table 5.9a TMN classification in non-small-cell lung cancer

Tis	Carcinoma-*in-situ*
TX	Positive cytology but no visible tumour
T1	Tumour < 3.0 cm
T2	Tumour > 3.0 cm and > 2.0 cm distal from carina, may invade visceral pleura, atelectasis extending to the hilar region
T3	Tumour any size with direct extension into chest wall, mediastinal pleura or pericardium
T4	Tumour any size with invasion into mediastinum, including heart, great vessels, trachea, oesophagus, carina, vertebral body or malignant effusion
N0	No metastases to regional lymph nodes
N1	Metastases to peribronchial or ipsilateral hilar region
N2	Metastases to ipsilateral mediastinal and subcarinal lymph nodes
N3	Metastases to contralateral mediastinal and hilar lymph nodes, scalene or supraclavicular lymphadenopathy
MX	Presence or absence of distant metastases cannot be assessed
M0	Distant metastases absent
M1	Distant metastases present (brain, bone, liver, contralateral lung or hilar nodes, scalene or cervical nodes)

T = extent of primary tumour; N = extent of regional lymphadenopathy; M = presence of distant metastases.

Table 5.9b   Summary staging and management in non-small-cell lung cancer

Staging	TMN classification	Management
Occult carcinoma	TXN0M0	Surveillance
Stage 0	TisN0M0	
Stage IA	T1N0M0	Lung resection
Stage IB	T2N0M0	
Stage IIA	T1N1M0	Lung resection
Stage IIB	T2N1M0	
	T3N0M0	
Stage IIIA	T1N2M0	Potentially resectable in context of clinical trial, consider radiotherapy/chemotherapy
	T2N2M0	
	T3N1 or N2M0	
Stage IIIB	AnyT,N3M0	Non-resectable, consider radiotherapy/chemotherapy, palliation
	T4,anyNM0	
Stage IV	AnyT, anyN, M1	Non-resectable, consider radiotherapy/chemotherapy, palliation

into small-cell (SCLC) and non-small-cell (NSCLC) lung cancer, with NSCLC approximately four times more common than SCLC. NSCLC can be further subdivided into four major histological types. These are squamous carcinoma, adenocarcinoma, large-cell carcinoma and alveolar cell carcinoma. Squamous carcinoma remains the most common histological type in the elderly, although the incidence of adenocarcinoma and SCLC is increasing, particularly in elderly women.[4]

Non-small-cell lung cancer

Management

The management of patients with NSCLC is determined by a combination of disease stage (Table 5.9a and 5.9b), performance status (Table 5.8), associated comorbid conditions and cardiorespiratory reserve.[29]

Surgery

Patients with stage I and II disease, performance status 0–2 and adequate cardiorespiratory reserve should be considered for curative surgical resection.[4] Recent data suggest that age alone has no significant effect on surgical mortality in patients up to the age of 80 years, but it is recognised that advancing age increases perioperative morbidity and older patients require intensive perioperative support. [30–32] The presence of comorbid conditions, particularly cardiovascular disease, increases both mortality and morbidity in patients at thoracotomy. Good studies of surgical management of stage I and II cancer in patients over 80 years of age are lacking. Current best practice would suggest that such patients should only be considered for lobectomy or wedge resection [32] with stage I disease, good performance status, adequate cardiorespiratory reserve and no significant comorbid conditions. [33, 34]

Radiotherapy

Patients medically unfit or who decline a surgical procedure may be suitable for radical radiotherapy. The current role of radical radiotherapy in the elderly with stage I and II lung cancer is controversial and its precise impact on survival and quality of life is unknown. [4] Currently elderly patients with small peripheral tumours, medically unfit for resection, may derive greatest benefit from this modality of treatment. Further studies are required to define the precise role of radical radiotherapy in the elderly. The majority of radiotherapy treatments administered in lung cancer are for palliation of symptoms in patients who have incurable disease. Two fractions are effective in controlling symptoms, including local and metastatic musculoskeletal pain, haemoptysis and cough. [4]

Chemotherapy

The role of chemotherapy in patients with NSCLC is controversial. No role for neoadjuvant chemotherapy has yet been established in patients with stage I or II lung cancer. Studies are currently underway to evaluate the role of neoadjuvant chemotherapy in stage IIIa disease and the results are awaited. In advanced NSCLC (stage IIIb, IV) almost no randomised studies comparing cisplatin-based combination chemotherapy with best supportive care have recruited elderly patients, resulting in little data for this group. [8] In younger patients with advanced NSCLC, the administration of cisplatin-based chemotherapy is associated with improved survival and symptom control when compared with best supportive care [35, 36] but responses are reported in only 30–50% of patients, are generally short-lived and often not linked with quality-of-life data. Recent data have suggested that advancing age may be associated with

Table 5.10 Chemotherapy in advanced non-small-cell lung cancer

Regimen	Drug	Dose and route	Days	Regimen	Comments
MVP	Mitomycin	8 mg/m² IV (alternate courses)	1	Six cycles given at 3-weekly intervals Monitor for objective response and symptom relief	30–50% response rate Patients with good performance status with weight loss < 10% body weight Toxicity more common in the elderly with cisplatin Reduce dose of cisplatin in renal impairment Lower cisplatin dose does not alter efficacy
	Vinblastine	6 mg/m² IV (maximum 10 mg)	1		
	Cisplatin	50 mg/m² IV	1		
MIC	Mitomycin	6 mg/m² IV	1	Four cycles at 3-weekly intervals Monitor for objective response and symptomatic relief	
	Ifosfamide	3 g/m² IV	1		
	Cisplatin	50 mg/m² IV	1		

IV = Intravenously.

higher response rates but has no influence on survival or symptom relief.[36] Older patients with comorbid conditions are more likely to develop toxicity in light of reduced hepatic and renal clearance and bone marrow failure.

Five drugs have previously been shown to produce significant responses in NSCLC. These are ifosfamide, mitomycin, cisplatin, vinblastine and vindesine.[35] Response rates can be increased when combinations of these drugs are administered. Commonly administered drugs in advanced NSCLC and their doses and potential toxicity are shown in Table 5.10. Newer drugs, such as paclitaxel, both as single agent and in combination, are currently undergoing phase III clinical trials and may result in further improvements in survival, quality of life and symptom relief when compared to regimens currently in use. Information about their role in the elderly is not yet available. Current practice suggests that only elderly patients with good performance status and no comorbid conditions should be considered for chemotherapy.

Small-cell lung cancer

Management

SCLC accounts for approximately 20% of cases of lung cancer.[8] It is accepted in many cases that at presentation wide dissemination with clinically undetectable micrometastases will already have occurred.[5] The mainstay of treatment is therefore combination chemotherapy. Patients can be subdivided into those with limited disease – tumour confined to one hemithorax including evidence of pleural effusion and/or involvement of the ipsilateral supraclavicular fossa – and those with extensive disease – evidence of tumour beyond one hemithorax.

In patients with limited disease, good performance status, normal haematology and biochemistry, treatment with up to six cycles of combination chemotherapy offers the best chance of prolonged survival.[29] Commonly used regimens are included in Table 5.11. Patients with good-prognosis SCLC who achieve a good response to chemotherapy should be considered for consolidation mediastinal radiotherapy and prophylactic cranial radiotherapy.[29]

Patients with extensive disease and poor performance status in addition to abnormal biochemistry and haematology have the poorest prognosis. These patients, however, still benefit from combination chemotherapy, to a maximum of four cycles in the light of cumulative toxicity causing myelosuppression and reduced quality of life.[29] Patients

Table 5.11 Chemotherapy for small-cell lung cancer

	Drug	Dose and route	Days	Regimen	Comments
ACE	Doxorubicin	40 mg/m^2 IV	1	Four to six cycles at 3-weekly intervals	Toxicity common
	Cyclophosphamide	1 g/m^2 IV	1	Consider adjuvant radiotherapy in	Marrow failure, vomiting,
	Etoposide	120 mg/m^2 IV	1 and 2	patients under 70 years with complete	cardiotoxicity and hair loss
		240 mg/m^2 orally	3	response	
PE	Cisplatin	80 mg/m^2 IV	1		Toxicity more common in the
	Etoposide	120 mg/m^2 IV	1 and 2		elderly with cisplatin
		240 mg/m^2 orally	3		Reduce dose in renal impairment
					Highly emetogenic regimen
VICE	Carboplatin	300 mg/m^2 IV	1	Six cycles at 4-weekly intervals	Reduce carboplatin dose in renal
	Ifosfamide	5 g/m^2 IV	1	Consider adjuvant radiotherapy in	failure
	Etoposide	120 mg/m^2 IV	1 and 2	patients under 70 years with complete	Coadminister mesna 10 mg/m^2
		240 mg/m^2 orally	3	response	over 24 h
	Vincristine	1 mg/m^2 IV	14	Only used in patients with limited	Trial regimen at present
		(maximum 2 mg)		disease and good performance status	

IV = Intravenously.

who relapse or decline chemotherapy should be considered for radiotherapy for control of local symptoms as SCLC is radiosensitive.

It is recognised that older patients tolerate chemotherapy for SCLC less well due to comorbidity, reduced renal function and poor bone marrow reserve.[4] These patients are also less likely to achieve a response. Some physicians advocate the use of single-agent chemotherapy with oral etoposide.[4] Such regimens result in lower levels of toxicity and survival figures which are similar to elderly patients who have been treated with combination chemotherapy.

Venous thromboembolism

Introduction

Venous thromboembolism (VTE) is common and the incidence increases with age. Postmortem studies have shown that 37% of patients who die in hospital have evidence of VTE and age is an important risk factor.[38] A number of age-specific risk factors have been identified for VTE. These include immobility for any reason, loss of calf muscle bulk resulting in decreased venous return, increased procoagulant activity and reduced fibrinolysis.[5] Other risk factors identified for VTE, not linked to age, are recent trauma, surgery, medical illness, previous thromboembolism, malignancy, heart failure and nephrotic syndrome.[39] VTE in the elderly is more severe due to a higher incidence of comorbid conditions. The presence of illnesses such as ischaemic heart disease and COPD compromise cardiorespiratory reserve, reducing the ability to cope with any additional vascular insult. Diagnostic tests in VTE include ventilation–perfusion lung scanning, Doppler ultrasound of leg veins or venography, d-dimers and in some circumstances pulmonary angiography or computed tomography of the pulmonary vasculature.[40] Despite these investigations VTE remains difficult to diagnose, particularly in the elderly where comorbid conditions make investigations difficult to interpret. All tests must therefore be interpreted in the light of pretest clinical suspicion.

Management

In acute VTE hypoxia should be corrected with controlled oxygen therapy and adequate analgesia administered to control pain. Non-steroidal anti-inflammatory drugs should, where possible, be avoided concurrently with anticoagulants to reduce the risk of major gastrointestinal bleeding. In patients with massive thromboembolism complicated by cardiovascular collapse, thrombolytic therapy should be considered. Streptokinase, urokinase or alteplase increase clot lysis and restore normal circulation faster than heparin alone and are associated with a better outcome.[39]

In acute VTE, not complicated by cardiovascular collapse, the administration of heparin remains the mainstay of treatment. Traditionally, unfractionated heparin has been given intravenously for 5–7 days (patients should receive an initial loading dose of 5000 U followed by a maintenance infusion of 1000–1500 U/h) to maintain the activated partial thromboplastin time (APTT) ratio between 1.5 and 2.5. Infusion rates should be altered according to the APTT ratio and local nomograms. The major adverse effects of heparin include bleeding, which is more likely when the APTT ratio is greater than 2.5, and thrombocytopenia. The full blood count should be monitored regularly while the patient is receiving heparin.

Recently low-molecular-weight heparins have started to replace unfractionated heparin in the acute management of VTE. Dalteparin and enoxaparin are licensed for deep venous thrombosis and tinzaparin and enoxaparin are licensed for treatment of both VTE and deep venous thrombosis.[40] These drugs have numerous advantages over unfractionated heparin, including once-daily dosing, absence of the need for daily monitoring of APTT and a lower incidence of bleeding. There is some evidence to suggest that they may reduce mortality when compared to patients treated with unfractionated heparin.[40] Thrombocytopenia is as common as with unfractionated heparin, therefore monitoring of platelet count is still advised. Oral anticoagulation with warfarin should be commenced at the same time as heparin and should be continued for a minimum of 3 months. The international normalised ratio (INR) of prothrombin time should be maintained between 2.0 and 3.0. The INR should be monitored daily initially and then every 6 weeks when stable.

Patients should be counselled on their increased tendency to bleed and made aware of possible drug interactions with warfarin, particularly when coadministered with analgesics and antibiotics. A warfarin warning card must be supplied to all patients. After 3 months of therapy patients should be reassessed for ongoing risk factors. Where none exist therapy should be stopped and where these persist, long-term anticoagulation should be considered. In patients where the risk of bleeding is significant with anticoagulants, or pulmonary embolism has recurred despite an adequate INR or who bleed during treatment with anticoagulants, consideration should be given to the insertion of an inferior vena caval filter.[40]

Diffuse parenchymal lung disease

Introduction

The diffuse parenchymal lung diseases (DPLD) are a group of more than 200 heterogeneous conditions which affect the lung parenchyma. It is beyond the scope of this chapter to consider these illnesses in great detail and readers are referred to the BTS guidelines on the diagnosis, assessment and treatment of DPLD in adults.[41] Little information is available on the incidence of DPLD in the general population but it is estimated that they account for 15% of a respiratory specialist's workload. Prevalence data from Mexico suggests an incidence of 31.5 per 100 000 in men and 26.1 per 100 000 in women.[41] There is however considerable variation in the prevalence, mortality and age at presentation between conditions. For example, the incidence and mortality of cryptogenic fibrosing alveolitis increase with age, unlike sarcoidosis which tends to present at a younger age and has a better prognosis.[41]

History and presentation

The presentation of DPLD may be acute, episodic or chronic and it should be noted that there is considerable overlap between conditions. Typical presenting symptoms include breathlessness and non-productive cough. The chest X-ray often demonstrates a pulmonary infiltrate, although it may be normal. It is important in patients with suspected DPLD to take an extensive history as this often provides important clues as to the aetiology of the underlying pulmonary disease. Factors to be included in the history are occupational exposure to dusts and allergens, domestic and hobby-related dust exposure, cigarette smoking, family history of respiratory or connective tissue disorder and drug history. Previous history of cancer, radiotherapy and drugs used during chemotherapy should be noted.[41] Symptoms associated with underlying connective tissue disease, including arthralgia, Raynaud's phenomenon, rashes and eye symptoms, should also be sought. Every effort should be made to review previous X-rays and investigations as they may provide important information about the duration and rate of progression of DPLD.

Investigation

The majority of patients will already have had a chest X-ray at presentation to a respiratory specialist and these are usually abnormal. Simple investigations are worthwhile in almost all patients. A number of serological tests may be useful in establishing an underlying cause for DPLD. These include full blood count with eosinophil count, erythrocyte sedimentation rate, renal function, liver function, serum calcium, immunopathology (rheumatoid factor, antinuclear antibody, antineutrophil cytoplasmic antibody, anti-basement membrane antibody), circulating precipitins to suspected environmental allergens, serum angiotensin-converting enzyme level and serum electrophoresis. Simple urine testing may be abnormal when there is associated renal involvement.

Pulmonary function testing, exercising testing and arterial blood gas estimation will provide important information about the degree of respiratory impairment. High-resolution computed tomography (HRCT) of the chest in DPLD has increased the likelihood of a diagnosis without the need for invasive tests. HRCT may also predict disease activity and the likelihood of response to immunosuppressive therapy in some conditions.

More invasive tests which may be required where the diagnosis remains in doubt following non-invasive tests include flexible fibreoptic bronchoscopy with bronchoalveolar lavage and transbronchial biopsy. Open-lung biopsy, which requires a general anaesthetic and mini-thoracotomy, will provide a large quantity of material for histological purposes but is associated with increased mortality and morbidity.[41] When planning invasive investigations of this nature the physician must be confident that the benefits of obtaining a more secure histological diagnosis outweigh the risks of the procedure. This risk–benefit ratio is particularly difficult to interpret in the elderly where there is a perception that they have higher complication rates from invasive investigations and disease that is more indolent.

Management

Management strategies are aimed at treating the underlying cause. In aspiration pneumonia the physician should consider percutaneous endoscopic gastrostomy (PEG) tube feeding, while addressing the underlying cause for aspiration. Where organic or inorganic dust exposure has been implicated in the development of DPLD, further exposure should be avoided. In drug-induced DPLD the offending drugs should be discontinued and where infection is suspected appropriate antibiotics should be administered.

Few data from placebo-controlled studies of immunosuppression in DPLD are available. It is however well recognised that there is considerable variation in corticosteroid response rates between conditions. Cryptogenic organising pneumonia, extrinsic allergic alveolitis, eosinophilic pneumonia and sarcoidosis are clearly corticosteroid-responsive. Other conditions such as asbestosis, pneumoconiosis and silicosis are not and corticosteroids currently have no role in their management.

Most data are available for cryptogenic fibrosing alveolitis. Response rates of 10–40% have been reported with high-dose oral corticosteroids.[41] It is reported however that older patients are significantly less likely to respond.[42] The decision to commence treatment is difficult, particularly in the elderly, who exhibit low response rates and have a higher incidence of comorbidity. Current BTS guidelines suggest combined treatment with prednisolone (0.5 mg/kg per day) and azathioprine (2–3 mg/kg per day) with assessment after 1 and 3 months and tapering of the prednisolone dose after 1 month. Complications of high-dose corticosteroids in the elderly include hyperglycaemia, fluid retention, hypertension, neuropsychiatric manifestations, osteoporosis, cataracts and Cushing's syndrome. Azathioprine may be associated with hepatitis and bone marrow failure, requiring monitoring of full blood count and liver function tests. The role of colchicine, penicillamine, ciclosporin and methotrexate in the treatment of cryptogenic fibrosing alveolitis is unclear. In the elderly patient the toxicity of this regimen is likely to outweigh any potential benefits in terms of improvement in lung function and symptoms.[41]

Drug-induced pulmonary disease

Drug-induced pulmonary disease can range in severity from mild to severe. The incidence of drug-induced pulmonary disease is largely unknown. This may be due to underreporting, especially in less severe cases where morbidity is low. A number of drugs have been implicated in the development of pulmonary diseases. These are included in Table 5.12.[43, 44]

While there may be many factors which predispose patients to respiratory complications from these drugs, few mention age as a specific predisposing factor, except for bleomycin which has an increased incidence of pneumonitis in the over-70 age group. Other factors which predispose patients to pulmonary side-effects include the total cumulative dose of the drug, coexisting renal impairment and administration of other drugs which affect the respiratory system. The coadministration of radiotherapy increases the incidence of drug-induced pulmonary disease in patients receiving chemotherapy.[44]

Table 5.12 Drug-related causes of respiratory problems

Respiratory problem	Drug
Cough or bronchospasm	Aspirin, NSAIDs, ACE inhibitors, vinca alkaloids, β-blockers, inhaled agents (pentamidine, metered-dose inhalers), contrast media
Pneumonitis	NSAIDs, methotrexate, gold salts, penicillamine, vinca alkaloids, azathioprine, bleomycin, melphalan, radiotherapy
Pulmonary oedema	Aspirin, vinca alkaloids, methotrexate, opiates
Bronchiolitis obliterans	Penicillamine, gold salts
Pulmonary renal syndrome	Penicillamine
Pulmonary fibrosis	Amiodarone, nitrofurantoin, radiotherapy, combination chemotherapy
Impaired respiratory muscle function:	
Central hypoventilation	Narcotics, sedatives, alcohol
Motor neuropathies	Phenytoin, isoniazid, gold, amiodarone, captopril, vincristine, vaccines
Neuromuscular blockade	Aminoglycosides, macrolides, calcium channel blockers
Myopathies	Diuretics, corticosteroids

NSAIDs = Non-steroidal anti-inflammatory drugs; ACE = angiotensin-converting enzyme.

Drug interactions

Drug interactions in the elderly are an important cause of morbidity. These patients are often on multiple therapies, increasing the risk of the co-prescription of interacting drugs. Table 5.13 is not an exhaustive list of interacting drugs, but concentrates on common and clinically significant interactions.[45, 46]

Conclusion

Respiratory illnesses in the elderly are common and are often underinvestigated and inadequately managed. With appropriate investigation and management the elderly can show a significant clinical response and an improved quality of life.

Table 5.13 Drug interactions

Drug	Interacting drug	Outcome	Notes
Theophylline	β-Agonists	Increased risk of hypokalaemia Reduction in theophylline levels	Important in patients on high-dose theophylline or oral salbutamol
	Calcium channel blockers	Increased theophylline level with diltiazem and verapamil	May be of little clinical significance
	Macrolides	Increased theophylline level Decreased effect of erythromycin	Important in patients on high-dose theophylline Newer macrolides may have a less profound effect
	Cimetidine	Theophylline level increased by 30% or more Decrease dose by 30–50%	Other H_2-blockers do not appear to share this interaction
	Isoniazid	Increased theophylline level	Important in long-term therapy
	Rifampicin	Decreased theophylline level	
	Quinolones	Increased theophylline level Increased risk of seizures	Effect most pronounced with ciprofloxacin and less likely with the newer agents
	Smoking	Decreased theophylline levels	Dose reduction may be required in patients who stop smoking
	Leukotriene inhibitors	Increased theophylline levels	Single case report
β_2-Agonists	Potassium-depleting drugs	Increased risk of hypokalaemia	Committee on Safety of Medicines warning
Corticosteroids	Non-steroidal anti-inflammatory drugs	Increased risk of gastrointestinal ulceration and bleeding	

References

1. Information and Statistics Division, National Health Service in Scotland. *Scottish Health Statistics 1998*. Edinburgh: Common Services Agency, 1999.
2. The British Thoracic Society, the National Asthma Campaign, the Royal College of Physicians of London in association with the General Practitioner in Asthma Group, the British Association of Accident and Emergency Medicine, the British Paediatric Respiratory Society, the Royal College of Paediatrics and Child Health. The British guidelines on asthma management. 1995 Review and position statement. *Thorax* 1995; 52: S1–S21.

3.   The COPD Guidelines Group of the Standards of Care Committee of the BTS. BTS guidelines for the management of chronic obstructive pulmonary disease. *Thorax* 1997; 52 (suppl 5): 1S–27S.

4.   Connolly M J, ed. *Respiratory Diseases in the Elderly Patient*, 1st edn. London: Chapman and Hall Medical, 1996.

5.   Fein M, ed. *Clinics in Chest Medicine. Pulmonary Disease in the Elderly*. London: W B Saunders, 1993.

6.   Thurlbeck W. The internal surface of the non-emphysematous lungs. *Am Rev Respir Dis* 1967; 95: 765–773.

7.   Kronenberg R S, Drage C W. Attenuation of the ventilatory and heart responses to hypoxia and hypercapnia with aging in normal men. *J Clin Invest* 1973; 52: 1812–1819.

8.   Brewis R A L, Corrin B, Geddes D M, Gibson G J. *Respiratory Medicine*, 2nd edn. London: W B Saunders, 1995.

9.   Cotton M M, Bucknall C E, Dagg K D *et al*. Early discharge for patients with exacerbations of chronic obstructive pulmonary disease: a randomised controlled trial. *Thorax* 2000; 55: 902–906.

10. Crockett A. Screening older patients for obstructive airways disease. *Thorax* 1999; 54: 472–473.

11. Jones P W, Bosh T K. Quality of life changes in COPD patients treated with salmeterol. *Am J Respir Crit Care Med* 1997; 155: 1283–1289.

12. Burge P S, Calverley P M A, Jones P W *et al*. Randomised, double blind, placebo controlled study of fluticasone propionate in patients with moderate to severe chronic obstructive pulmonary disease: the ISOLDE trial. *BMJ* 2000; 320: 1297–1303.

13. Pauwels R A, Lofdahl C G, Laitinen L A *et al*. Long-term treatment with inhaled budesonide in persons with mild chronic obstructive pulmonary disease who continue smoking. *New Engl J Med* 1999; 340: 1948–1953.

14. Report of the Medical Research Council working party. Long term domicilary oxygen therapy in chronic hypoxic cor pulmonale complicating chronic bronchitis and emphysema. *Lancet* 1981; i: 681–686.

15. Nocturnal Oxygen Therapy Trial Group. Continuous or nocturnal oxygen therapy in hypoxemic chronic obstructive lung disease: a clinical trial. *Ann Intern Med* 1980; 93: 391–398.

16. Anthionisen N R, Connett J E, Kiley J P *et al*. Effects of smoking intervention and the use of an inhaled bronchodilator on the rate of FEV_1. The lung health study. *JAMA* 1994; 272: 1497–1505.

17. Raw M, McNeill A, West R. Smoking cessation guidelines for health professionals. A guide to effective smoking cessation interventions for the health care system. *Thorax* 1998; 53: S1–S19.

18. Gravil J H, Al-Rawas O A, Cotton M M *et al*. Home treatment of exacerbations of chronic obstructive pulmonary disease by an acute respiratory assessment service. *Lancet* 1998; 351: 1853–1855.

19. Smyrnios N A. Asthma: a six-part strategy for managing older patients. *Geriatrics* 1997; 52: 36–44.

20. Sherman C B. Late-onset asthma: making the diagnosis, choosing drug therapy. *Geriatrics* 1995; 50: 24–33.

21. Bucknall C E, Slack R, Godley C G *et al*. Scottish Confidential Inquiry into Asthma Deaths (SCIAD), 1994–6. *Thorax* 1999; 54: 978–984.

22. Ullah M I, Newman G B, Saunders K B. Influence of age on response to ipratropium and salbutamol in asthma. *Thorax* 1981; 36: 523–529.

23. Lipworth B J. Leukotriene-receptor antagonists. *Lancet* 1999; 353: 57–62.

24. Tsang K W, Lam W K, Ip M *et al*. Inability of physicians to use metered-dose inhalers. *J Asthma* 1997; 34: 493–498.

25. Taylor D, Tunstell P. Metered dose inhalers: a system for assessing technique in patients and health professionals. *Pharm J* 1991; 246: 626–627.

26. Doll R, Peto R, Whestley K *et al*. Mortality in relation to smoking: 40 years observations on male British doctors. *BMJ* 1994; 309: 901–910.

27. Muers M F, Haward R A. Management of lung cancer. *Thorax* 1996; 51: 557–560.

28. Brown J S, Eraut D, Trask C, Davison A G. Age and the treatment of lung cancer. *Thorax* 1996; 51: 564–568.

29. Scottish Intercollegiate Guidelines Network. *Management of Lung Cancer*. Edinburgh: SIGN, 1998.

30. Kristerson S, Lindell S, Svanberg L. Prediction of pulmonary function loss due to pneumonectomy using ^{133}Xe-radiospirometry. *Chest* 1972; 62: 694–698.

31. Boysen P G, Harris J O, Block A J, Olsen G N. Prospective evaluation for pneumonectomy using perfusion scanning. *Chest* 1981; 80: 163–166.

32. British Thoracic Society, Society of Cardiothoracic Surgeons of Great Britain, and Ireland Working Party. Guidelines on the selection of patients with lung cancer for surgery. *Thorax* 2001; 56: 89–108.

33. Mitsudomi T, Mizoue T, Yoshimatsu T *et al*. Postoperative complications after pneumonectomy for treatment of lung cancer, multivariate analysis. *J Surg Oncol* 1996; 61: 218–222.

34. Holden D A, Rice T W, Stelmach K, Meeker D P. Exercise testing, 6 min walk and stair climb in the evaluation of patients at high risk of pulmonary resection. *Chest* 1992; 102: 1774–1779.

35. Cullen M H, Joshi R, Chetiawardana A D, Woodroffe C M. Mitomycin, ifosfamide and cisplatin in non-small-cell lung cancer: treatment good enough to compare. *Br J Cancer* 1988; 58: 359–361.

36. Ellis P A, Smith I E, Hardy J R *et al*. Symptom relief with MVP (mitomycin C, vinblastine and cisplatin) chemotherapy in advanced non-small-cell lung cancer. *Br J Cancer* 1995; 71: 336–370.

37. Hickish T F, Smith I E, Ashley S, Middleton G. Chemotherapy for elderly patients with lung cancer. *Lancet* 1995; 346: 580.

38. Nordstrom M, Lindbald B. Autopsy-verified venous thromboembolism within a defined urban population in the city of Malmo Sweden. *APMIS* 1998; 106: 378–384.

39. Turkstra F, Koopman M W, Buller H R. The treatment of deep vein thrombosis and pulmonary embolism. *Thromb Haemost* 1997; 78: 489–496.

40. Scottish Intercollegiate Guidelines Network. *Antithrombotic Therapy*. Edinburgh: SIGN, 1999.

41. The Diffuse Parenchymal Lung Disease group. The diagnosis, assessment and treatment of diffuse parenchymal lung disease in adults. *Thorax* 1999; 54: S1–S30.
42. Turner-Warwick M, Burrows B, Johnson A. Cryptogenic fibrosing alveolitis: clinical features and their influence in survival. *Thorax* 1980; 35: 171–180.
43. Belton K J, Lee A. Drug induced respiratory disorders. *Pharm J* 1997; 259: 412–417.
44. Cooper J A D, ed. *Clinics in Chest Medicine*. London: W B Saunders, 1990.
45. Parfitt K, ed. *Martindale: The complete drug reference*, 32nd edn. London: Pharmaceutical Press, 1999.
46. Stockley I H. *Drug Interactions*, 5th edn. London: Pharmaceutical Press. 1999.

6

Psychiatry and the elderly

Barbara Baigent

Many people become mentally ill for the first time late in life, partly because of life changes such as bereavement and failing physical health causing them to feel depressed and partly because of organic changes in the brain leading to delirious confusion and to the dementias. They are more likely than younger people to present their mental distress as physical symptoms, therefore cognitive as well as physical assessment is essential, and since the elderly are often unwilling to come to a surgery or to an outpatient clinic, domicilary visits are important.

At the time of the visit it is important to check the medications in the house, whether being taken currently or previously by the patient or by anyone else in the house. Many elderly have carers who should be interviewed particularly about their knowledge of the patient's illness and medication, whether they oversee this and whether they are aware of available support services.

Elderly patients are often confused about what different medications are for and with the multiplicity of their physical ailments are often taking several prescribed drugs plus over-the-counter remedies which they have purchased. On the whole they will take analgesics more readily than antipsychotics; they are very fearful of becoming addicted to antidepressants; but will take benzodiazepine hypnotics which are still being prescribed by many general practitioners and which add to the confusion, drowsiness and falling to which the elderly are prone.

Depression

Depression is often the most common reason for the referral of an elderly person today. The prevalence of depressive symptoms far exceeds that of depressive illness. Major depression affects 2–4% of older people but 10–20% suffer less severe depression which is under-diagnosed and should be treated. The prevalence of depression among people aged over 65 has been reported to be 15% in the general community, 25% in general practice patients and more than 30% in community homes.[1]

How does depression differ in elderly people from its presentation in younger people? Depressive delusions concerning poverty and nihilistic delusions that the body is empty or not functioning are common. Older people have more thoughts of death and a greater preoccupation with the wish to die, although not significantly so; but are less likely to report memory problems.[2] Hallucinations of an obscene or accusing kind may occur.

Another study did *not* find symptoms which reliably differentiated older people with major depression from younger ones.[3] However there are identifiable factors which may alter or obscure the presentation of depression in the elderly, some of which are: overlap of physical and somatic psychiatric symptoms; disproportionate complaints associated with physical disorder, or somatisation of the physical disorder; medically trivial deliberate self-harm; pseudodementia (i.e. severe depression can mimic dementia); depression superimposed on dementia; or late-onset alcohol dependence syndrome.

Some of the symptoms of bereavement overlap with those of depressive illness but those which point more clearly to depression and therefore to a trial of antidepressant use are slipping back for no apparent reason after making progress for a few months; suicidal thoughts; pervasive guilt (not merely over what might have been done to prevent the death) and maintaining grief by keeping everything unchanged.[4]

The important biological symptoms are reduced sleep and early-morning wakening; loss of appetite and weight loss; diurnal mood variation (worse in mornings); constipation; physical and mental slowing and suicidal thoughts.

Predisposing factors to depression in the elderly are poor physical health such as stroke and idiopathic Parkinson's disease; also the fact that some biological changes associated with the ageing brain are similar to those of depression, e.g. decreased brain concentrations of serotonin (5-HT), dopamine and noradrenaline (norepinephrine) and increased monoamine oxidase B activity.[5]

In all age groups women are more prone to depression than men (7 : 3 female to male) and in the elderly the risk factor for depression in first-degree relatives is much lower (8%) than in early-onset depression (20%).[6]

Precipitating factors are life events such as loss or threatening circumstances in the previous year, in common with all age groups;

in the elderly, recent grave physical illness or a chronically disabling disorder plays a greater part.[7]

Most problems with outcome were associated with disability, loss of spouse and lack of support – emotional, tangible and family support. The role of the carer is an important one and carers need support. Recently several studies have shown a better outcome in elderly depressed patients than in younger ones.[8] Others have found the outcome to be at least as good.[9]

Elderly people are over-represented in suicide statistics; the incidence in people over 65 years is three times that of the 15–24-year age group.[10] The rate rises in the over-80s, particularly men. Two-thirds of elderly attenders have a psychiatric disorder, mainly severe depression. Others have chronic painful physical health or suffer from loneliness.

Treatment

Successful treatment of depression in the elderly will include psychological and social as well as medical skills. Hurdles to be overcome are patients' belief that tablets are not the answer because they are not suffering a true illness – only a moral weakness or becoming senile – and their fear of becoming addicted to the tablets. Current research has not shown clear superiority of one group of antidepressants over another in terms of efficacy, therefore the choice of treatment remains controversial and should be made after consideration of such factors as previous tolerability and response; type of depression (agitated or retarded); concurrent drug treatment and interactions; compliance; concurrent physical illness and liability to side-effects such as postural hypotension, cognitive impairment and sedation.

Drug treatment will take time – weeks rather than days – and this should be explained to the patient and carer, otherwise they may lose heart and give up on treatment. Also the drugs should be continued in all age groups for at least 4–6 months after the depression has resolved, otherwise they will relapse.[11] For the elderly this might need extending to 12 months and some may need to take the tablets for 2 years or more.

ECT

Electroconvulsive therapy (ECT) remains the most effective treatment for depressive illness at any age, with recovery rates around 80%. It is the first choice of treatment for those who are suicidal or dehydrated through refusing food and drink or experiencing delusions.[12] The elderly respond well, especially when the picture is dominated by anxiety (unlike in younger people), but memory impairment is worse, which is why unilateral placement of the electrodes is often used. Others feel that it is more important to use bilateral electrodes which give a better therapeutic outcome. For the elderly a course of six ECTs may not be enough and they may need up to 12, at two per week.

Tricyclic antidepressants

Tricyclic antidepressants act by inhibiting the reuptake of both noradrenaline and 5-HT presynaptically and were once the conventional choice of antidepressant medication with dosulepin (dothiepin) as the preference over amitriptyline or imipramine. However some side-effects are troublesome, such as dry mouth, constipation, sweating, drowsiness, tremor and vivid dreams, and others can be clinically problematic in the elderly, for example, dizziness on standing up, postural hypotension, urinary hesitancy, worsening of delirium or of epilepsy and risk of overdose. A tricyclic, such as dosulepin, should be started at the lowest dose and raised at 25-mg increments every 7 days to the highest tolerated dose (up to 150 mg daily). The blood pressure should be checked weekly, lying and standing.

Lofepramine, a newer tricyclic, has reduced cardiotoxicity and fewer sedative and anticholinergic effects but may still cause orthostatic hypotension.

Selective serotonin reuptake inhibitors (SSRIs)

SSRIs only prevent the reuptake of 5-HT, not of noradrenaline. They are not free from side-effects but they have several advantages over the tricyclics for some patients, especially those who are at risk of suicide; or those who have poor left ventricular function; or who experience clinically relevant cardiac arrhythmias on tricyclic medication; or who are taking antihypertensive medication (which may interact with tricyclics). Another advantage is that the dose of an SSRI does not generally require to be altered from the initial dose, which improves compliance and means that the effective dose can be reached sooner.

The main side-effects of SSRIs are nausea, diarrhoea, insomnia and anxiety/agitation, especially in those who were already agitated. Weight gain rarely occurs. They are safer than the tricyclics in overdose because they are less cardiotoxic; however, they can cause convulsions in overdose. They are involved in far fewer drug interactions than the tricyclics are, which is useful for the elderly who may be taking a number of medications.

Fluoxetine   The long half-life of this SSRI may make it less suitable for the elderly; however, it could be used to advantage by giving the tablet on alternate days at a day hospital to a person whose compliance was in doubt. The daily dose for all ages is 20 mg.

Dose reduction is recommended in patients with reduced hepatic metabolism and poor renal function. There has been only one death reported (after ingestion of 6 g fluoxetine) whereas the number of deaths per million prescriptions of amitriptyline was 38.94 for the years 1987–1992. Fluoxetine has been shown to improve the quality of life both physically and mentally in the elderly. There are no problems with sudden withdrawal because it has such a long half-life but this also means that when changing to a different antidepressant this should be borne in mind.

Paroxetine   The advantage of this drug is its shorter half-life; it can be given once a day, but its disadvantage is problems on sudden withdrawal such as anxiety, dizziness, agitation, sleep disturbance, tremor, paraesthesia, nausea, sweating and confusion. The drug dose should be tapered slowly down using alternate-day dosing if necessary. The maximum daily dose in the elderly is 40 mg. There have been reports of orofacial dystonias with paroxetine.

Sertraline, fluvoxamine and citalopram These are similar drugs to paroxetine.

Sertraline causes fewer drug interactions because it does not affect the cytochrome P450 system. The dose does not need to be reduced in normal elderly patients.

Fluvoxamine produces nausea in a high percentage of patients and interacts with many other drugs, such as theophylline, carbamazepine, clozapine, phenytoin, terfenadine and astemizole.

Citalopram has a maximum daily dose in the elderly of 40 mg and causes fewer problems on sudden withdrawal but there have been some fatalities in overdose. Interactions with other drugs are fewer than those of the other SSRIs.

Newer antidepressants

The newer antidepressants should probably be reserved for resistant depression.

Venlafaxine, for example, which inhibits reuptake of both nora-drenaline and 5-HT, is safer to use than combining a tricyclic with an SSRI. The dose is unchanged in the elderly but if the dose is 200 mg daily or more, the blood pressure should be checked.

Mirtazapine increases the appetite and causes weight gain.

Nefazodone has a maximum daily dose in the elderly of 200 mg twice a day.

Reboxetine is not recommended in the elderly.

A consensus statement from the United States National Institute of Mental Health (1998) lists venlafaxine, mirtazapine and nefazodone as being useful in senile depression[13] together with SSRIs.

Monoamine oxidase inhibitors (MAOIs)

The MAOIs have virtually been superseded by newer antidepressants which are safer because the patient does not have to avoid cheese and other tyramine-containing foods. Moclobemide is a reversible inhibitor of monoamine oxidase Type A and, although a restrictive diet is not nec-essary, it would be safer not to eat excessive amounts of cheese. It may be useful for depressive illness but is not for atypical depression, for which the older MAOIs were used.

Problems with drug treatment

Hyponatraemia

One of the most frequent side-effects of antidepressant treatment in the elderly is hyponatraemia due to inappropriate antidiuretic hormone (ADH) secretion. It has occurred with all classes of antidepressants and should be suspected if the patient develops drowsiness, confusion or convulsions on treatment. The drug should be stopped but it is impossible to predict whether a drug from an alternative class will cause it to recur.

Resistant depression

Sometimes the older patient just does not respond to either a tricyclic alone or to an SSRI alone. Each drug should be tried for a 6-week course. Venlafaxine or mirtazapine could be tried next, or augmentation could be considered. Lithium can be added to either a tricyclic or (with caution) to an SSRI. However, it should be remembered that lithium may worsen the extrapyramidal side-effects of an antipsychotic or an antidepressant; and if the patient has poor renal function or is on diuretic or non-steroidal anti-inflammatory drug (NSAID) treatment, or has a poor memory for taking tablets, he or she will be liable to lithium toxicity.

Response rates have been shown to be much lower (20%) in older than in younger adults[14] but there have been no double-blind controlled trials of lithium augmentation therapy in elderly patients to date.

Mania and manic-depressive illness

Mania is not thought to be fundamentally different from unipolar depression; indeed, many elderly people have had many years of multiple depressive episodes which have converted to mania in later years. They are then said to suffer from a bipolar disorder, i.e. manic-depressive illness. An average psychogeriatric inpatient unit can expect to treat 8 patients per year suffering from mania which is severe enough to require hospitalisation. This is 12% of all elderly cases of affective disorder and there is a female to male ratio of 2 : 1. The summary of the ICD-10[15] criteria for a manic episode is shown in Table 6.1.

There is a significant association between brain disease and mania. In 20–40% of elderly the manic episode will be secondary to cerebrovascular disease, chronic alcohol misuse, head injury or a right-sided lesion to the brain (stroke).[16] Alzheimer's disease does not appear to

Table 6.1 Summary of ICD-10 criteria[15] for a manic episode

Without psychotic symptoms
Elevated mood or irritability
Increased energy and overactivity
Pressure of speech
Decreased sleep
Social disinhibition
Poor attention and marked distractibility
Grandiose or overoptimistic ideas
Extravagant schemes and overspending
Aggressive or amorous episodes

With psychotic symptoms
As above plus:
Severe and sustained excitement
Flight of ideas
Mood-congruent delusions or hallucinations

give rise to mania.[17] Very few elderly people with mania will have become manic before the age of 40 years, in contrast to figures for the general population which show mania occurring in 20- and 30-year-olds with bipolar affective disorder. The mean age for the elderly is about 55 years, with some manic cases occurring for the first time when patients are well into their 80s.

The clinical features are not as severe as those in young people, but include decreased sleep, physical hyperactivity, flight of ideas, thought disorder, overspending, grandiose delusions, irritability and hypersexuality.

The prognosis for mania in old age has improved over the last generation. A study showed that after 5–7-year follow-up, 72% of survivors were symptom-free and 80% of survivors were living independently.[18] Survival in elderly patients with mania and a matched group with unipolar depression has also been examined.[16] After a follow-up period of 3–10 years, 50% of patients with mania had died, compared with only 20% with depression. The high mortality is of concern but may mean that mania results from a more severe disruption of the central nervous system.

Drug treatment

Drugs are used both to control acute attacks and to prevent recurrence but few data are available concerning the treatment of mania in the elderly.

Lithium

Lithium treatment remains the first option but more research is needed to confirm the safe blood levels and dosage in old age. Whereas in younger people the blood level should be 0.4–0.8 mmol/l for prophylactic long-term treatment and 0.8–1.0 mmol/l for manic episodes, in the elderly a blood level of 0.3–0.6 mmol/l is probably sufficient and will be reached by doses of 300–450 mg/day.[19] The dangers of lithium treatment are all concerning the kidney, i.e. poor renal function will lengthen the half-life; excessive sweating, vomiting or diarrhoea will lower sodium and therefore raise lithium levels in the blood; a change in diet where less sodium is taken will also raise lithium levels. Perhaps more importantly, most NSAIDs (taken for arthritis) except aspirin will be excreted preferentially to lithium and therefore will raise lithium levels, as will diuretics, because they cause sodium loss. Loop diuretics are safer than thiazides, which should be avoided. When either group of drugs (loop diuretics or NSAIDs) are combined with lithium, the dose of lithium should be halved and a blood level taken after 5 days. Its excretion may be reduced by angiotensin-converting enzyme inhibitors and neurotoxicity may occur with calcium channel blockers, although plasma lithium concentrations are normal.

The adverse effects of lithium are a fine tremor which becomes coarse in toxicity states; initial nausea, vomiting and diarrhoea, which also recur in toxicity; polyuria, weight gain and oedema. Other signs of toxicity are muscle weakness, central nervous system disturbance – drowsiness, giddiness and lack of coordination – and eventually convulsions and coma.

Treatment should be preceded by renal function tests and after the initial lithium blood tests, the level should be checked at least every 6 months (*British National Formulary* no. 41[20] states 3-monthly). Lithium should never be stopped abruptly except in toxicity. It may impair glucose tolerance of diabetics on oral hypoglycaemic treatment.

The mechanism by which lithium acts is not completely understood but certainly it does affect calcium channels, as do drugs such as nifedipine and diltiazem. These drugs, often used in later life, have been reported to cause depression.[21, 22]

Carbamazepine and sodium valproate

Carbamazepine and sodium valproate are both widely used in mania but little is known of their use in the elderly.[23]

Carbamazepine is known to be useful in rapid cycling (more than three episodes of mood disorder in 1 year). The dose in younger people is 200–300 mg twice a day.

Valproate has been found to be well tolerated in the elderly as an adjunct to lithium[24] but it does not have a product licence for mood stabilisation in the UK. The dose in younger people is 600 mg twice a day. There is danger of neurotoxicity with all these drugs, especially in combination.

Semisodium valproate is now licensed for short-term treatment of manic episodes. Although its kinetics are altered in the elderly, this has little clinical significance.

Antipsychotics

In severe mania it may be necessary to add an antipsychotic drug because the mood stabilisers take about 5 days to act. There are dangers in adding haloperidol to lithium because a condition similar to neuroleptic malignant syndrome has occurred. Clopixol Acuphase injection of zuclopenthixol acetate requires a reduced dose in the elderly, although some centres use it for rapid tranquillisation of younger adults. It is an aqueous suspension which has effects for about 72 h. It may cause excessive sedation and a fall in blood pressure.

Lithium exacerbates the extrapyramidal side-effects of all antipsychotics. Carbamazepine will reduce the plasma concentrations of haloperidol and risperidone, also of theophylline, levothyroxine (thyroxine) and warfarin (relevant to the elderly). Conversely, a course of erythromycin will raise the plasma concentration of carbamazepine and could cause toxicity, manifest as drowsiness.

Schizophrenia

In elderly people the term 'paraphrenia' is used. There are at present two conflicting views about 'late paraphrenia'. Some believe that it is merely an expression of schizophrenia in the elderly;[25] others believe that the paranoid symptoms of late life are genetically different from schizophrenia and arise from various pathogenic factors associated with old age.[26] In either case the symptoms are delusions, usually persecutory, in 90% of patients; and hallucinations, usually auditory, in 75% of patients, with visual hallucinations less common (16–60%). Other schizophrenic symptoms also differ in the elderly from those found in early-onset schizophrenia. Thought disorder, negative features (e.g. reduced speech and facial expression) and catatonia are very uncommon in late-onset cases.

Since ICD-10[15] does not identify 'late paraphrenia', people have to be classified either under 'schizophrenia' or under 'delusional disorder', but this is often inappropriate because it excludes prominent hallucinations[27] (Table 6.2).

Table 6.2 Divisions of patients with late paraphrenia[29]

ICD-10 *diagnosis*	%
Delusional disorder	31
Paranoid schizophrenia	61
Schizoaffective disorder	8

The prevalence among the elderly living in the community is 0.1–4% and of the elderly in psychiatric hospitals it is 10%. Only 1.5% of all those diagnosed with schizophrenia are over 60 years of age.[26] The incidence is higher in women than in men (unlike early-onset schizophrenia, with a predominance in men). Other risk factors are sight and hearing loss, social isolation, brain disease and family history.

Drug treatment

The use of antipsychotic medication is widely accepted although no controlled trials have been reported. A study found that 60% of patients made a complete response to treatment with 10–30 mg/day of trifluoperazine or 40–500 mg/day of thioridazine and 9% made no response,[28] but more recently less optimistic results have been reported, e.g. 42% showed no response to medication after 3 months of treatment.[29] Thioridazine is now licensed only for second-line treatment of schizophrenia in the UK.

Undoubtedly, neuroleptics benefit a majority of patients but side-effects are a great problem. Doses must be kept very low and a newer antipsychotic such as risperidone, may be more acceptable than the conventional phenothiazines and other classes of drugs.

Adverse effects of antipsychotic medication

Antipsychotic medications are generally dopamine receptor-blocking drugs with varying degrees of affinity to block other receptors as well. There are dopamine receptors in both the limbic area of the brain, related to psychoses, and in the striatal areas, related to motor function. This is why, by blocking dopamine in all areas of the brain, the conventional antipsychotics cause movement disorders like dyskinesias and dystonias. If they also block acetylcholine and α-adrenoceptors, adverse effects like postural drop, body sway and falls will occur. These, coupled with sedation from histamine blockade, can be dangerous in the elderly. Conventional antipsychotics also blunt thermo-regulatory mechanisms in the hypothalamus so that the body fails to cool down in heat or to warm up in the cold. This can lead to accidental hypothermia in the elderly.

Neuroleptic malignant syndrome   This is a poorly recognised condition which can occur with any neuroleptic or when levodopa is suddenly withdrawn. It is often associated with lithium as an additional treatment. There is no firm guidance as to which treatment can be restarted once the condition has improved. The syndrome involves hyperthermia, muscle rigidity, fluctuating consciousness and autonomic disturbance such as labile blood pressure, sweating and tachycardia. The patient should be transferred to an acute hospital, treated with dantrolene and possibly bromocriptine, and held psychiatrically on diazepam alone for 2 weeks.

Extrapyramidal adverse effects   These fall into four categories in all age groups:

1. Akathisia or restlessness. This is incessant movement, inability to sit still, the feeling of wanting to move about. It occurs 30–75 days after treatment has commenced and is difficult to treat. Changing the drug or reducing the dose or adding propranolol (not a good idea in the elderly) are possibilities.
2. Dystonias occur when particular muscles go into spasm, mainly the neck or tongue, throat or eye (oculogyric crisis). They occur up to 48–72 h after the dose has been given and should be treated immediately with oral or intramuscular procyclidine, benzatropine, trihexyphenidyl (benzhexol) or orphenadrine.
3. Drug-induced parkinsonism. This syndrome resembles idiopathic Parkinson's disease with tremor, rigidity, drooling and shuffling gait. It also takes weeks or months to develop and should be treated with oral anticholinergic medication as under dystonias. Levodopa cannot be used since it liberates dopamine and the patient is receiving antipsychotic medication, which is dopamine receptor-blocking medication.
4. Tardive dyskinesia. This consists of irregular movements, usually orofacial, such as chewing movements of the jaw, rolling or smacking of the tongue and twisting of the fingers. Although it is distressing to observe, patients never complain of it and appear untroubled. It is late in onset, often after many years of neuroleptic treatment, but can also occur when high doses are suddenly lowered or when an antipsychotic is suddenly stopped. Treatment with antiparkinsonian drugs such as procyclidine hinders rather than helps and such drugs should be stopped. This is because tardive dyskinesia is thought to be caused by a supersensitivity to the patient's own dopamine, thus the only remedy would be to restart the antipsychotic or raise the dose in order to block more dopamine receptors. But these are not clinically good suggestions; some clinicians have had success with sodium valproate (acting on γ-aminobutyric receptors) and others with vitamin E (acting on free radicals).

Phenothiazines and other conventional antipsychotic drugs

Although low-dose chlorpromazine has been widely used in the elderly because it produces fewer extrapyramidal side-effects (e.g. tremor, rigidity and dyskinesias), it actually produces more anticholinergic side-effects which are not good in the elderly, leading to orthostatic hypotension and falls.

Haloperidol 1.5 mg (a butyrophenone) or trifluoperazine 2 mg would be better choices, giving rise to less sedation, hypotension and cardiac effects, but are limited by their adverse extrapyramidal effects.

Whilst some psychiatrists will not use depot injections in the elderly, others feel that 10–20 mg Depixol (flupentixol decanoate, a thioxanthene) 2-weekly or monthly will dampen down the symptoms without producing side-effects and without the need for patient compliance with tablets or syrup, which is often a problem.[29]

Newer classes of drugs

Sulpiride is often used in the elderly; it causes less tardive dyskinesia but can still produce the other extrapyramidal symptoms such as tremor and rigidity; also the tablets are quite large to swallow.

The true atypical or newer antipsychotics have various characteristics so that at present no one is sure what contributes to being 'atypical'. Is it blockade of 5-HT-receptors as well as dopamine? Is it that the drug has no effect on the pituitary gland, or that it does not produce extrapyramidal symptoms, or that it does not give rise to tardive dyskinesia or that it improves negative as well as positive symptoms of schizophrenia?

Clozapine use is limited by the number of blood tests required and, like olanzapine, by sedation, but it is the antipsychotic drug which does produces least extrapyramidal side-effects. Low doses (50 mg/day) are being used to improve psychosis in patients with Parkinson's disease.[30]

Risperidone is well tolerated by the elderly but will antagonise the effect of levodopa in parkinsonism. It is not sedative; rather it may cause insomnia and agitation. The dose should start at 0.5 mg twice a day, adjusted gradually to 2 mg twice a day. Orthostatic hypotension may be a problem.

Anxiety

In all age groups there is extensive comorbidity between anxiety and depression. In the past benzodiazepines were prescribed when in fact antidepressants would have been the preferred treatment. It is very difficult to separate out a pure anxiety disorder from depression.

ICD-10[15] recognises phobic disorders, panic disorder and generalised anxiety disorder among other neurotic, stress-related and somatoform disorders. One-year prevalence studies in 1991[31] found that, in the elderly, 5% of males and nearly 8% of females suffered from phobic disorder; 2% from generalised anxiety and less than 0.1% from panic disorder. Many important physical disorders may be presented as anxiety, especially in males; conversely, an episode of physical illness may be a frightening experience for elderly patients and in vulnerable people this may result in generalised anxiety or phobic withdrawal. Clinical, but not community studies, have found significant levels of anxiety in the early stages of dementia.[32]

Panic disorder is less common and less severe than in younger people; is more common in women and widows; and is often mistaken for cardiac or gastrointestinal problems.[33]

In phobic disorder the irrational fears of going out, public transport and heights are similar to those in younger age groups; however, often they are dismissed in the elderly as being rational fears, especially, for example, the fear of crime in an inner-city area. The phobia is often accompanied by depression which then dominates the picture.[34]

Treatment

Psychological treatment

Cognitive-behavioural therapy is the most favoured and is of proven effectiveness in phobic disorder in the elderly as well as in younger people. Anxiety management training is also important in the elderly.

Antidepressant treatment

If depression is a prominent feature then a course of antidepressant treatment should always be considered. Some of the SSRI drugs (e.g. citalopram and paroxetine) have a product licence (PL) for panic disorder and the PL for clomipramine includes phobias.

Benzodiazepines

Benzodiazepines should only be used in acute situations, preferably for days rather than weeks. There have been relatively few controlled trials of benzodiazepines in elderly people although they are the largest consumers of this class of drugs, particularly as hypnotics. Because of accumulation of active metabolites, a short-acting drug like oxazepam should be used for anxiety and, if the condition does not improve, the drug should be slowly withdrawn. It is well known that abrupt withdrawal produces withdrawal symptoms which are the converse of the drug's actions, i.e. rebound anxiety, rebound insomnia, increased muscle tone and twitching and (rarely) convulsions.

The adverse effects of this class of drugs in the elderly are persistent drowsiness, falls, incontinence, delirium and amnesia, and long-term use can result in physical dependence, cognitive impairment and paradoxical excitement.[35] In addition the effect of a benzodiazepine on the respiratory centre may be compounded in respiratory illness.

When respiratory-depressant drugs are contraindicated, hydroxyzine, an antihistamine, may be useful for anxiety in the elderly. Buspirone may also be useful; thus far it has not been associated with rebound problems, dependence or misuse. It takes 3 weeks to have an effect so is not suitable for acute anxiety. These drugs are for short-term use.

Organic brain syndromes

Delirium

This is a common clinical picture in old age originating in a cerebral metabolic disturbance as a result of a physical illness or of a toxic dose of medication. Otherwise known as an acute confusional state, it may occur in one-fifth of patients in an elderly ward.

The predisposing factors are pre-existing dementia, defective hearing and vision, Parkinson's disease and advanced age.

The precipitating causes include pneumonia, infection, stroke, hypoxia and medication (Table 6.3).

Table 6.3 Drug treatment which can precipitate delirium

Alcohol use, misuse and withdrawal
Benzodiazepines and their withdrawal
Anticholinergics: tricyclic antidepressants, some antipsychotics, antiparkinsonian drugs used in psychiatry
Dopamine agonists: levodopa, bromocriptine, amantadine, selegiline
Anticonvulsants: phenytoin, barbiturates
Cardivascular: digoxin, diuretics, β-blockers
Miscellaneous; lithium carbonate, cimetidine, non-steroidal anti-inflammatory drugs

The primary clinical feature is impaired consciousness (reduced awareness of the environment); other features may vary between patients. Some will be restless, oversensitive to stimuli and with psychotic symptoms; others will be lethargic and quiet with few psychotic symptoms. Repetitive, purposeless movements are common; thinking is slow and muddled but rich in content. Visual hallucinations may occur with fantastic content and, less often, auditory or tactile hallucinations. Some patients are frightened and agitated; others are perplexed. Anxiety, depression or labile mood is common. Afterwards there is usually amnesia about most of the illness.

General management of the patient is aimed at relieving the distress and reducing the disorientation. It includes allowing friends and relatives to visit frequently; having as few nursing staff changes as possible; nursing the patient in a single room and giving repeated explanations of his/her condition and where he/she is.

Treatment

The fundamental treatment is directed to the physical cause. As few drugs as possible should be given, avoiding any that may further impair the consciousness. However if the patient requires to be calmed in the day time, haloperidol is the drug of choice since it causes the least drowsiness, hypotension and cardiac side-effects. Low doses 3–5 mg should be given because of the risk of extrapyramidal symptoms such as dystonia or dyskinesia. Although short-acting benzodiazepines may be given to promote sleep at night, any daytime sedation will increase the disorientation. They are safer in liver failure; whereas clomethiazole, which is a useful drug in the elderly for calming and sedation, is very dangerous in liver failure and with alcohol.

The dementias

Dementia is a generalised impairment of intellect, memory and personality with no impairment of consciousness. It usually presents with impairment of memory; other features could include mood disorder, hallucinations and delusions. Behaviour is often disorganised, inappropriate, distractible and restless, and changes in behaviour may include sexual disinhibition, shop lifting and sudden explosions of emotion such as anger.

Thinking becomes impoverished with impaired judgement, false ideas – often persecutory in content, disturbed speech with nouns muddled or forgotten (nominal dysphasia). As dementia worsens patients neglect themselves and social conventions. They become disoriented for time, place and person. Insight is lacking.

In the elderly, dementia can be divided into three groups:

1. Dementia of the Alzheimer type. This is the most common type of dementia in old age.
2. Vascular dementia, often associated with multiple infarcts.
3. Dementia due to other causes, such as Lewy body disease, parkinsonism, alcohol abuse (Korsakoff's dementia with Wernicke's encephalopathy), Huntington's disease and prion dementias (these include Creutzfeldt–Jakob disease (and BSE in cows)).

The prevalence rates for dementia are summarised in Table 6.4. The EURODEM project pooled data from a number of studies around Europe in 1991.[36] Prevalence doubles after 5 years so that at 75 years it is 5%; around 80 years it is 10%; and at 90 years, 20%. About two-thirds of patients would have Alzheimer's-type and one-third vascular dementia.

Vascular dementia

This is slightly more common in men than in women and geographically there are higher rates in China, Japan and Russia than in the rest of the world. It may follow a cerebrovascular accident or be associated with hypertension. Depression and emotional lability are common, as are behavioural retardation and anxiety. Insight may be retained to a late stage. The survival is shorter (4–5 years) than for Alzheimer's disease and patients usually die from ischaemic heart disease or cerebral infarction.

Table 6.4 EURODEM prevalence rates for dementia

Age band (years)	%
65–69	1
70–74	4
75–79	6
80–84	13
85–89	22
90–94	32
95–99	35

Dementia with Lewy bodies

Lewy bodies are frequently found in the substantia nigra of some patients with Parkinson's disease and have been found in the cortex of some people with Alzheimer's disease. When this is the case, the dementia includes rapid fluctuations in cognitive function and visual hallucinations. Treatment with standard antiparkinsonian drugs will improve the motor symptoms but worsen the hallucinations and confusion. Antipsychotic drugs, given to reduce the hallucinations, may cause marked side-effects such as dystonias and dyskinesias even at very low doses, and will of course worsen the parkinsonism.

Alzheimer's disease

It is important in view of possible treatments to diagnose the kind of dementia as accurately as possible, since the newer drugs are only for Alzheimer's dementia. Examination of the brain by computed tomographic scan shows cell loss and enlarged lateral ventricles, and serial examination may reveal evidence of progressive disease. Magnetic resonance imaging scans, positron emission tomography and single-photon emission computed tomographic blood flow studies will reveal deficits in specific areas such as the hippocampus, parietal and temporal cortex.

Silver staining of the brain after death shows senile plaques through the cortical and subcortical grey matter; also neurofibrillary tangles which may predict neuronal degeneration and death and whose number correlates with the degree of cognitive impairment. The senile plaques contain β-amyloid peptide which is a derivative of the β-amyloid precursor protein for which there is a gene located on chromosome 21.[37] This accounts for one-quarter of early-onset cases of Alzheimer's disease. The other three-quarters are accounted for by mutations found on chromosome 14.[38]

In late-onset Alzheimer's disease, on the other hand, there is an association with the E4 allele of apolipoprotein E which is found in both plaques and tangles and the gene for which is located on chromosome 19. This may be a predisposing factor for Alzheimer's but is also a predisposing factor for coronary artery disease and hypercholesterolaemia. This is interesting, because some people have a mixed dementia of both Alzheimer's and vascular type.

The suggestion that aluminium may be an environmental contributory cause[39] is controversial. Studies have failed to agree whether or not aluminium is present in the plaques and tangles. However, aluminium can promote the phosphorylation of τ protein and lead to the formation of amyloid peptide, which suggests that it could play a role in the development of Alzheimer's disease.

More importantly, neurochemical studies have shown widespread loss of neurotransmitters, particularly of choline acetyltransferase due to loss of cholinergic nerve cells which results in low levels of acetylcholine and is associated with decreased cognitive function. It is in this area that treatment is emerging.

Treatment

Until recently treatment was limited to psychiatric and behavioural symptoms, rather than treating the underlying process. Depressive symptoms should be treated with antidepressants (see section on depression above); hallucinations should be treated with antipsychotic drugs (but see adverse effects above in the section on schizophrenia and beware in dementia with Lewy bodies); and in vascular dementia low-dose aspirin is recommended to slow the progression of the disease, whilst risk factors such as smoking and hypertension should be addressed.

Cognition-preserving drugs   The recent advances in treatment are cognition-preserving drugs which inhibit the action of acetylcholinesterase to break down acetylcholine. As has been seen above, the reduction of acetylcholine results in the cognitive impairment seen in Alzheimer's disease. Thus these drugs are only useful in Alzheimer's and Lewy body dementia with no effect in vascular dementia. The patient must be suffering only from mild to moderate dementia (this is about 50% of all patients with Alzheimer's disease). Accurate diagnosis is essential. Only 40–60% of patients will benefit from the memory improvement which the drugs offer. The drugs are reversible inhibitors of acetylcholinesterase so that if and when the drug is stopped, there will be deterioration.

The three drugs currently marketed are donepezil, galantamine and rivastigmine but there are other drugs in various stages of pre-marketing. They are generally well tolerated, the main adverse effects being nausea, vomiting, diarrhoea, headache, dizziness and fatigue. Caution is advised if there is a history of asthma or obstructive airways disease, gastric ulcers or cardiac conduction disorders. There have been recent reports of seizures, bradycardia and bladder outflow obstruction problems; also of agitation, hallucinations and aggressive behaviour with donepezil.

The main concern is the cost of these drugs in view of the numbers of patients involved and the fact that unless the treatment is continued long-term, there is little advantage in beginning it. The treatment is symptomatic; there are no substantial data to support the hypothesis that the disease is modified, i.e. that the progress of the disease is delayed; and the improvement in the carer-rated quality of life was not a dramatic increase.[40] Additional costs will include the cost of accurate diagnosis and brain scans. It has been suggested that part of the cost could come from the money saved from residential care. To date, many health authorities in the UK are not funding these drugs.

NSAIDs Recently the possibility has been raised that NSAIDs may inhibit the onset and slow the progress of Alzheimer's disease. Postmortem studies have shown a chronic inflammatory state in the brains of people with this disease, possibly due to neuronal death, the accumulation of debris and toxic products which lead to further neuronal death and inflammation. By reducing inflammation, the NSAID may inhibit further neuronal death. In one study, patients taking NSAIDs for other reasons had a slower progression of Alzheimer's disease;[41] and in another, it was predicted that an NSAID might delay the onset of the disease by 5–7 years.[42] There is a reluctance to treat the elderly with NSAIDs because of the side-effects of gastric bleeding and ulceration, therefore more clinical trials are needed to determine the best drug and the minimum dose to achieve desired results.

References

1. Macdonald A J D. Mental health in old age. *BMJ* 1997; 315: 413–417.
2. Blazer D G, George L, Lauderman R. The phenomenology of late life depression. In: Bebbington P E, Jacoby R, eds. *Psychiatric Disorders of the Elderly*. London: Mental Health Foundation, 1986: 143–152.
3. Musetti L, Perugi G, Soriani A *et al*. Depression before and after age 65: a re-examination. *Br J Psychiatry* 1989; 155: 330–336.
4. Baldwin R. Depression. In: Butler R, Pitt B, eds. *Seminars in Old Age Psychiatry*. London: Royal College of Psychiatrists, 1998: 102–124.
5. Veith R C, Raskind M A. The neurobiology of aging; does it predispose to depression? *Neurobiol Aging* 1988; 9: 101–117.
6. Mendelwicz J. The age factor in depressive illness: some genetic considerations. *J Gerontol* 1976; 31: 300–303.
7. Murphy E. Social origins of depression in old age. *Br J Psychiatry* 1982; 141: 135–142.
8. Meats P, Timol M, Jolley D. Prognosis of depression in the elderly. *Br J Psychiatry* 1991; 159: 659–663.

9. Alexopoulos G S, Meyers B S, Young R C *et al*. Recovery in geriatric depression. *Arch Gen Psychiatry* 1996; 53: 305–312.

10. Barraclough B M. Suicide in the elderly. In: Kay D W K, Walk A, eds. *Recent Developments in Psychogeriatrics*. Ashford: Headley, 1971: 87–97.

11. Old Age Depression Interest Group. How long should the elderly take antidepressants? A double blind placebo-controlled study of continuation/ prophylaxis therapy with dothiepin. *Br J Psychiatry* 1993; 162: 175–182.

12. Benbow S B. The role of electroconvulsive therapy in the treatment of depressive illness in old age. *Br J Psychiatry* 1989; 155: 147–152.

13. Lebowitz B D, Pearson J L, Schneider L S *et al*. Diagnosis and treatment of depression in later life. Consensus statement update. United States National Institute of Mental Health. *JAMA* 1997; 278: 1186–1190.

14. Flint A J, Rifat S L. A prospective study of lithium augmentation in antidepressant-resistant geriatric depression. *J Clin Psychopharmacol* 1994; 14: 353–356.

15. *The ICD-10 Classification of Mental and Behavioural Disorders. Clinical Descriptions and Diagnostic Guidelines*. Geneva: WHO, 1992.

16. Schulman K, Tohen M, Satlin A *et al*. Mania compared with unipolar depression in old age. *Am J Psychiatry* 1992; 149: 341–345.

17. Snowdon J. A retrospective case note study of bipolar disorder in old age. *Br J Psychiatry* 1991; 158: 485–490.

18. Dinghra U, Rabins P V. Mania in the elderly: a 5–7 year follow-up. *J Am Geriatr Soc* 1991; 39: 581–583.

19. Schulman K, Mackenzie S, Hardy B. The clinical use of lithium carbonate in old age: a review. *Prog Neuropsychopharmacol* 1987; 11: 159–164.

20. Mehta D K, ed. *British National Formulary*, vol. 41. London: British Medical Association/Royal Pharmaceutical Society of Great Britain, 2001.

21. Biriell C, McEwan J, Sanz E *et al*. Depression associated with diltiazem. *BMJ* 1989; 299: 796.

22. Hullett F J, Potkin S G, Levy A B *et al*. Depression associated with nifedipine-induced calcium channel block. *Am J Psychiatry* 1988; 145: 1277–1279.

23. McElroy S, Keck P, Pope H *et al*. Valproate in the treatment of bipolar disorder: literature review and clinical guidelines. *J Clin Psychopharmacol* 1992; 12: (suppl1) 42S–52S.

24. Kando J C, Tohen M, Castillo J *et al*. The use of valproate in an elderly population with affective symptoms. *J Clin Psychiatry* 1996; 57: 238–240.

25. Grahame P S. Schizophrenia in old age (late paraphrenia). *Br J Psychiatry* 1984; 145: 493–495.

26. Almeida O P, Howard R, Forstl H *et al*. Late paraphrenia: a review. *Int J Geriatr Psychiatry* 1992; 7: 543–548.

27. Howard R, Almeida O P, Levy R. Phenomenology, demography and diagnosis in late paraphrenia. *Psychol Med* 1994; 24: 397–410.

28. Post F. *Persistent Persecutory States of the Elderly*. Oxford: Pergamon Press, 1966.

29. Howard R, Levy R. Which factors affect treatment response in late paraphrenia? *Int J Geriatr Psychiatry* 1992; 7: 667–672.

30. Parkinson Study Group. Low dose clozapine for the treatment of drug-induced psychosis in Parkinson's disease. *N Engl J Med* 1999; 340: 757–763.

31. Robins L N, Regier D A. *US Epidemiologic Catchment Area (ECA) Study. Psychiatric Disorders in America*. New York: Free Press, 1991.
32. Ballard C, Boyle A, Bowler C *et al*. Anxiety disorders in dementia sufferers. *Int J Geriatr Psychiatry* 1996; 11: 987–990.
33. Beitman B D, Kushner M, Grossberg G T. Late onset panic disorder: evidence from a study of patients with chest pain and normal cardiac evaluations. *Int J Psychiatry Med* 1991; 21: 29–35.
34. Lindesay J. The Guys/Age Concern survey: physical health and psychiatric disorder in an urban elderly community. *Int J Geriatr Psychiatry* 1990; 5: 171–178.
35. Fancourt G, Castleden M. The use of benzodiazepines with particular reference to the elderly. *Br J Hosp Med* 1986; 5: 321–325.
36. Rocca A, Hofman A, Brayne C *et al*. Frequency and distribution of Alzheimer's disease in Europe. *Ann Neurol* 1991; 30: 381–390.
37. Goate A, Chartier-Harlin M C, Mullen M *et al*. Segregation of a missense mutation in the amyloid precursor protein gene with familial Alzheimer's disease. *Nature* 1991; 349: 704–706.
38. Sherrington R, Rogaev E, Liang Y. Cloning of a gene bearing missense mutations in early onset familial Alzheimer's disease. *Nature* 1995; 375: 754–760.
39. Martyn C, Barker D, Osmand C *et al*. Geographical relation between Alzheimer's disease and aluminium in drinking water. *Lancet* 1989; 1: 59–62.
40. Flicker L. Acetylcholinesterase inhibitors for Alzheimer's disease. *BMJ* 1999; 318: 615–616.
41. Rich J B, Rasmusson D X, Folstein M F *et al*. Nonsteroidal anti-inflammatory drugs in Alzheimer's disease. *Neurology* 1995; 45: 51–55.
42. Breitner J C S, Welsh K A, Helms M J *et al*. Delayed onset of Alzheimer's disease with nonsteroidal anti-inflammatory drugs and histamine H_2 blocking drugs. *Neurobiol Aging* 1995; 16; 523–530.

7

Treatment of neurological disease in the elderly

Soraya Dhillon

Parkinson's disease

Parkinson's disease is the most common neurodegenerative disease after Alzheimer's disease, with an estimated incidence of 20/100 000 and a prevalence of 150/100 000. Population-based epidemiological studies indicate that the risk of Parkinson's disease is approximately doubled in first-degree relatives whilst hospital-based studies suggest a higher risk.[1,2] It is characterised clinically by asymmetric onset of brady-kinesia, rigidity, and in most cases resting tremor. The cause of the most common clinical features is the progressive deterioration and death of dopaminergic neurons in the substantia nigra of the midbrain. Lewy bodies (characteristic eosinophilic inclusion bodies) are present in a pro-portion of surviving neurons. In terms of pathology there is overlap with other neurodegenerative disorders, including Alzheimer's disease, and this has been used to support the view that these diseases may share some common pathogenic mechanisms.

Parkinson's disease causes substantial morbidity and results in a shortened life span. It also has considerable economic consequences, including loss of earnings, cost of care and cost of drug treatment. This is particularly important since Parkinson's is primarily a disease of the elderly and there is some evidence for a recent rise in mortality of affected individuals.[3] The main challenges in the treatment of Parkinson's disease are therefore firstly, to protect dopaminergic neurons so that either the disease is prevented or its progression is slowed and secondly, to provide treatment early to 'rescue' neurons which are at risk.

Despite extensive research the cause still remains unknown. However there is evidence for a genetic component in the cause of Parkinson's disease. The population-based studies showing an increased risk (two- to threefold) of developing Parkinson's disease in first-degree relatives of patients and mutations in the α-synuclein gene on chromosome 4 and the parkin gene on chromosome 6[4,5] have been identified in families showing autosomal-dominant and recessive parkinsonism respectively. The families show atypical disease. A further gene (on chromosome 2), again causing autosomal-dominant parkinsonism, has shown an effect in several members of the different families with features characteristic of idiopathic Parkinson's disease, including age of onset, symptoms and clinical course.[6]

There is also some evidence for an environmental component in the aetiology of the condition. Exposure to areas of high pesticide use in Canada multiplied the incidence by a factor of seven, compared to people living in areas where pesticides were little used.[7] These results have not been confirmed by other investigators, but the effects of the neurotoxin 1-methyl-4-phenyl-1,2,3,6-tetrahydropyridine (MPTP), a contaminant of designer street drugs which can produce irreversible parkinsonian effects, show that there are synthetic chemicals which can elicit such symptoms. Parkinson's disease was unknown in medical literature before the industrial revolution and this constitutes support for an environmental cause.

Clinical features

Early diagnosis is an important feature in the clinical management of Parkinson's disease. Around half of the patients will present with tremor and it is important also to look for early bradykinesia such as loss of arm swing or micrographia. Many patients with essential or familial tremor are misdiagnosed as having Parkinson's disease. To confirm diagnosis clinicians need to make sure that the apparent rest tremor is not worse with the arms outstretched. If it is and the tremor is bilateral and has a long history then the likely diagnosis in an essential tremor. Parkinson's disease patients can present with tremor of the outstretched arms, but it is rarely as marked as the resting component, and under these circumstances the additional sign of bradykinesia or rigidity is important to confirm the diagnosis.

In addition, patients may show loss of facial expression. Depression and constipation are sometimes very prominent, even right at the beginning. Aches and pains are also surprisingly common. A general slowing up, including mental slowing, can often be attributed by the patient and relatives to ageing, and such patients are often diagnosed rather late when there is no tremor evident.

If a patient has a gait disorder with typical festination (short accelerating steps), the diagnosis is usually clearly of Parkinson's. However, in elderly patients, particularly if they have vascular risk factors or have previously had a stroke, the gait apraxia of diffuse vascular disease is particularly diagnostic, especially if there are no other signs of Parkinson's disease.

The management of Parkinson's disease is usually in the hands of a general practitioner unless the patient is under 55 years of age, the diagnosis is uncertain or there is poor response to initial treatment.

For most elderly patients the diagnosis and management of uncomplicated Parkinson's disease can occur in primary care. However, if the diagnosis is in doubt or if there are complicating factors, or the patient fails to respond to standard first-line therapy then a second opinion is required. In addition, for complications such as dyskinesia, the on/off syndrome or confusion, a referral to a geriatrician or neurologist would be indicated.

In primary care there is a need for pharmaceutical care since an understanding of the pharmacological approach to management is important as the disease progresses. Dosage titration and monitoring are important as well as drug selection and use of more complicated drug delivery systems. In elderly patients it is important to assess iatrogenic disease and review the patient's other drug therapy. This is an area which is as yet poorly developed by pharmacists.

Drug therapy

Drug therapy for Parkinson's disease is centred around the use of levodopa. The management was revolutionised by the introduction of levodopa in 1969.[8] However, despite dramatic efficacy initially, a major drawback is the premature wearing-off of the effect of the drug, and extensive swings in symptom control. This long-term effect has an incidence of 10%. In general with levodopa therapy, the management of the condition is good and offers patients an improved quality of life. Some controversies do exist however, e.g. it is not known whether levodopa has some underlying neurotoxicity, despite the symptomatic benefit. This provides a logical argument for delaying treatment or for levodopasparing tactics, for example using dopamine agonists (see below) either alone or in combination with a lower dose of levodopa, accepting that the symptomatic benefit given by agonist drugs is usually not so good.

It is particularly important in elderly patients to aim for the best drug regimens for maximal symptomatic benefit and minimal polypharmacy.

Drug treatment

Levodopa is the most commonly used treatment for Parkinson's disease. It is always combined with a dopa-decarboxylase inhibitor (see below) which gives a dose-sparing effect by reducing peripheral metabolic inactivation and thus ensuring that more levodopa reaches the site of action.

Direct-acting dopamine agonists have been available for some years, but some evidence suggests that those developed more recently have better efficacy and are associated with fewer side-effects.[9]

Selegiline is an inhibitor of the enzyme monoamine oxidase B and prolongs the action of dopamine at the synapse. There is evidence that the early use of selegiline delays a patient's need for additional treatment by 9–12 months. Concerns about the safety of selegiline however remain controversial following the publication by the UK Parkinson's disease research group findings of an increase in mortality in the group who were prescribed selegiline and levodopa;[10] despite criticism of the study design, a smaller report from the same group has shown a small excess in mortality in patients taking selegiline.[11]

The newly developed catechol-O-methyltransferase (COMT) inhibitors increase the availability of levodopa to the brain, and their action is complementary to that of the dopa-decarboxylase inhibitors. Two drugs were licensed: tolcapone and entacapone. Due to the problems of hepatotoxicity of tolcapone it was withdrawn, whereas entacapone, another COMT-inhibitor, appears to have a safer profile. Amantadine remains a viable alternative to dopamine-related drugs, as their use is often limited by side-effects and tolerance.

Another group of drugs active in Parkinson's disease are the anticholinergics such as trihexyphenidyl (benzhexol), orphenadrine and procyclidine. These are used more sparingly, if at all, in elderly patients because the risk of confusion or bladder disturbance is high. Moreover the benefit that can be expected from these agents is small.

Levodopa

Levodopa remains the mainstay of therapy for the treatment of Parkinson's disease. To reduce the incidence of cardiovascular (hypotension) and gastrointestinal (nausea, anorexia) effects it is

Table 7.1 Available levodopa preparations

Product name	Dose form	Formula	Specific use
Co-beneldopa 62.5 (Madopar)	Co-beneldopa 12.5/50 capsules	Benserazide 12.5 mg Levodopa 50 mg	
Co-beneldopa 125 (Madopar)	Co-beneldopa 25/100 capsules	Benserazide 25 mg Levodopa 100 mg	
Co-beneldopa 250 (Madopar)	Co-beneldopa 50/200 capsules	Benserazide 50 mg Levodopa 200 mg	
Co-beneldopa 62.5 dispersible (Madopar Dispersible)	Co-beneldopa 12.5/50 dispersible tablets	Benserazide 12.5 mg Levodopa 50 mg	Rapid onset of effect needed or swallowing difficulty
Co-beneldopa 125 dispersible (Madopar Dispersible)	Co-beneldopa 25/100 dispersible tablets	Benserazide 25 mg Levodopa 100 mg	Rapid onset of effect needed or swallowing difficulty
Co-beneldopa (Madopar CR)	Co-beneldopa 25/100 modified-release capsules	Benserazide 25 mg Levodopa 100 mg	Fluctuations in response related to plasma concentrations or dose timing
Co-careldopa (Sinemet-110)	Co-careldopa 10/100 tablets	Carbidopa 10 mg Levodopa 100 mg	
Co-careldopa (Sinemet-275)	Co-careldopa 25/250 tablets	Carbidopa 25 mg Levodopa 250 mg	
Co-careldopa (Sinemet-62.5, previously known as Sinemet-LS)	Co-careldopa 12.5/50 tablets	Carbidopa 12.5 mg Levodopa 50 mg	To achieve full inhibition of peripheral dopa-decarboxylase at low doses of levodopa
Co-careldopa (Sinemet-Plus)	Co-careldopa 25/100 tablets	Carbidopa 25 mg Levodopa 100 mg	To achieve full inhibition of peripheral dopa-decarboxylase at low doses of levodopa
Co-careldopa (Half Sinemet CR)	Co-careldopa 25/100 modified-release tablets	Carbidopa 25 mg Levodopa 100 mg	Fluctuations in response related to plasma concentrations or dose timing
Co-careldopa (Sinemet CR)	Co-careldopa 50/200 modified-release tablets	Carbidopa 50 mg Levodopa 200 mg	Fluctuations in response related to plasma concentrations or dose timing

available as combinations with dopa-decarboxylase inhibitors, giving two groups of preparations: co-beneldopa, containing levodopa plus benserazide, and co-careldopa, containing levodopa plus carbidopa (Table 7.1). Central side-effects such as dyskinesias and psychiatric disturbances may however occur earlier in treatment.

Current management involves starting with low doses (50 mg levodopa), usually three times a day increasing slowly over a few weeks to 100 mg levodopa three or four times a day. In most patients during the early years this management is effective. This slow upward titration of dosage should avoid dyskinesia initially, although such symptoms may be unavoidable as the disease progresses.

The dispersible form of co-beneldopa is occasionally useful to achieve a rapid response, particularly in early-morning stiffness and in some patients where swallowing may be difficult.

Controlled-release preparations used as sole therapy will tend to cause dyskinesia as the day progresses, limiting their usefulness.

Co-beneldopa or co-careldopa three or four times a day is useful as standard therapy, but as symptom fluctuations start to appear some patients will need to take them more frequently.

Selegiline

This drug may have limited symptomatic benefit and slight smoothing-out action, but because of the recent possible increase in mortality seen in some patients, the drug is of limited use in the elderly.

Dopamine agonists

These drugs directly stimulate the undamaged receptor and hence have theoretical advantages over levodopa. In practice the symptomatic benefit is not as good as levodopa and the drug regimens are somewhat more complicated, particularly if one has to use levodopa as well. In the UK the use of dopamine agonists is relatively restricted and has limited value as first-line medication in the elderly.

In younger patients, e.g. those in their 40s, some neurologists may wish to try an agonist first, and if necessary supplement with levodopa. Although the evidence to support such a practice is somewhat controversial, this age group is more likely to tolerate polypharmacy well than the elderly.[12]

Bromocriptine in doses of 10–40 mg daily (after slow initial titration) may be effective. Other examples are lisuride, pergolide and ropinirole.

These drugs may be of value in patients with wearing-off and on/off phenomena, though the results are variable and usually require a reduction in the amount of levodopa; they are best managed by a specialist team. In patients who have a great deal of problems with the on/off effect the agonist apomorphine is of value. Treatment is started in hospital after 3-day premedication with domperidone to avoid severe vomiting. Apomorphine is available in a prefilled pen containing 3 ml apomorphine in a concentration of 10 mg/ml. The usual dose range is 3–30 mg/day by subcutaneous injection. If more than 10 injections a day are needed, the drug is best given by subcutaneous infusion using a syringe driver.

Psychiatric effects

Depression can be a problem in patients with Parkinson's disease and this will often respond to an antidepressant. It is important to avoid neuroleptics, because of their dopamine-blocking effects in the central nervous system (CNS). In the elderly it is important to recognise changes in mood and a recent deterioration in physical and mental state should be looked for. Choice of antidepressant is important in the elderly patient to avoid iatrogenic disease (see also Chapter 6).

Surgery

Surgery can be considered in Parkinson's disease, especially in those patients where therapeutic management becomes ineffective. Patients with severe tremor unresponsive to therapeutic intervention may undergo stereotactic thalamotomy or pallidotomy. Some patients with very severe dyskinesia may be considered for pallidotomy. Fetal nigral implants do improve the symptoms and postmortem inspection of the brains of the recipients did seem to confirm this method of restoring synaptic communication.[13] The elderly patient with Parkinson's disease is not likely to be a good risk for major brain surgery, however.

Research initiatives: long-term prospects

Neuroprotection may be defined as preventing neuronal cell death and maintaining function without necessarily affecting the underlying biochemical mechanisms involved in pathogenesis. Reducing progression of the disease is an important consideration in Parkinson's disease.

Neurorescue is a mechanism which aims to reverse established metabolic abnormalities and restore normal neuronal function and hence prolong survival. Clinically, this would result in an improvement in symptoms as well as reducing disease progression. Inevitably, there will be some overlap between neuroprotection and neurorescue, and their relative benefits will vary according to the stage of disease. Research currently focuses on these two approaches.

Neuroprotection is perhaps best exemplified by strategies designed to prevent cells undergoing apoptosis. Upregulating apoptosis defence genes, such as *bcl–2*, or downregulating apoptosis-promoting genes, such as *bax*, may be useful if effects can be targeted to nigral neurons. The role of the mitochondrion in the apoptotic pathway as a possible site at which to direct neuroprotective agents has been described.[14] Ciclosporin inhibits opening of the mitochondrial megapore, which is associated with loss of membrane potential and the start of apoptotic cell death. Both low-dose ciclosporin and its non-immunosuppressant analogue, *N*-methyl-4-valine ciclosporin, prevent the cell death *in vitro* induced by toxins that cause parkinsonism, while selegiline and its desmethyl metabolite have antiapoptotic properties.[15] In a review based on the current knowledge of pathogenesis in Parkinson's disease, drugs were identified which prevent or reduce free radical damage or enhance mitochondrial energy production.[16]

Epilepsy

Management

Clinical management of an older patient with epilepsy should include a good deal of reassurance and information. These patients need to be told that fits do not generally indicate serious brain damage and that the majority of patients can be controlled with therapeutic interventions. Lifestyle changes and implications for employment need to be handled sympathetically, for example issues such as driving and responsibility for notifying the DVLC. For an elderly patient this can be devastating. Fits can also have severe effects on confidence and self-restriction of activities. In an older person, this may precipitate the downward spiral of diminishing mobility and increasing dependence.

Elderly-onset epilepsy is much more common than in the younger population.[17,18] This is to some extent a reflection of an increased incidence of stroke,[19] head injury[20] and CNS infection[21] in old age. Additionally, predisposing metabolic conditions such as uraemia, hyponatraemia and hypoglycaemia are frequently encountered in old age. Postictal states (recovery) may be very prolonged in the elderly; 24 h of confusion is not uncommon and the person may be affected for up to a week.[22] There is also a greater risk of premature death or injury due to accidents during a seizure, or to the seizure itself.[23] Postictal hemiparesis is not uncommon in the elderly and may result in a mis-diagnosis of stroke.[24]

Seizure types

In mature individuals the main types are:

- generalised (whole-brain) tonic–clonic seizures (formerly known as grand mal)
- partial (part of brain) seizures which may be:
  — simple, without loss of consciousness
  — complex, with some loss of consciousness
  — secondarily generalised (partial seizure leading to a generalised tonic–clonic seizure)

Absence seizures (formerly known as petit mal) are generalised seizures which are common in childhood but extremely rare in adults. Generalised tonic–clonic seizures involve loss of consciousness, usually for several minutes, with convulsive movements of limbs and body, followed by a recovery phase of confusion and fatigue.

Drug treatment

The clinical use of medications involves an evidence-based approach to management in choosing the best drug treatment for patients with epilepsy. The choice of treatment needs to be matched to the patient and the type(s) of seizure they experience. Many of the newer drugs act by affecting the brain levels of γ-aminobutyric acid (GABA), one of the main inhibitory neurotransmitters of the CNS.

Established drugs

Carbamazepine Carbamazepine is used for patients with partial seizures, generalised tonic–clonic seizures, or both.[25] It acts by blocking sodium channels in CNS cells and by membrane stabilisation. It must be introduced gradually; tolerability is relatively good but in the elderly it can cause blurred vision and gastrointestinal disturbances. If further

seizures occur, the dose is titrated upwards until the seizures are controlled or the patient starts to have side-effects of unsteadiness or
drowsiness that necessitate limiting the dose; this is particularly a
problem in more elderly patients. Routine monitoring of the drug serum
concentration may not be very useful, as the patient's actual symptoms
offers the most appropriate dosing end-point. With high doses, elderly
patients may complain of transient double vision or blurred vision.
These adverse effects can often be alleviated by changing to the
modified-release formulation of the drug, which minimizes serum level
fluctuations. Modified timing of doses can also help. A suppository is
available for short-term use for patients who are temporarily unable to
swallow. There may however be differences in bioavailability between
the various formulations and brands of carbamazepine. Changeover
should be careful and may be helped by serum level measurements.

Carbamazepine can cause an allergic rash in some patients, but
dose-related symptoms are not usually severe. However, idiosyncratic
effects on blood and liver cells may rarely cause serious problems.
Carbamazepine causes enzyme induction, which may result in drug
interactions, and this is particularly important in patients on other
medications. Carbamazepine is associated with drug interactions that
arise through enzyme inhibition (for example, with erythromycin),
hence choice of antibiotics is important. Dosage should be reduced in
advanced liver disease.

Sodium valproate   Valproate is the first-line agent in a range of seizure
types; it is particularly effective in generalised tonic–clonic seizures and
partial seizures. Its mechanism of action has not been fully elucidated but
probably depends in part on its structural similarity to GABA. It can be
used to treat a wider range of seizure types than carbamazepine[25] and is
the drug of choice for absences and myoclonic seizures. Dosage should be
titrated upwards slowly according to the patient's response. The upper
end of the recommended dosage range is 2.5 g/day, but patients are
likely to complain of unacceptable side-effects such as sedation, weight
gain or tremor well before this dose is reached. In the elderly patient
tremor can be a dose-related factor influencing the choice of the drug.
Sodium valproate is an enzyme inhibitor, which is an important factor to
consider when using this drug in the elderly. However it is a drug of
choice for seizures in elderly people.[26] A modified-release formulation
(Epilim Chrono) offers the convenience of a single daily dose, but claims
that this improves compliance compared with a twice-daily regimen may
be exaggerated. Valproate should be avoided in liver disease, if possible.

Phenytoin   Phenytoin has been used extensively since the mid-1930s and, because of medical reluctance to attempt a switch to a more modern therapy, is still used in a number of the elderly.[25] It acts mainly by stabilising membranes and as a sodium channel blocker. The main problems are side-effects such as hirsutism, gum hypertrophy and, during chronic use, osteomalacia even in patients whose phenytoin concentration is in the therapeutic range. The second problem is that phenytoin has unusual pharmacokinetic properties. Dose adjustments produce disproportionately large changes in blood concentrations and its metabolism varies considerably between individuals.

Therapeutic drug monitoring (TDM) is very important if the drug is to be used optimally. Serum blood phenytoin concentrations must be monitored at the start of therapy and during continued treatment. The drug is also implicated in a large number of drug interactions.[27]

The drug is now not first choice for the elderly but it will still be encountered because of reluctance to change.[28] Doctors still need to know enough about phenytoin to be able to adjust the dose correctly and it may still have a place in severe epilepsy when other 'kinder' treatments have failed. Its effects on physical appearance are less evident in elderly people, among whom it seems to be as well tolerated as valproate.[25] A dose reduction may be needed in liver disease.

Drug targeting: newer agents

In the UK the past decade has seen the emergence of a new range of drugs which have been developed using a drug-targeting approach. Five new drugs for epilepsy (vigabatrin (Sabril), lamotrigine (Lamictal), gabapentin (Neurontin), topiramate (Topamax) and tiagabine (Gabitril)) have been licensed.

These new drugs were licensed as adjunctive (add-on) treatments and are still used as such, but lamotrigine is now licensed as mono-therapy for all main seizure types. The use of these newer agents is mainly for treatment of patients with partial seizures, with or without secondarily generalised tonic–clonic seizures, who have not responded to the first-line agents sodium valproate or carbamazepine.

Limited trials currently exist which compare these drugs, and there is no scientific basis for stating that one is more effective than another.

Lamotrigine   Lamotrigine has been on the UK market for several years. It acts primarily by blocking sodium channels. One of the main advantages of lamotrigine is that it causes little cognitive impairment or overt sedation compared with other treatments. It sometimes has an arousing or alerting effect. In some patients, mainly elderly people, this may manifest itself as unwanted agitation. Lamotrigine has a wide spectrum of activity. The chief drawback is the risk of skin rashes, which are usually mild but may progress to Stevens–Johnson syndrome or toxic epidermal necrolysis. Rash may also occur as part of a more generalised reaction, with facial swelling, lymphadenopathy and liver and kidney abnormalities. These occur less often than is the case with carbamazepine, but they are more often severe and can be life-threatening, although this is rare.[29] More recently it has been stated that there often seems to be synergy between lamotrigine and valproate, over and above that expected from the pharmacokinetic interaction.[30] Lamotrigine is very useful in some elderly patients, and quite low doses may be optimum in this age group.[30] The drug is primarily inactivated by hepatic metabolism and the manufacturer advises that it should not be used in liver disease.

Vigabatrin   Vigabatrin, introduced in the late 1980s, was the first new antiepileptic drug to be licensed in the UK for many years. It acts by irreversibly inhibiting GABA transaminase, thereby increasing brain levels of GABA. Because it is licensed only as an adjunctive drug (apart from use as a single agent for infantile spasms) it has been added to therapy for many patients with long-standing epilepsy. Permanent visual loss has been reported and the UK Committee on Safety of Medicines has advised restrictions on its use.[31] The drug is inactivated by renal excretion, not metabolism, and dose reduction will be needed if there is any renal impairment.

Gabapentin   The mechanism of action of gabapentin remains obscure at the moment. The overall impression of the balance of efficacy and toxicity, compared with the other newer drugs, is that gabapentin seems less effective, but also less toxic. Gabapentin may come into its own when it is used earlier in treatment and (when licensed) as monotherapy.[30] This drug is also inactivated by renal excretion, not metabolism, and dose reduction will be needed if there is any renal impairment.

Topiramate   Topiramate is used as an adjunctive treatment for partial seizures with or without secondary generalisation. It acts by blocking sodium channels in CNS cells. It has now been on the market for a few years, and its effects seem to be at the other end of the spectrum from those of gabapentin; that is, it is more potent and more toxic.[30]

Topiramate has side-effects which affect personality or induce cognitive changes, sometimes accompanied by difficulty in finding words, and this can be a major problem in elderly patients, affecting self-confidence. In addition, topiramate has to be stopped in some patients who are otherwise tolerating it well, because of weight loss. There is also a significant incidence of nephrolithiasis. For the moment topiramate remains a treatment to be prescribed by the experienced neurologist.[30]

Tiagabine Tiagabine is currently the newest antiepileptic drug on the market in the UK. It is licensed as adjunctive therapy for partial seizures, whether or not secondarily generalised. It blocks the reuptake of GABA into CNS cells, thus enhancing GABAergic effects. Similar side-effects to topiramate (dizziness, cognitive slowing, fatigue) tend to limit its use in the elderly. A dose reduction will be needed in moderate liver impairment, but the drug should be avoided in severe liver disease.

Drug therapy management

The aim should be monotherapy in all older patients, to minimise the incidence of side-effects and drug interactions and to increase patient compliance. Many adult patients with epilepsy can be controlled with a single drug, and if satisfactory control cannot be achieved with one antiepileptic, then it is worth trying monotherapy with another[32] as the response to different antiepileptic drugs can vary with the individual.

Carbamazepine (Tegretol) and sodium valproate (Epilim) may all be considered broad-spectrum antiepileptics and are likely to be equally effective in common seizure types encountered in the elderly. Sodium valproate can now be administered in a single daily dose as a controlled-release formulation. Use of phenytoin tends to be reserved for more resistant epilepsy and would not be considered first-line.

Side-effects

Elderly patients with declining intellectual function or motor impairment may be especially susceptible to dose-related neurological side-effects, including ataxia, dysarthria, dizziness and visual disturbance.

Of the many non-neurological side-effects, the one most relevant to the older population is osteomalacia, since older people may already be at risk due to a reduction in vitamin D dietary intake and reduced exposure to sunlight. Enzyme inducers such as carbamazepine and phenytoin accelerate vitamin D metabolism, but valproate does not.

Carbamazepine can cause the syndrome of inappropriate antidiuretic hormone secretion (SIADH) which shows itself as hyponatraemia. Susceptibility to this effect increases with age and this is especially relevant to the many elderly patients on diuretics, which may necessitate changing either carbamazepine or the diuretic.

New antiepileptics

Two of the new-generation antiepileptics may be particularly beneficial to elderly patients as adjunctive therapy: gabapentin (Neurontin), because of its efficacy, its comparatively favourable side-effects profile and its lack of interaction with other drugs,[33] and lamotrigine (Lamictal), because of its efficacy and side-effect profile.[34]

However, at present they should only be used when satisfactory control of seizures is not being achieved and hence on the advice of a specialist. Studies are underway to investigate their potential as first-line monotherapy in newly diagnosed cases of epilepsy in elderly patients.

Dosage considerations

Age-related changes in drug handling may influence the availability of drugs and consequently the relationship between prescribed dosage and serum levels. Albumin levels tend to be lower in older people, which may reduce plasma protein binding, resulting in higher free concentrations of certain drugs, especially phenytoin and valproate. In older people, a greater proportion of the total body mass is fatty tissue which leads to an increased volume of distribution for lipid-soluble drugs. This effect, combined with reduced clearance, leads to increased persistence in the body and particularly applies to phenytoin.

In general treatment should be started at the bottom of the recommended dose range, and the dose then tailored to the needs of the individual patient.

Concomitant diseases and medication

Iatrogenic disease is an important consideration in the elderly. Some of the established drugs already have a large range of interactions, hence this is an important consideration for choice of agent and monitoring of the clinical effectiveness of the drug. Elderly patients will have multiple pathologies and thus be taking other drugs: monitoring for drug interactions is important.

Phenytoin and valproate are highly bound to albumin, so conditions that lead to a reduction in albumin, such as liver failure, will affect the handling of antiepileptics.

Other drugs may alter the absorption, distribution and metabolism of antiepileptics. Examples include: cimetidine and propranolol increasing the serum concentration of phenytoin and erythromycin and calcium channel blockers such as diltiazem increasing the serum concentration of carbamazepine. In addition, antiepileptics may affect the metabolism of other agents, resulting in a decline in target response. Interactions with warfarin and angiotensin-converting enzyme (ACE) inhibitors such as enalapril are particularly important. Phenytoin and carbamazepine reduce the effectiveness of warfarin, haloperidol and theophylline.

Monitoring of patients is important and assessing the patient's clinical response is vital. TDM is a helpful tool if used appropriately. It is however important to interpret the results with caution since the published therapeutic ranges were not established in elderly patients, and it is possible that toxicity may occur at levels that fall within the normal ranges determined on younger subjects. In patients who are currently fit-free, doses which are apparently subtherapeutic should not be adjusted to bring drug levels into a 'therapeutic' range. Monitoring is particularly useful with phenytoin because of its kinetics, whereby small adjustments in dose may bring about large changes in drug levels.

Seizure control with carbamazepine may be achieved throughout a very wide range of concentrations because of the variable metabolism of its active metabolite and individual pharmacodynamic variability. The values given for the therapeutic range should therefore be treated with caution and a single measurement may be meaningless; both peak (3–4 h after a dose) and trough (at time of next dose) levels may be measured.

There is little correlation between sodium valproate concentration and its pharmacological effect and so the place of monitoring valproate levels is uncertain and probably not very helpful, although it can be useful for checking compliance.

Optimal care of older patients with epilepsy includes careful dose selection, cautious use of other medication and to some extent the use of serum antiepileptic level monitoring, especially where there is uncertainty about toxic effects, where control is poor and where compliance is uncertain. However, with judicious management it is possible to achieve satisfactory seizure control in most older patients with epilepsy.

Nausea and vomiting

Nausea and vomiting in most patients is a self-limiting illness that does not require specific treatment other than attention to fluid balance (see also Chapter 14). In the elderly, however, it may lead to hospital referral, particularly if symptoms persist and if dehydration and weight loss occurs.

It is important to assess the underlying cause. The differential diagnosis is wide and ranges from surgical conditions to metabolic, drug-induced and psychogenic causes. While gastrointestinal causes such as gastroenteritis, peptic ulceration and gallbladder disease tend to predominate, less common causes, e.g. raised intracranial pressure (ICP) and Addison's disease, must not be forgotten. Common causes are:

- infective
- food poisoning, gastroenteritis, hepatitis
- peptic ulcer
- intestinal obstruction
- pyloric stenosis
- Crohn's disease
- gallstones, tumour
- motion
- labyrinthitis
- meningitis
- uraemia
- diabetes
- drugs.

Mechanism of nausea and vomiting

The feeling of nausea can be triggered by a wide variety of stimuli, including visceral pain, labyrinthine stimulation and psychological distress. The precise neurological pathways involved remain uncertain, but nausea does appear to represent a low-level activation of the vomiting pathway. Vomiting results from complex integration of signals in the vomiting centre. The process of vomiting involves initial inhibition of gastric contractions, relaxation of the lower oesophageal sphincter and, usually, orally migrating contractions of the small intestine.

The vomiting centre may be activated by afferent vagal neurons or by stimulation of the chemoreceptor trigger zone (CTZ). The CTZ can be stimulated by a variety of mechanisms which include: vagal or splanchnic afferent stimulation, e.g. visceral pain, gastrointestinal mucosa irritants and bacterial toxins; circulating emetic substances or by exogenous emetic agents (morphine, levodopa, digitalis, chemo-therapeutic agents and radiation). In the elderly this may be due to prescribed drugs, as shown in Table 7.2.

Irrespective of the specific trigger, vomiting is mediated through a common final pathway involving muscarinic, dopaminergic (D_2), histaminergic (H_2) and serotonergic ($5-HT_3$) receptors. Currently, drugs available to help control nausea and vomiting work on these receptors.

Identifying the cause

Persistent vomiting may be due to obstruction, which should be excluded. Ultrasound examination may be helpful in identifying biliary and pancreatic causes. In the elderly uraemia and diabetes should be excluded while history, fundoscopy and measurement of pulse and blood pressure can help exclude raised ICP. Delayed gastric emptying is a feature of many acute infections causing nausea and vomiting, as well as more chronic diseases such as Parkinson's disease and diabetes.

Drug treatment

The approach to the management of nausea and vomiting is to treat the underlying cause; however, antiemetics may be given for symptomatic relief. The two most commonly used drug groups are those that act on the gastrointestinal tract (the prokinetic agents) by speeding up gut transit time and those that act centrally (phenothiazines and antihistamines).

Table 7.2 Drugs that commonly cause nausea and vomiting

Thiazides
Theophylline
Allopurinol
Non-steroidal anti-inflammatory drugs
Antibiotics
Opi oids
Cytotoxics
Penicillamine
Digoxin
Quinidine
Gold
Sulfasalazine
Iron
Levodopa

The prokinetic agents are useful for both drug-induced nausea and vomiting as well as intestinal motility disorders, e.g. gastroparesis and pseudo-obstruction. Centrally acting drugs are particularly useful for motion sickness.

Prokinetic agents

Metoclopramide

Metoclopramide is very useful in preventing nausea and vomiting from many causes, including drug-induced vomiting. A wide range of formulations are also available: oral, intravenous and subcutaneous administration.

Metoclopramide blocks central and peripheral dopamine D_2-receptors, while in high doses it also acts on central and peripheral 5-HT_3-receptors, which accounts for its enhanced antiemetic efficacy. Metoclopramide has prokinetic effects on the upper gastrointestinal tract that include an increase in tone in the lower oesophageal sphincter and increased contraction in the gastric antrum with relaxation of the pylorus and duodenum. Clinically these effects combine to reduce oesophageal reflux and enhance gastric emptying and are useful in treating the gastric hypomotility found in migraine, diabetic neuropathy and after surgery.

Metoclopramide is rapidly absorbed after oral administration and is distributed into most tissues crossing both the blood–brain barrier and placenta. Hepatic first-pass metabolism reduces bioavailability to about 75%. The plasma half-life is about 4–6 h with 30% of the dose excreted unchanged by the kidneys and the remainder eliminated in urine and bile after hepatic metabolism.

Side-effects occur in approximately 10% of patients and are usually mild, transient and reversible on discontinuation of therapy. CNS side-effects include dizziness, drowsiness, anxiety and depression, which can be a particular problem in the elderly. Extrapyramidal symptoms occur in up to 9% of patients. Acute dystonic reactions are however more frequent in young patients, particularly when high doses are used: they include trismus, torticollis, opisthotonos and oculogyric crises. Parkinsonian reactions may occur with long-term treatment. The neurological side-effects will resolve on drug withdrawal and can be minimised with low dosage.

Domperidone
Domperidone possesses both antiemetic and prokinetic properties. Its effects on gastrointestinal motility are similar to those of

metoclopramide but are not antagonised by atropine. Following oral administration domperidone is rapidly absorbed and metabolised in the liver with a half-life of about 8 h. Since domperidone does not cross the blood–brain barrier to any appreciable extent, it causes little CNS toxicity and mainly affects D_2-receptors. However, since the CTZ is accessible without penetration of the blood–brain barrier, it does have central antiemetic effects.

It has minimal extrapyramidal side-effects and is less sedating than metoclopramide and therefore is used to treat gastrointestinal symptoms in patients with Parkinson's disease where it prevents the nausea and vomiting associated with levodopa and bromocriptine (Parlodel). Orally it seems to be as effective as metoclopramide, but the parenteral form was withdrawn because of cardiotoxicity associated with high-dose intravenous therapy. It is generally well tolerated, with dry mouth, headache (migraine) or skin rash occurring in fewer than 2% of patients.

Cisapride Cisapride was used clinically to treat gastro-oesophageal reflux, diabetic gastroparesis, intestinal pseudo-obstruction and systemic sclerosis. The product licence has been suspended by the Committee on Safety of Medicines as cisapride can prolong the QT interval, which may lead to rare but life-threatening ventricular arrhythmias.[35]

Antiemetic drugs

Phenothiazines Phenothiazines, e.g. prochlorperazine and trifluoperazine, are used as oral and intramuscular antiemetics. They act on the CTZ and vomiting centre as well as being sedative and can be used in a wide range of circumstances.

Long-term use is limited by side-effects including extrapyramidal reactions (which may persist despite drug withdrawal) and anticholinergic effects. Sedation can be troublesome and patients should be warned about drowsiness during early treatment and advised not to drive or operate machinery. Side-effects include hypotension, cholestatic jaundice, skin rash, leukopenia and, rarely, agranulocytosis. The sedative effects are potentiated by alcohol and other sedative drugs. Hypotensive agents are also potentiated.

Antihistamines (H₁-receptor antagonists) Antihistamines such as promethazine act on the vestibular apparatus and CTZ and are useful in motion sickness and vomiting due to vestibular disease. Sedation and anticholinergic effects are common. They potentiate other CNS depressants such as alcohol, phenothiazines and benzodiazepines. Cyclizine is less likely to cause drowsiness and has a short duration of action of about 4 h.

Selective 5-HT$_3$-antagonists These drugs were developed after it had been shown that the improved antiemetic effect of high-dose metoclopramide was related to blockade of 5-HT$_3$-receptors in addition to dopamine antagonism. Use of high-dose metoclopramide is limited by unacceptable toxicity due to lack of selectivity.

The 5-HT$_3$-antagonists ondansetron, tropisetron and granisetron act on peripheral and central 5-HT$_3$-receptors blocking emetogenic stimuli via the vagus nerve while also acting on the CTZ. These drugs are mainly used to treat nausea and vomiting in patients on highly emetogenic chemotherapy, e.g. cisplatin.

Ondansetron is available in both oral and intravenous formulations; a single intravenous dose of 8 mg is recommended immediately before chemotherapy. If vomiting is not adequately controlled it should be continued orally or intravenously at a dose of 8 mg 12-hourly for up to 5 days. Granisetron has just recently become available as an oral as well as an intravenous preparation; adverse effects include constipation and headache. These drugs are expensive.

References

1.   Marder K, Tang M X, Mejia H *et al*. Risk of Parkinson's disease among first degree relatives, a community based study. *Neurology* 1996; 47: 155–160.
2.   Seidler A, Hellenbrand W, Rober B P *et al*. Possible environmental, occupational and other etiologic factors for Parkinson's disease. A case control study in Germany. *Neurology* 1996; 46: 1275–1284.
3.   Lilenfield D E, Chan E, Ehland J *et al*. Two decades of increasing mortality from Parkinson's disease. *Arch Neurol* 1990; 47: 731–734.
4.   Krüger R, Kuhn W, Muller T *et al*. Ala30Pro mutation in the synuclein in Parkinson's disease. *Nat Genet* 1998; 18: 106–108.
5.   Kitada T, Asakawa S, Hattori N *et al*. Mutations in the parkin gene cause autosomal recessive juvenile parkinsonism. *Nature* 1998; 392: 605–608.
6.   Gasser T, Müller-Myhsok B, Wszolek Z *et al*. A susceptibility locus for Parkinson's disease maps to chromosome 2p13. *Nat Genet* 1998; 18: 262–265.
7.   Lewin R. Parkinson's disease: an environmental cause? *Science* 1985; 229: 257–258.
8.   Larner A J, Farmer S F. Recent advances. Neurology. *BMJ* 1999; 319: 362–366.
9.   Schapira A H V. Parkinson's disease. *BMJ* 1999; 318: 311–314.

10. Ben-Schlomo Y, Churchyard A, Head J *et al.* Investigation by Parkinson's Disease Research Group of United Kingdom into excess mortality seen with combined levodopa and selegiline treatment in patients with early, mild Parkinson's disease: further results of randomised trial and confidential inquiry. *BMJ* 1998; 316: 1191–1196.

11. Thorogood M, Armstrong B, Nichols T, Hollowell J. Mortality in people taking selegiline: observational study. *BMJ* 1998; 317: 252–254.

12. Williams A. Guide to GP management of Parkinson's disease. *Prescriber* 1997; 8: 39–46.

13. Olanow C W, Kordower J H, Freeman T B. Fetal nigral transplantation as a therapy for Parkinson's disease. *Trends Neurosci* 1996; 19: 102–109.

14. Seaton T A, Cooper J M, Schapira A H V. Free radical scavengers protect dopaminergic cell lines from apoptosis induced by mitochondrial complex I inhibitors. *Brain Res* 1997; 777: 110–118.

15. Mytilineou C, Radcliffe P M, Olanow C W. L-(–)-desmethylselegiline, a metabolite of selegiline [L-(–)-deprenyl], protects mesencephalic dopamine neurons from excitotoxicity in vitro. *J Neurochem* 1997; 68: 434–436.

16. Schapira A H V, Gu M, Taanman J-W *et al.* Mitochondria in the aetiology and pathogenesis of Parkinson's disease. *Ann Neurol* 1998; 44 (suppl 1): S89–S98.

17. Hauser W A, Annegers J F, Kurland L T. Incidence of epilepsy and unprovoked seizures in Rochester, Minnesota, 1935–1984. *Epilepsia* 1993; 34: 453–468.

18. Sander J W, Hart Y M, Johnson A L, Shorvon S D. National General Practice Study of Epilepsy: newly diagnosed epileptic seizures in the general population. *Lancet* 1990; 336: 1267–1271.

19. Broderick J P, Phillips S J, Whisnant J P *et al.* Incidence rates of stroke in the eighties: the end of the decline in stroke? *Stroke* 1989; 20: 577–582.

20. Cooper K D, Tabaddor K, Hauser W A *et al.* The epidemiology of head injury in the Bronx. *Neuroepidemiology* 1983; 2: 70.

21. Nicolosi A, Hauser W A, Beghi E, Kurland L T. Epidemiology of central nervous system infections in Olmstead County, Minnesota 1950–1981. *J Infect Dis* 1986; 154: 399–408.

22. Godfrey J W, Roberts M A, Caird F I. Epileptic seizures in the elderly: 2 Diagnostic problems. *Age Ageing* 1982; 11: 29–34.

23. Guberman A H, Bruni J. Epidemiology. In: Guberman A H, Bruni J. *Essentials of Clinical Epilepsy*, 2nd edn. Boston: Butterworth Heinemann, 1999: 6.

24. Norris J W, Hachinski C. Mis-diagnosis of stroke. *Lancet* 1982; 1: 328.

25. Brodie M J, Dichter M A. Established antiepileptic drugs. *Seizure* 1997; 6: 159–174.

26. Craig I, Tallis R. Impact of valproate and phenytoin on cognitive function in elderly patients: results of a single-blind comparative study. *Epilepsia* 1994; 35: 381–390.

27. Richens A, Perucca E. Clinical pharmacology and medical treatment. In: Laidlaw J, Richens A, eds. *A Textbook of Epilepsy*, 4th edn. Edinburgh: Churchill Livingstone, 1993: 508–509.

28. Roberts S J, Feely M, Bateman D N. Prescribing of anti-epileptic drugs in the northern and Yorkshire region 1992–1995. *Seizure* 1998; 7: 127–132.

29. Stephen L J, Brodie M J. New drug treatments for epilepsy. *Prescribers' J* 1998; 38: 98–106.

30. Feely M. Drug treatment of epilepsy. *BMJ* 1999; 318: 106–109.

31. Committee on Safety of Medicines, Medicines Control Agency. Vigabatrin (Sabril) and visual field defects. *Curr Probl Pharmacovigilance* 1998; 24: 1.

32. Dhillon S, Sander JWAS, eds. Epilepsy. In: Walker R, Edwards W, eds. *Clinical Pharmacy and Therapeutics*. Edinburgh: Churchill Livingstone, 1999: 435–453.

33. The US Gabapentin Study Group no. 5. Gabapentin as add-on therapy in refractory partial epilepsy: a double-blind placebo-controlled, parallel-group study. *Neurology* 1993; 43: 2292–2298.

34. Fitton A, Goa K L. Lamotrigine. An update of its pharmacology and therapeutic use in epilepsy. *Drugs* 1995; 50: 691–713.

35. Anon. Changes. In: Mehta D K, ed. *British National Formulary*, vol. 40. London: British Medical Association/Royal Pharmaceutical Society of Great Britain, 2000: viii.

8

Anti-infective therapy in the elderly

Caroline Bradley

At the extremes of age, susceptibility to infection and to its complications is at a maximum. The large growth in the numbers of old people in the industrial societies of the world means that the treatment of infection in such patients presents a commonplace medical occurrence. The morbidity and mortality associated with infections in the aged is significantly higher than in younger patients.[1] Elderly patients with infectious processes often present with masked or atypical symptoms compared to young patients and may not have leukocytosis. The inflammatory response to infection may be attenuated or chronic disease states may obscure the diagnosis. Additional acute pathology such as renal impairment due to dehydration or cardiac failure further complicates the treatment of an infectious process. Specific infecting organisms differ from those affecting the younger population.

Underlying or chronic disease affects resistance to infection and ability to mount an adequate immune response. The higher rate of invasive procedures and devices in the older population additionally contributes to the greater risk of infection. Elderly patients living in residential or nursing homes present special problems related to cross-infection.

Age-related degeneration of organ status is not uniform across the population. Biological variation means that, while some elderly individuals may have organ function equivalent to a young adult, a similarly aged individual may have severely impaired function. The difference in biological variability will often be greater than the effect of age itself on the immune system.

Immune function has been shown to decrease with age, with the acquired immune system specifically affected. The incidences of infections, cancers and vascular diseases increase with age as immune function wanes. T-cell function declines to a greater extent than B-cell and macrophage function.[2] T cells modulate immune function by promoting or suppressing production of immunoglobulins. Suppressor T cells prevent the immune system from attacking the host's own tissues. Promotor T cells enhance the production of immunoglobulins targeted against invading pathogens. The T cells of old individuals elicit reduced production of interleukins-2 and 3, and this is reflected in an impaired response to antigenic stimulation.[2]

Cutaneous hypersensitivity is delayed, which may result in a false-negative response to the tuberculin test. With the decline in the functioning of T cells, the ability to mount an adequate antibody response to vaccines is reduced and the level and duration of protection are attenuated with age. With advancing age there are increased levels of auto-antibodies, as evidenced by increased vascular and connective tissue disease, and the incidence of benign and malignant monoclonal gammopathies similarly increases.[3]

Immune function and resultant resistance to infection are affected by nutritional status. Gross malnutrition is rare in old people living an independent life in their own homes, but it is common in those suffering from mental and physical incapacity and multiple pathology.[4] Ill health causes anorexia and impairs the physical ability to achieve adequate nutritional intake and also increases catabolism. It is therefore not uncommon for elderly patients to present with infection plus additional signs of protein-energy, mineral or vitamin deficiency. Nutritional supplementation in the malnourished person has a beneficial effect on mortality, morbidity and rehabilitation.

Because of the greater mortality and morbidity from infections in the elderly, rapid diagnosis and treatment of the infection are critical.[5] Empirical antibiotic therapy is frequently justified in the elderly, not only because of high mortality rates, but also because of the difficulty of interpreting non-specific signs and symptoms of infection.

The treatment of infection in the elderly population is likely to be complicated by the presence of impaired renal and hepatic function. This must be taken into account when administering antimicrobial agents; however, this will not be specifically addressed in this chapter. Research has indicated that the normal ageing process has little impact on the absorption, distribution and metabolism of most antibiotics,[6] however the age-related decline in renal function substantially influences the excretion of many antibiotics.

The decline in renal function may be made greater by disease states such as diabetes mellitus, congestive heart failure and hypertension that are more prevalent in the elderly. It is recognised that the elderly may experience more adverse drug-related events because of age-related decline in renal function, multiple disorders, severity of disease,

Table 8.1 Examples of adverse drug events associated with antibiotics which particularly affect the elderly

Antibiotic	Adverse event
Aminoglycosides	Nephrotoxicity
	Ototoxicity
Broad-spectrum agents	Antibiotic-associated pseudomembranous colitis
Co-amoxiclav	Acute liver injury
Co-trimoxazole	Blood dyscrasias
	Hyperkalaemia
Isoniazid	Hepatic injury
Tetracycline or doxycycline	Oesophageal ulcers and strictures
Quinolones	Seizures

concomitant medications and inappropriate compliance. Examples of age-associated adverse drug events are given in Table 8.1. In particular the elderly are at risk of drug interactions because they are usually on multiple drug therapy. Compliance with treatment regimes may be an issue in the elderly and this may lead to suboptimal therapy and treatment failure.

Genitourinary tract infections

Urinary tract infections

These are among the most common infections of old age. They are especially prevalent in long-stay facilities. In early life urinary tract infection (UTI) is a predominantly female disease; it is uncommon in males until the seventh decade when the incidence increases in both sexes but especially in males. The incidence of this condition is approximately 10% in women over the age of 65 and 20% in men in the same age group.[7] The rate is greater in the more impaired elderly, especially those with indwelling catheters.

The increase in the occurrence of UTIs with age is due to multiple factors. Decline in immunological function, increased residual urine volume post voiding due to poor muscle function, pelvic floor laxity in women or the use of antimuscarinic drugs; incapacity or immobility leading to poor perineal hygiene, increased incidence of catheterisation and glycosuria have all been cited as causes of the increased incidence. In addition contributing causes are age-related changes in the genital tract such as oestrogen deficiency and vaginal atrophy in the female leading to colonisation with pathogenic organisms and prostatism in the male causing outflow obstruction.

UTI is generally classified by the anatomical site of infection. Lower UTI includes infections of the bladder and urethra, upper UTI or pyelonephritis refers to infection (or inflammation) of the kidneys. UTI may also be classified into uncomplicated and complicated types. Uncomplicated infections are generally considered to be those in adult females with no anatomical abnormalities. Complicated UTI includes infections at sites other than in the bladder, infections in men and those with obstruction, catheters or other additional factors.

Most UTIs are caused by bacteria and only rarely by fungi or viruses. The presentation is generally of cystitis or acute pyelonephritis. Symptoms of cystitis are dysuria, frequency and urgency of urination; those of acute pyelonephritis are flank pain and fever, often with nausea, vomiting, malaise or symptoms of cystitis. However, elderly patients with upper UTI may not present with classical symptoms. Mental state changes such as confusion or gastrointestinal disease such as nausea, vomiting and abdominal tenderness or alternatively respiratory symptoms may be strongly suggestive of the diagnosis. Unpleasant-smelling urine may be an additional indicator.

Asymptomatic bacteriuria is the finding of significant numbers of bacteria in urine without symptoms. Asymptomatic bacteriuria is a dynamic and common finding in the elderly female or in the very elderly male and is found in 15–20% of women aged 65–70 years. It does not appear to impair renal function or shorten life[8,9] and treatment with antibiotics often results in rapid reappearance of bacteriuria once the course is finished, often with different organisms. There is no evidence to support the treatment of asymptomatic bacteriuria in the elderly;[1] exceptions are those undergoing urological surgery.

Community-acquired urinary tract infections in women

Diagnosis of UTI is usually made on the history and clinical signs. The urine can be dip-tested for nitrites (produced by bacteria converting nitrates to nitrites) and leukocyte esterase to detect white blood cells. On the basis of these investigations treatment is usually started empirically but if the dip tests are negative, urine may be sent for culture. It is important that the urine sample is fresh (or is refrigerated to prevent overgrowth) and collected with the labia apart to prevent contamination. The current cut-off point for definition of infection is a level of 10^5 organisms per ml.[10] A lower count may indicate early infection but mixed growth usually indicates contamination or growth in transport. Treatment is usually initiated before the results of culture are known.

The causative organism in uncomplicated community-acquired UTI in elderly women is *Escherichia coli* 50–70%,[9] most of the rest being caused by *Proteus mirabilis*, *Klebsiella pneumoniae* and enterococci. Elderly patients who have had prior antibiotic therapy may have infections with other Gram-negative organisms such as *Enterobacter* or *Pseudomonas* species. The ideal characteristics of a drug used to treat UTI are given in Table 8.2.

Renal function is often impaired in the elderly and this should be taken into account when selecting the drug, dose and frequency of administration. Trimethoprim is usually considered first-line treatment[11] and is effective against 70% of urinary pathogens.[12, 13] An alternative agent is a first-generation cephalosporin; nitrofurantoin is generally not recommended in the elderly because it is contraindicated in those with a creatinine clearance of less than 50 ml/min. Co-amoxiclav and quinolones should be reserved for more complicated cases or where resistance to first-line agents is an issue. Amoxicillin is generally ineffective due to a high incidence of resistance by *Escherichia coli*.

In younger women, 3 days of therapy is considered adequate and is as effective as 5–7 days.[11] Older women have poorer outcome to short-course therapy, although the majority of women over 65 years without evidence of invasive infection when treated for 3 days will be cured of infection.[14] Single-dose therapy should not be used because of likely treatment failure and recurrent infection, which is thought to be secondary to persistent colonisation from faecal and vaginal reservoirs. If symptoms fail to respond to 3 days of treatment, urine should be sent for culture and sensitivity testing.

If UTI involving the upper renal tract is suspected, duration of treatment should be for 10–14 days and in the event of treatment failure

Table 8.2 Ideal characteristic of antibiotics for use in urinary tract infections

High urinary excretion in active form
Activity against usual pathogens
Minimal effect on vaginal and bowel flora
Low potential to induce bacterial resistance
Ease of administration
Safe
Good patient tolerance

Table 8.3 Antimicrobials commonly used to treat urinary tract infections and precautions

Drug	Action	Urinary pathogens covered	Dose	Renal impairment dose (creatinine clearance (CrCl) ml/min)	Side-effects and precautions
Trimethoprim	Bacteriostatic Folate antagonist	Escherichia coli Klebsiella spp. Enterobacter spp. Streptococcus spp. Staphylococcus epidermidis	200 mg twice daily	CrCl 10–50 200 mg every 18 h CrCl < 10 200 mg/day	Nausea, rash, Stevens–Johnson syndrome, fever, thrombocytopenia, agranulocytosis, especially on long-term use: counselling is required. Unsafe in porphyria
Amoxicillin	Bactericidal Cell wall lysis	Streptococcus spp. Proteus spp. 50% of E. coli are resistant 90% of Staphylococcus aureus are resistant	250 mg three times a day or two 3 g doses 12 h apart	CrCl 10–50 250 mg twice daily CrCl < 10 250 mg/day	Nausea, rash, diarrhoea. Rarely, antibiotic-associated diarrhoea
Co-amoxiclav	Bactericidal with β-lactamase inhibitor	Streptococcus groups ABCG Staphylococcus spp. E. coli Klebsiella spp. Enterobacter spp.	375 mg three times a day	CrCl 10–50 375 mg twice daily CrCl < 10 375 mg/day	Allergic reactions, rash, diarrhoea. Cholestatic jaundice, especially in over 65 years of age: limit treatment to < 14 days. (Committee on Safety of Medicines warning)

Drug	Action		Spectrum	Dose	Renal adjustment	Adverse effects/cautions
First-generation cephalosporin, e.g. cefradine	Bactericidal	Cell wall lysis	*Streptococcus* spp. *Staphylococcus* spp. *E. coli*	250 mg four times a day or 500 mg 12-hourly	CrCl 10–50 250 mg two to three times daily CrCl < 10 250 mg/day	Allergic reaction: 10–20% cross-allergy with penicillins. Diarrhoea
Quinolones, e.g. norfloxacin	Bactericidal		Moderate activity against *Streptococcus* and *Enterococcus* spp. Broad-spectrum Gram-negative action including antipseudomonal	400 mg twice daily	CrCl < 50 400 mg once daily	Dizziness, headache, visual disturbance, seizure, central nervous system disturbance, gastro-intestinal upset, Stevens–Johnson syndrome, photosensitivity, increased abnormal liver function tets.Tendon damage, especially in elderly and those taking corticosteroids (Committee on Safety of Medicines advice). Caution in patients with a history of convulsions and glucose-6-phosphate dehydrogenase deficiency. Serious drug interactions

longer courses may be required. Elderly patients with pyelonephritis are likely to have bacteraemia and hypotension. Patients who are vomiting, confused, generally unwell or requiring rehydration should be admitted to hospital for administration of intravenous antibiotics and supportive care. The choices of intravenous antibiotics include trimethoprim, a second-generation cephalosporin, a quinolone or – with caution due to risk of renal toxicity – gentamicin. Treatment should be switched to suitable oral antibiotics when possible once temperature and symptoms settle, usually after 2–3 days. Persistence of symptoms may indicate inadequate treatment or a lesion requiring draining.

Table 8.3 gives the drugs commonly used to treat UTI with sensitivity and special precautions for use in the elderly.

Community-acquired urinary tract infections in men

After the age of 60 years the prevalence of UTI in men increases; this is thought to be related to urinary outflow obstruction due to prostatic hypertrophy or increasing rates of debilitation.

The presentation and causative organisms in male UTI are similar to that in females. Treatment choice is as for females, but males should receive 10–14 days of therapy. Consideration should be given to underlying structural abnormality such as enlarged prostate causing bladder outflow obstruction. Relapse is common in men and usually relates to a sustained focus within the prostate that has not been eradicated.

Treatment of complicated urinary tract infections

Complicated UTI includes infections associated with indwelling catheters, structural abnormalities, hospital-acquired infections, or, in men, those associated with prostatitis. Ciprofloxacin is a good choice of antibiotic in complicated infections in males because of good tissue penetration and broad Gram-negative spectrum of activity; however, trimethoprim may be used and culture and sensitivity results will usually guide choice of therapy. Sustained therapy for 4–6 weeks may be required in relapsing cases. In cases which continue to relapse, continuous suppressive antibiotic therapy may be required or alternatively prostatectomy may be indicated.

In hospital or long-stay facilities UTI is the most common nosocomial infection;[15] it leads to 30–40% of Gram-negative bacteraemias and is most commonly associated with indwelling urological catheters. The risk of morbidity increases with the duration of catheterisation and chronic catheter use should be avoided if at all possible. Persistent infection associated with catheter use will lead to renal damage; however, this is less of an issue in frail elderly patients who commonly have multiple pathologies.[4] Because repeated antibiotic use will select resistant organisms, catheter-associated bacteriuria should only be treated in those patients who are symptomatic.

Treatment of complicated UTI should include appropriate surgical intervention and therapy with broad-spectrum antibiotics which will cover the relatively resistant bacteria found in patients with previous antibiotic exposure or in the institutional or hospital environment. Suitable choices of antibiotics include ciprofloxacin, a third-generation cephalosporin or gentamicin, with due caution with regard to renal function and toxicity. Antibiotic therapy should be adjusted according to culture and sensitivity results. Treatment in a catheterised patient may need to provide antistaphylococcal therapy and should include the removal of the catheter because biofilm build-up will impair antibiotic action.

Table 8.4 gives details of the antibiotics used in the treatment of complicated UTI.

Renal tuberculosis

The genitourinary tract is the leading site of the 10% of human tuberculosis (TB) infection which is not pulmonary. Renal TB is a disease of the elderly, which mirrors the higher rate of TB in the elderly. Renal TB is usually the result of blood-borne dissemination from a primary focus elsewhere in the body.[15] Infection in the elderly is often the result of reactivation of dormant TB acquired in early life. The infection usually starts as small foci in the renal cortex which expand and spread to cause necrosis of the kidney. Calcification may develop leading to nephrolithiasis and renal damage may result in secondary hypertension.

Caseous material is produced which is irritant to the urethra and bladder and the disease may spread to the urethra, prostate, fallopian tubes or other genitourinary organs. Symptoms are usually similar to UTI, with flank and back pain, although fever and constitutional symptoms are usually absent. Culture of urine by standard methods will usually be sterile but large numbers of leukocytes will be present in the specimen. Cystoscopy, X-ray, ultrasound and computed tomography scan investigations will usually show structural changes in the affected tissues. Once diagnosis is confirmed, treatment is with standard anti-TB

Table 8.4 Antimicrobials used to treat complicated urinary tract infection

Drug	Urinary pathogens covered	Dose	Renal impairment dose (creatinine clearance (CrCl) ml/min)	Side-effects and precautions
Co-amoxiclav IV	*Streptococcus* *Staphylococcus* *Escherichia coli* *Klebsiella* *Proteus* spp.	600 mg 8-hourly	CrCl 10–50 600 mg 12-hourly CrCl < 10 600 mg 24-hourly	Allergic reactions, rash, diarrhoea. Cholestatic jaundice, especially in those over 65 years of age: limit treatment to < 14 days (Committee on Safety of Medicines warning)
Second- or third-generation cephalosporin, e.g. cefuroxime	*Streptococcus* *Staphylococcus* *E. coli* *Klebsiella* *Proteus* spp. Ceftazidime is also effective against *Pseudomonas*	750 mg 8-hourly	CrCl 10–50 750 mg 12-hourly CrCl < 10 750 mg 24-hourly	Allergic reaction: 10–20% cross-allergy with penicillins. Diarrhoea, *Clostridium difficile* diarrhoea, fever, arthralgia, toxic epidermal necrolysis, transient hepatitis
Quinolone, e.g. ciprofloxacin IV	Moderate activity against *Streptococcus* and *Enterococcus* Broad-spectrum Gram-negative action, including antipseudomonal	200–400 mg 12-hourly	CrCl 10–50 200 mg 12-hourly CrCl < 10 200 mg 24-hourly	Dizziness, headache, visual disturbance, seizure, central nervous system disturbance, gastrointestinal upset, Stevens–Johnson syndrome, photosensitivity, increased liver functions. Tendon damage, especially in elderly and those taking corticosteroids (Committee on Safety of Medicines advice). Caution in patients with a history of convulsions and glucose-6-phosphate dehydrogenase deficiency. Serious drug interactions
Aminoglycoside, e.g. gentamicin	*Staphylococcus* Broad-spectrum Gram-negative, including antipseudomonal action	120 mg 12-hourly	Adjust dose in any degree of renal impairment according to renal function	Renal impairment, ototoxicity, nausea, vomiting, rash. Serum level monitoring recommended. Extreme caution in renal failure and the elderly

IV=intravenously

therapy for 9 months, but men with overt genital disease usually receive an additional 3–6 months of therapy.[16] For details of drug therapy see the section on TB under respiratory infections, below. Surgery is reserved for complications of renal TB, including secondary hypertension.

Genital infections

Female genital infections

Postmenopausal changes in the female genital tract have a large effect on the incidence and presentation of infections in this organ system. The increase in the pH of the vagina changes the flora from lactobacilli and permits overgrowth with organisms from the perineum such as coliforms and streptococci. Treatment of atrophic vaginitis is by the use of oestrogen cream which restores the acid environment and permits re-establishment of lactobacilli. Vulvovaginal candidiasis in the elderly occurs more commonly in patients receiving corticosteroids or those with poorly controlled diabetes. The signs of vaginal candidiasis are a watery discharge and creamy deposit on the mucosa. Treatment with imidazole pessaries and cream is usually effective.

Pyometra is an accumulation of pus in the womb which may result from inadequate drainage. Infective organisms commonly include anaerobic organisms such as *Bacteroides* spp. The patient may present with septicaemia and shock requiring supportive care. Treatment of the infection is with dilatation of the cervix, leaving a drain in place. If the patient displays signs of systemic infection, systemic broad-spectrum antibiotics such as cefuroxime plus metronidazole should be started, and then tailored to the results of culture and sensitivity tests.

Male genital infections

Balanitis is an inflammation of the glans penis which is more common amongst uncircumcised men.[17] It is common in the elderly male and in those with diabetes. Infection may be by fungi such as *Candida albicans* or with bacteria such as *Bacteroides* spp (most commonly) or possibly streptococci and staphylococci. Infection presents as a tender and swollen foreskin and tip of penis with discharge. Treatment should be topical imidazole or oral fluconazole for *Candida* infection or, for bacterial infections, metronidazole plus ampicillin.

Epididymitis may develop in elderly men as a result of UTI. The predominant organisms are Enterobacteriaceae, especially *E. coli*. Initial treatment choice is usually ciprofloxacin or ofloxacin which have good tissue penetration. Alternative agents include ceftriaxone or cefotaxime. Metronidazole should be added if anaerobic infection is suspected. Duration of treatment is usually for 10–21 days.

Fournier's gangrene is necrotising fasciitis of the perineum and genitalia. Infection is usually polymicrobial and a broad-spectrum agent such as piperacillin/tazobactam, meropenem or a combination of ceftazidime plus metronidazole is usually indicated. Surgery and skin grafting may be required for recovery of affected areas.

Respiratory infections

The elderly patient has a higher risk of developing a respiratory tract infection than younger individuals. The mortality and morbidity from such infections are higher because of the increased incidence of comorbid conditions such as chronic lung disease, heart failure and pulmonary oedema, decreased immune function and predisposing conditions such as stroke and aspiration.

Influenza

Each year 3000–4000 deaths are attributed to influenza in the UK in non-epidemic years.[18] Most of the people affected are elderly and those with underlying chronic medical conditions. Immunisation of those at high risk prevents hospitalisation in about 70% of cases and mortality due to influenza-related complications by 80%. Department of Health guidelines[19] specify routine immunisation of all those with underlying disease which puts them at special risk from influenza and all those over the age of 65 years. Groups recommended for vaccination are given in Table 8.5.

Vaccination should be given in October or early November and repeated annually. Influenza vaccine is prepared each year based on inactivated virus strains similar to those likely to be circulating in the coming winter months. The two types of vaccine, the split virion and the surface antigen, are equivalent in efficacy and adverse effects. The adult dose is a single 0.5 ml intramuscular or deep subcutaneous injection. Mild local reaction occurs in 20% of cases and this subsides in 48 hours. Egg protein sensitivity is extremely rare but may result in bronchospasm, urticaria and angioedema. Vaccination is contra-

Table 8.5 Groups recommended for influenza vaccination

Chronic heart disease
Chronic lung disease
Chronic renal disease
Diabetes mellitus
Immunosuppression due to disease or treatment
Long-stay care residents
Everyone aged over 65 years

indicated in pregnancy, acute illness and previous sensitivity or known sensitivity to egg products.

The antiviral drug amantadine is licensed in the UK for the treatment and prophylaxis of influenza A, but it should not be used for both purposes in the same household. It is recommended that it is only used for prophylaxis in unimmunised patients in at-risk groups while the vaccine takes effect (as in Table 8.5), or at-risk patients in whom immunisation is contraindicated or in health care workers and other key personnel during an epidemic. It is recommended that the dose be reduced in the elderly to less than 100 mg/day or 100 mg at intervals of greater than 1 day. Duration of therapy for treatment is 4–5 days, and 6 weeks for prophylaxis or for 2–3 weeks when given with vaccination in at-risk groups.

The drug zanamivir inhibits the enzyme neuroaminidase which has a role in the infectivity and replication of influenza A and B viruses. Zanamivir is licensed in the UK for the treatment of influenza A and B within 48 hours of the onset of symptoms; it is reported to reduce the duration of symptoms by about one day in otherwise healthy individuals. The use of zanamivir is controversial and the National Institute for Clinical Excellence (NICE) recommends restricting its use to the treatment of at risk adults who present within 36 hours of the onset of influenza-like illness.[20] At risk adults are defined as those who meet any of the following criteria:

- age over 65 years
- having chronic respiratory disease
- having significant cardiovascular disease
- being immunocompromised
- having diabetes mellitus.

However these recommendations are disputed because of lack of evidence of efficacy in preventing morbidity and mortality in at-risk patients.[21] Zanamivir has poor oral bioavailability and is administered

Table 8.6 Bacterial causes of community-acquired pneumonia (CAP)

Pathogen	Frequency implicated	Population affected and risk factors	Antibiotic sensitivities
Streptococcus pneumoniae (*Pneumococcus*)	40–60%	All age groups. More common in winter. Epidemics may occur in closed communities	Penicillin is antibiotic of choice. Resistance rates 1–5% in UK but much higher in rest of world. Resistance is often intermediate and may be overcome by high doses. Pneumococcal vaccine should be given to at-risk groups
Mycoplasma pneumoniae	10–20%	Transmitted by droplets. Occurs in 4-year epidemics, predominantly in young adults; may be less common in elderly. Appearance on X-ray may be atypical or typical. Can cause immune complications such as Guillain–Barré syndrome and Stevens–Johnson syndrome	Macrolide such as erythromycin is the antibiotic of choice. Also sensitive to quinolones and tetracyclines
Haemophilus influenzae	10%	Occurs mainly in those with underlying chest disease such as COPD, bronchiectasis, or in alcohol abuse and smoking	Amoxicillin first choice: resistance rates in the UK are about 20% but much higher in other parts of the world. Consider co-amoxiclav if resistance is a problem. Alternative agents are quinolones, trimethoprim, first- or second-generation cephalosporin, tetracycline or clarithromycin
Legionella spp.	5%	May cause mild to severe CAP or nosocomial pneumonia. 40% of patients have recently returned from overseas travel, hence peak incidence in autumn. Found in warm still water; air conditioners are an important source of infection. Infection is often in a predisposed host such as smoker or with COPD	A macrolide ± rifampicin or quinolone in severe cases are the antibiotics of choice

Organism		Comments	Treatment
Staphylococcus aureus	5%	50% of cases are associated with prior influenza virus infection. May be more common in the elderly. Consider in severe CAP or when cavitation is present on chest X-ray	Flucloxacillin ± rifampicin or fusidic acid, depending on severity of infection. Vancomycin for methicillin-resistant *Staphylococcus aureus*
Moraxella catarrhalis		Usually in the presence of COPD	Co-amoxiclav or second- or third-generation cephalosporin
Tuberculosis		Consider if presenting history is long, pneumonia is mainly in the upper zone, cavitation is present or response to antibiotics is poor. See section on tuberculosis for predisposed individuals	Rifampicin + isoniazid + pyrazinamide ± ethambutol
Gram-negative enterobacteria	Rare	Mainly cause nosocomial pneumonia. More common in some parts of South Africa	Second- or third-generation cephalosporin ± aminoglycoside. Ciprofloxacin, piperacillin with tazobactam, meropenem
Chlamydia psittaci	Rare	Usually acquired from exotic birds, but can be from ducks and turkeys and occasionally sheep	Tetracycline
Chlamydia pneumoniae	Associated with 20%	Commonly a bacterial co-pathogen: role needs clarification. Spread directly from human to human	Tetracycline or erythromycin
Coxiella burnetii (Q fever)		Causes variable infection which may include pneumonia. Acquired from sheep, therefore more common in sheep-rearing areas	Tetracycline Macrolide
Influenza viruses A and B		Occurs in epidemics in winter. High morbidity and mortality in elderly or underlying disease	Vaccination most effective. Amantadine if given within 48 h
Varicella-zoster		Usually only causes pneumonia in adults and this may be severe; associated rash	Aciclovir
Parainfluenza and adenovirus		May occasionally cause pneumonia in the elderly	

COPD = Chronic obstructive pulmonary disease.

by means of a dry powder for inhalation, which should be used with caution in those with chronic pulmonary disease because of the risk of bronchospasm. It has been shown that many elderly patients are unable to use the inhaler device to deliver the zanamivir which may make the treatment ineffective.[22] The dose of zanamivir is 10 mg twice daily for 5 days given by inhalation of powder.

Pneumonia

In the UK there are 40–80 cases of lower respiratory tract infection per 1000 adults per year, of which 1 in 25 cases are pneumonia.[23] Lower respiratory tract infections are most common in the young and elderly. Pneumonia is a more severe illness than lower respiratory tract infection and there are 25 000 deaths in people aged over 65 years per year in the UK.[24] Most patients with pneumonia are managed by their general practitioner, with 1 in 6 being admitted to hospital. The rate of nosocomial (hospital-acquired) pneumonia is about 10% of patients over 70 years of age. The overall mortality for community-acquired pneumonia (CAP) managed in hospital is 5% and for nosocomial pneumonia or CAP requiring intensive care it is 30%.

Pneumonia is an accumulation of secretions and inflammatory cells in the alveolar spaces of the lung and is caused by infection. The resulting inflammation and consolidation result in disturbance of gas exchange and may permit bacterial invasion of the blood stream (bacteraemia) and subsequent sepsis. The lower airways are normally sterile and pneumonia is usually associated with conditions which disrupt the natural defences such as chronic lung disease, compromised immunity or viral respiratory tract infections which allow secondary bacterial infections.

It is useful to categorise pneumonia by the likely origin of infection because the causative organisms vary and therefore the treatment varies:

- community-acquired
- nosocomial (hospital-acquired)
- in immunosuppressed patients.

Community-acquired pneumonia

This typically presents with fever, rigors and often pleuritic chest pain; however, in the elderly the symptoms may not be respiratory and the patient may present with confusion, incontinence or falls. A history should be taken to point to sources of infection and narrow the causative possibilities, for example contact with birds (possible psittacosis) or recent foreign travel (possible legionnaires' disease).

The causes of CAP are given in Table 8.6. The most common cause of CAP is *Streptococcus pneumoniae* (60%). It occurs most commonly in the winter and may cause severe pneumonia with high mortality. Bacteraemia develops in approximately 20% of patients and, of these, 20% will die.

In order to aid treatment the severity of the pneumonia should be assessed as mild, moderate or severe according to the British Thoracic Society guidelines.[25] The features of severe pneumonia are given in Table 8.7.

Patients with two or more of the features are considered to have severe pneumonia and increased risk of death.

The classification of pneumonia by severity is usually as follows:

Mild

- Age less than 65 years
- No pre-existing cardiopulmonary disease
- No major constitutional symptoms

Moderate

- Any patient who is not mild or severe

Severe

- Presence of two of the risk factors for increased death given in Table 8.7

When two or more of the following three factors are present, the patient is at a greatly increased risk of death and should be considered for intensive care:

- Respiratory rate > 30 breaths/min
- Diastolic blood pressure < 60 mmHg
- Serum urea > 7 mmol/l

Table 8.7 Features of severe pneumonia associated with increased risk of death: patients with two or more of the features are considered to have severe pneumonia and an increased risk of death

Clinical	Laboratory
Mental confusion	Serum urea > 7 mmol/l
Respiratory rate ⩾ 30 breaths/min	Serum albumin < 35 g/l
Diastolic blood pressure ⩽ 60 mmHg	$PaO_2 < 8$ kPa
New atrial fibrillation	White blood cell count $< 4 \times 10^9$ or
Multilobar involvement	$> 20 \times 10^9$ per litre
	Bacteraemia

Mild-to-moderate CAP may be treated at home with therapy, which is usually empirical and based on clinical diagnosis. Investigations such as chest X-ray and sputum culture and sensitivities may be useful in those who fail to respond to treatment. For moderate-to-severe CAP treated in hospital a chest X-ray is obtained to confirm diagnosis and aid the severity assessment and a white blood cell count and urea and electrolyte screen are carried out to assist diagnosis and monitor for organ function impairment. Oximetry or arterial blood gas is indicated in the severely ill to assess requirement for intensive care. Microbiological investigation is usually carried out in severe pneumonia to direct or modify antibiotic treatment. In patients requiring intensive care and ventilator support, fibreoptic bronchoscopy is often performed to obtain lower respiratory tract samples for culture and sensitivity.

In all cases, antibiotic treatment should be started promptly and not delayed for the results of tests. In moderate-to-severe pneumonia or in patients unable to tolerate oral medications, antibiotics should be given parenterally. As the patient improves treatment can be switched to the oral route. The current recommendations for empirical antibiotic therapy in pneumonia are:

Mild

- Amoxicillin
- Macrolide in those who are allergic to penicillin

Moderate CAP

- Amoxicillin or co-amoxiclav
- Plus a macrolide if *Mycoplasma* is suspected

or:

- First- or second-generation cephalosporin with optional macrolide

Severe CAP

- Second- or third-generation cephalosporin plus macrolide

However, these guidelines are currently being reviewed due to the increase in *Clostridium difficile* diarrhoea associated with increased broad-spectrum cephalosporin use. Acquired antibiotic resistance of common respiratory bacterial pathogens is acknowledged by the British Thoracic Society working group as a concern, but is currently considered a rare cause of clinical failure in the UK. The major change is expected to be:

Moderate CAP

- Amoxicillin plus a macrolide given to all patients (erythromycin oral or clarithromycin intravenously)

Or alternative:

- β-Lactam plus oral clarithromycin

Or alternative:

- Fluoroquinolone with Gram-positive activity (e.g. ofloxacin) may be considered as monotherapy
- Step-down oral regimen should be amoxicillin plus erythromycin

Severe CAP

- First choice: co-amoxiclav plus clarithromycin with optional rifampicin

Or alternative:

- Second- or third-generation cephalosporin plus clarithromycin with optional rifampicin

Or alternative:

- Fluoroquinolone with Gram-positive activity as monotherapy
- Step-down oral regimen as for moderate CAP

Pneumococcal vaccination is recommended as a preventive measure for patients who are at increased risk of contracting pneumonia or for those with increased mortality. Table 8.8 gives the groups recommended to receive pneumococcal vaccination. The vaccine can be given at any time during the year and should be repeated at 5-year intervals.

Nosocomial pneumonia

This is pneumonia diagnosed after at least 3 days of hospitalisation. It occurs mostly among patients admitted with medical problems or recovering from abdominal or thoracic surgery.[26] The highest incidence occurs in mechanically ventilated patients. Nosocomial pneumonia is

Table 8.8 Department of Health recommendations on which groups should be given pneumococcal vaccination

Asplenic or with severe dysfunction of the spleen	Human immunodeficiency virus infection at any stage
Coeliac syndrome	Chronic heart failure
Symptomatic sickle cell disease	Chronic lung disease (including emphysema
Chronic renal failure	emphysema, chronic bronchitis, asthma
Immunodeficiency or immunosuppression due to either disease or therapy	and bronchiectasis)
	Chronic liver disease, including cirrhosis
	Diabetes mellitus
Nephrotic syndrome	

Table 8.9 Bacterial causes of nosocomial pneumonia

Pathogen	Population affected and risk factors	Antibiotic choice
Staphylococcus aureus	Especially associated with ventilator-acquired pneumonia in intensive care. Also associated with coma, head trauma, diabetes mellitus and renal failure	Flucloxacillin Vancomycin if methicillin-resistant Staphylococcus aureus is suspected ± rifampicin or fusidic acid
Streptococcus pneumoniae	More likely if pneumonia occurs within 5 days of hospital admission	Penicillin (high dose if intermediate resistance)
Haemophilus influenzae	More likely if pneumonia occurs within 5 days of hospital admission	Cefradrine or cefuroxime Co-amoxiclav
Enteric Gram-negative bacilli: Enterobacter spp. Escherichia coli Klebsiella spp.	Common cause of nosocomial pneumonia. Within 72 h of hospital admission the upper respiratory tract becomes colonised with enteric Gram-negative bacilli which have	Cefuroxime Cefotaxime Quinolone
Enterobacteriaceae: Proteus spp. Serratia marcescens	antibiotic resistance patterns reflective of the hospital	
Acinetobacter spp. Xanthomonas spp.	Occasional causes of epidemic nosocomial pneumonia, especially ventilator-associated pneumonia in intensive care	Often very resistant
Pseudomonas aeruginosa	Should be considered in patients with prolonged stay in intensive care, on steroids, previous antibiotics, with structural lung disease	Ceftazidime Ciprofloxacin Piperacillin Aminoglycoside is often added to above Carbapenem
Anaerobic bacteria	Usually following aspiration or associated with recent abdominal surgery	Metronidazole

mostly caused by Gram-negative enterobacteria and reflects the colonis-ation of the oropharynx by hospital-acquired resistant organisms within 48 h of admission to hospital. It is microaspiration of these virulent organisms usually in patients with impaired host defences which then leads to pneumonia. Table 8.9 gives the common causes. Mortality from nosocomial pneumonia is high because of the severity of the infection, the resistant nature of the infecting organisms and often because of the underlying condition of the patient.

Aspiration pneumonia

This is an important cause of pneumonia in the elderly due to reduced gag reflex from such causes as stroke or general debilitation. Aspiration pneumonia occurs when oropharyngeal contents pass into the lungs. In the community anaerobic mouth bacteria such as *Bacteroides*, *Prevotella* and *Peptostreptococcus* spp. are the usual cause. Treatment is with penicillin plus metronidazole or co-amoxiclav. In hospitalised patients antibiotic cover will additionally need to be effective against resistant Gram-negative organisms.

Pulmonary tuberculosis

This occurs most commonly in the elderly as reactivation of a primary focus. It may however also occur as infection from other patients in a care setting or in the community. TB is transmitted through droplet inhalation. The risk of TB is increased in heavy smokers or those with high alcohol consumption. TB occurs more commonly in conditions which lead to immunosuppression such as extreme age, diabetes or malignancy or those taking immunity-suppressing drugs such as corti-costeroids or cytotoxic agents. TB is on the increase in the UK due to the ageing population, and increase in poverty and immigration from areas of the world with a high incidence of TB.[27] Rates of TB in England and Wales in 1998 were 10.9 per 100 000 people.

The main causative organism in the UK is *Mycobacterium tuber-culosis* but atypical mycobacteria such as *M. xenopi*, *M. kansasii* and *M. avium intracellulare* may cause disease in those who are immuno-compromised (such as human immunodeficiency virus (HIV)-positive people) or have damaged lungs, for example from previous TB or severe bronchiectasis.[28]

The signs and symptoms of TB are weight loss, anorexia, malaise and fever and in pulmonary TB, cough, sputum production and haemoptysis. Investigations include a chest X-ray which will typically

Table 8.10 Characteristics of first- and second-line antituberculous drugs

Drug	Side-effects	Adjustment for renal or hepatic failure
First-line treatments		
Rifampicin	Nausea, dyspepsia, vomiting, skin rashes, hepatitis, fever, jaundice, eosinophilia, red staining of body secretions. Flu-like syndrome, especially with intermittent treatment regimens. Enhances metabolism of drugs at CYP3A4 enzyme: adjust dose of affected drugs to compensate	Decrease dose in hepatic impairment. Take especial care in alcoholics, those with liver disease and the malnourished. Monitor LFTs and stop if 5 × upper limit of normal; reintroduce carefully once recovered
Isoniazid	Nausea, dyspepsia, vomiting, skin rashes, hepatitis (especially in alcoholics and pre-existing liver disease), peripheral neuropathy, encephalopathy. Drug interactions. Supplement with pyridoxine to prevent peripheral neuropathy, especially in malnourished or alcoholic patients	Decrease dose in severe renal or hepatic impairment. Take especial care in alcoholics and the elderly. Monitor LFTs and stop if serum aminotransferase or bilirubin 5 × upper limit of normal; reintroduce cautiously when recovered
Pyrazinamide	Nausea, dyspepsia, skin rash, hepatotoxicity, gout, arthropathy	Decrease dose in renal or hepatic impairment. Monitor LFTs and serum uric acid levels
Ethambutol	Optic neuritis: check vision before and during treatment. Hyperuricaemia	Decrease dose in mild renal impairment
Second-line treatments		
Streptomycin Amikacin Kanamycin Capreomycin	Ototoxicity, nephrotoxicity	Decrease dose in renal impairment
Ciprofloxacin	Gastrointestinal intolerance, seizures, photosensitivity, increased LFT, arthralgia, confusion. Avoid in children and pregnant and breast-feeding women	Decrease dose in moderate renal impairment. Caution in patients with history of seizures
Clarithromycin	Gastrointestinal intolerance, hepatitis, jaundice, ventricular tachycardia (caution with drug interactions)	Decrease dose in moderate renal impairment
Ethionamide Cycloserine Para-aminosalicylic acid Rifabutin	Nausea, vomiting, hepatotoxicity, drowsiness, rarely seizures Rash, convulsions, neuropathy, rarely seizures and psychosis Hepatitis, gastrointestinal disturbance, lupus-like syndrome As for rifampicin: drug resistance often cross-reacts with rifampicin	Caution in liver disease

LFTs = Liver function tests.

show cavitation, particularly in the upper lobes, a sputum smear for acid-fast bacilli and culture and sensitivity testing. In a proportion of cases it is not possible to grow the organism and diagnosis is made from typical clinical features and confirmed by a response to anti-TB therapy. The Mantoux and Heaf test only give an indication of the immune status of the patient; a positive test indicates current or previous infection and a negative test may indicate no previous exposure to TB or severe infection with inadequate immunological response.

TB is treated with combination therapy. Triple therapy consisting of rifampicin, isoniazid and pyrazinamide is given for 2 months with ethambutol added for those at risk of drug-resistant TB. Once response to therapy and sensitivity testing is available, therapy is reduced to rifampicin and isoniazid for a further 4 months in uncomplicated pulmonary TB. Longer treatment periods may be required for extrapulmonary TB, particularly of the central nervous system where a 12-month course of therapy may be required. If treatment is interrupted before the end of the course drug-resistant TB may develop.

Table 8.10 gives information on the main antitubercular agents with side-effects and monitoring parameters.

Gastrointestinal infections

Elderly people are particularly susceptible to infections of the gastrointestinal tract because of age-related reduction in gastric acid production which may lead to overgrowth with enteric Gram-negative organisms. In addition elderly individuals are often prescribed medication which may cause a reduction in salivary or gastric secretions or in gastrointestinal motility which may lead to constipation. Examples of drugs which may cause problems include antimuscarinics, antipsychotics, tricyclic antidepressants, opioids and antacids. Comorbidity such as diabetes or diverticulitis may increase susceptibility to gastric infections. There may be increased rates of non-invasive gastrointestinal infections such as oral candidal infections and increased rates of mortality from invasive infections such as salmonella and *E. coli*.

Parotitis

Suppurative parotitis occurs most commonly in elderly patients who have a dry mouth or are chronically ill with poor nutritional intake, or it may occur following general anaesthesia. Dry mouth may be the result of dehydration due to illness or drugs such as diuretics or antimuscarinics. Infecting organisms gain access usually from the mouth via the ducts to the salivary glands, so infecting organisms are usually pathogenic mouth flora such as *Staphylococcus aureus* and anaerobes. Onset is usually marked by fever, chills, unilateral swelling and pain. Gram stain, culture and sensitivity should guide antibiotic choice, which should include a penicillinase-resistant antibiotic such as flucloxacillin, or vancomycin if methicillin-resistant *Staphylococcus aureus* (MRSA) is suspected. Improved hydration and oral hygiene are important in treating and preventing further infection. An abscess which does not drain through the salivary duct may require surgical drainage. Complications include septicaemia, osteomyelitis and facial nerve palsy.

Candidiasis

Infections caused by *Candida* spp. have increased in recent years due to the increased numbers of patients who are immunocompromised.[29] Candidaemia is the fourth most common blood stream infection in the USA, with a higher rate in those aged over 65 years. Superficial candidal infections are also more common in the elderly because of increased exposure to precipitating factors.

Candida spp. are yeasts which often colonises gastrointestinal and genitourinary tracts. The most common species is *C. albicans*, but less frequent species include *C. glabrata*, *C. parapsilosis* and *C. tropicalis*. All *Candida* species can cause infection when interruption of normal host defences occurs. Neutrophils and monocytes provide defence against invasive disease and T cells against mucosal disease so invasive disease usually occurs in patients with neutropenia. In contrast, acquired immune deficiency syndrome (AIDS) patients commonly suffer from recurrent oral, oesophageal or vaginal candidiasis. Old age of itself is not a risk factor for the incidence of candidal infections, but it is associated with increased morbidity and mortality from both superficial and invasive types of such infection.

Oral candidiasis usually presents as white plaques which are present on the buccal, palatal or oropharyngeal mucosa. In addition, painful cracks may develop at the corners of the mouth (angular cheilitis). Factors which predispose to the development of oral candidiasis include dry mouth, the use of broad-spectrum antibiotics, inhaled corticosteroids and decreased cell-mediated immunity. Oral thrush in an elderly person without obvious cause may herald underlying immunosuppression in the form of malignancy or AIDS. Dry mouth, often due to medication, increases the rate of colonisation with yeast which predisposes to oral thrush. The underlying cause should be removed and treatment effected with nystatin or amphotericin pastilles or miconazole gel. Suspension is not as effective because of limited contact time. Treatment-resistant cases may be given fluconazole 50 mg orally for 7 days.

Denture stomatitis is a variation of oral candidiasis which presents as a chronic mucosal erythema beneath dentures. It may affect up to 65% of people who wear dentures, especially full sets or in those who do not remove them at night. The appearance is usually of diffuse erythema; plaques are not usually present so the diagnosis may easily be missed. Treatment is by denture removal at night, vigorous brushing and cleaning plus disinfecting of dentures. If this does not result in cure, treatment with antifungal pastilles or gel may be required or, in unresponsive cases, oral fluconazole 50 mg/day with appropriate hygiene measures.

Antibiotic-associated diarrhoea

The elderly are at particular risk of morbidity from diarrhoea because of reduced tolerance to fluid and electrolyte imbalance, reduced response of the elderly kidney to antidiuretic hormone (ADH) and reduced thirst stimulus. The elderly are more likely to become severely dehydrated and succumb to circulatory collapse.

Antibiotic therapy alters colonic flora which permits colonisation with pathogenic bacteria, in particular *Clostridium difficile*.[30] Most antibiotics have been implicated in causing *C. difficile* diarrhoea, but broad-spectrum agents with activity against enteric bacteria are the most frequent offenders. Antibiotics more commonly associated with diarrhoea include amoxicillin, clindamycin and cephalosporins, especially those of the second and third generation. Increased incidence has been correlated with increased use of the latter. The elderly are at particular risk of developing *C. difficile* diarrhoea because of increased use of antibiotics in this age group and increased incidence of hospital admission. Mortality in the frail elderly is 10–20%, largely due to profound dehydration.

Colonisation occurs by the oral–faecal route. Spores of *C. difficile* are heat-resistant and may persist in the environment for months or years, hence the infection may become endemic in long-stay institutions and hospitals. Infection results from ingestion of spores which survive the acid environment of the stomach and convert to vegetative forms in the colon. Toxin-producing strains cause diarrhoea and colitis. Toxins are believed to be proinflammatory, leading to colonic inflammation and colitis. The toxins are cytotoxic and cause epithelial necrosis in the colon and

Table 8.11 Treatment suggestions for infective diarrhoea

Infective cause	Comments	Treatment	Alternative
Clostridium difficile	Antibiotic-associated diarrhoea. Treat for 10 days. Relapse is common: spores may persist for months in environment. Vancomycin is reserved choice to prevent spread of vancomycin-resistant enterococcus	Metronidazole 400 mg t.d.s. orally. May be given IV if not able to tolerate oral	Vancomycin 125 mg q.d.s. orally. Not effective if given IV
Salmonella spp.	Very serious infection in elderly; should be treated with antibiotics in addition to rehydration. Quinolone first choice as most effective in preventing carrier state	Quinolone, e.g. ciprofloxacin 500 mg b.d. oral for 7–10 days or IV 200 mg b.d.	Trimethoprim 200 mg b.d.
Campylobacter spp.	Usually settles without antibiotics: treat severe cases. Carrier state does not usually develop	Ciprofloxacin 500 mg b.d. for 5 days	Erythromycin 250 mg q.d.s.
Shigella spp.	Older people more at risk of invasive disease: treat all but most mild cases with antibiotics	Ciprofloxacin 500 mg b.d. for 5 days	Trimethoprim 200 mg b.d. or Amoxicillin 500 mg t.d.s. or Co-amoxiclav
Toxin diarrhoea, e.g. Staphylococcus aureus	Toxin is heat-labile and destroyed with adequate cooking. Onset of symptoms is rapid but usually self-limiting as toxin is shed from gastrointestinal tract. Treatment is supportive		
Escherichia coli 0157	Use of antibiotic may increase release of toxin and increase risk of haemolytic–uraemic syndrome	In severe or prolonged diseases ciprofloxacin may be used	
Listeria monocytogenes	Associated with soft cheeses and precooked chilled meals. Not detected in stool culture	Ampicillin 500 mg q.d.s. IV or Amoxicillin 500 mg t.d.s oral	
Rotaviruses	Usually causes mild disease but may cause epidemic in institutions and fatalities in frail elderly. Treatment is supportive		

IV = Intravenously.

ulceration overlaid by a pseudomembrane of mucin, fibrin, leukocytes and cell debris. *C. difficile* diarrhoea may occur without pseudomembranes.

Infective diarrhoea

Other causes of diarrhoea are *Campylobacter*, *Salmonella*, *Shigella* spp., *E. coli*, in particular, strain O157 and rotaviruses. Most of these infections are associated with poor food-handling practices or contact with an infected individual or via the oral–faecal route.[31] The emergence of multidrug-resistant enteric pathogens such as *Campylobacter jejuni* and *Salmonella enterica* DT104 is associated with the use of antibiotics as growth promoters for poultry and pigs.[32] Bacterial resistance is a cause for concern, particularly in the elderly who have a high rate of morbidity from gastrointestinal infections and in whom treatment with antibiotics is more frequently indicated because of a higher incidence of invasive disease. Viruses such as small round structured virus (SRSV), astrovirus and calcivirus may cause diarrhoea. For those who have had recent overseas travel parasitic causes of diarrhoea such as giardiasis and amoebiasis should be considered.

Diarrhoea in the elderly may rapidly result in dehydration and electrolyte imbalance if not carefully managed. The elderly have a reduced renal tubular responsiveness to ADH and reduced ability to concentrate urine, and thirst may also be impaired in the elderly. Because of the laxity of aged skin the clinical indicators of decreased skin turgor and tongue dryness are less useful as a marker of dehydration. It is necessary to monitor serum electrolytes and urine output carefully. If the dehydration is mild and the patient is able to drink, electrolyte oral replacement fluid is suitable, but large volumes are required (2–3 l/ day). If dehydration is marked or fluid intake is poor, parenteral fluid is required. Care should be taken to prevent fluid overload, especially if cardiac impairment is an issue. If serum sodium levels rise above 160 mmol/l there is a risk of permanent neurological damage. When patients are rehydrated a rapid decrease in serum sodium should be avoided as this may cause further neurological damage. Antimotility agents should only be used in conjunction with fluid replacement and are contraindicated in *Clostridium difficile* diarrhoea. When infective diarrhoea is diagnosed, infection control measures should be instituted promptly to prevent spread; this is particularly important in long-stay institutions because the elderly and debilitated are at high risk of mortality.

Treatment suggestions for infective diarrhoea are given in Table 8.11.

Central nervous system infections

Delay in diagnosis of infections in the central nervous system (CNS) may occur in the elderly because the symptoms may be atypical or non-specific. Additionally, comorbidity such as mild dementia or drug therapy causing drowsiness or ataxia may confound the diagnosis.

Bacterial meningitis

Bacterial meningitis has a high mortality rate in older adults (38–80%).[33] The incidence of meningitis is highest in infants; however, there is a later peak of incidence among persons aged 60 years and older. The disease is more often fatal in the older adult, with 50% of all deaths from meningitis occurring in persons aged 60 years or older.

Streptococcus pneumoniae is the most common cause of meningitis in older adults,[34] accounting for 24–57% of all cases. In 40–50% of cases concurrent infection such as pneumonia or otitis will be present. Predisposing conditions are alcoholism, asplenia, chronic lymphocytic leukaemia or multiple myeloma.

Neisseria meningitidis is a less common cause of meningitis in the elderly, accounting for up to 19% of cases; this is in contrast with younger adults where it is more common. In 50% of cases petechiae or purpura may be present.

While uncommon in young adults, *Listeria monocytogenes* accounts for up to 25% of cases in the elderly. Diagnosis is more difficult because it does not Gram-stain easily, it produces a variable white blood cell count in cerebospinal fluid (CSF) and it is difficult to culture.

Gram-negative organisms infrequently cause meningitis in young adults but are more common causative agents in the elderly, accounting for 11–25% of all cases. Causal organisms include *Escherichia coli*, *Klebsiella* spp., *Proteus* spp., *Pseudomonas aeruginosa* and *Enterobacter* spp. Gram-negative meningitis is associated with head injury and neurosurgical procedures or it may be a haematogenously disseminated infection, e.g. from UTIs. The Gram-negative organism *Haemophilus influenzae*, which was common in children as a cause of meningitis before the advent of Hib vaccination, is rare in the elderly, accounting for 2–7% of cases. It is often associated with infections of the head and neck such as sinusitis, otitis or mastoiditis.

Less common causes of meningitis in the elderly include *Staphylococcus aureus* (4–11% of cases) and coagulase-negative staphylococci which may be associated with neurosurgical procedures. Group B streptococci may be the cause in patients with diabetes or chronic renal or liver failure.[35]

Bacterial meningitis typically presents with abrupt onset of fever, headache and meningismus; however presentation may be atypical in the elderly, manifesting as drowsiness, confusion and pyrexia or even hypothermia. Meningitis may also present in elderly as seizures, stroke syndromes, cranial nerve deficits or persistent alteration in mental status. Rigidity is not a useful sign in the elderly as it may be attributable to other disease states such as spondylosis or Parkinson's disease. CSF studies are important (unless contraindicated), to confirm diagnosis and identify causative organism by Gram stain, glucose, protein and white blood cell count and also culture and sensitivity.

CSF studies aid in the differential diagnosis of bacterial and viral causes of meningitis. Antigen testing of CSF for common bacteria is possible but expensive and is generally used when prior antibiotic treatment has prevented culture growth. However, commencement of broad-spectrum antibiotic treatment should not be delayed while awaiting the results of tests, empirical therapy should be started and adjusted on the basis of results. Treatment requires bactericidal antibiotics given in high dosages to achieve maximum CSF penetration. Suggested antibiotic choice is given in Table 8.12.[33, 34, 36]

Antibiotics should be given by injection to guarantee adequate serum levels and maintained at high dosages throughout, particularly since disease resolution reduces meningeal inflammation and reduces drug penetration to the CSF. Treatment duration is usually 10–14 days, except in the case of Gram-negative organisms, when longer may be required.

Even when promptly and appropriately treated, meningitis has a high mortality rate in the elderly, thus prevention by vaccination with polyvalent pneumococcal polysaccharide vaccine in those over 65 years of age or in previously indicated high-risk groups could be considered important (see vaccination recommendations for pneumonia). Chemoprophylaxis of close contacts of *Neisseria meningiditis* with rifampicin or ciprofloxacin is important.

Viral meningitis

Viral meningitis is rare in the elderly, the most common causative agent being enterovirus. Other causes include mumps virus, herpes simplex and herpes zoster. Treatment is supportive and the course is usually benign.

Table 8.12 Suggested antibiotics to treat bacterial meningitis in patients over 50 years of age

Pathogen	Patient factors	Suggested antibiotic choice	Comments
Initial blind therapy	Community-acquired	Cefotaxime 2 g 6-hourly or Ceftriaxone 2 g 12-hourly plus Ampicillin 2 g 6-hourly	Need to cover Listeria monocytogenes
Initial blind therapy	Impaired cellular immunity	Ampicillin 2 g 6-hourly plus Ceftazidime 2 g 6-hourly	Need to cover L. monocytogenes and Gram-negative bacilli
Initial blind therapy	Head trauma, neurosurgery or cerebrospinal fluid shunt	Vancomycin 1 g 12-hourly plus Ceftazidime 2 g 6-hourly	Need to cover staphylococci, Gram-negative bacilli or Streptococcus pneumoniae
Neisseria meningitidis	On culture of organism	Benzylpenicillin 2.4 g 4-hourly or Cefotaxime 2 g 6-hourly plus Rifampicin 600 mg b.d. for 2 days before discharge	Chloramphenicol 25 mg/kg IV 6-hourly for those with clear history of anaphylaxis to β-lactams
Streptococcus pneumoniae	On culture of organism	Cefotaxime 2 g 6-hourly or, if penicillin-sensitive: Benzylpenicillin 2.4 g 4-hourly or, if penicillin- and cephalosporin-resistant, add: Vancomycin 1 g 12-hourly plus Rifampicin 600 mg 12-hourly to cefotaxime	
Haemophilus influenzae	On culture of organism	Cefotaxime 2 g 6-hourly or Chloramphenicol 100 mg/kg 6-hourly	Reduce chloramphenicol dose as soon as clinically indicated; monitor for serious side-effects
Listeria monocytogenes	On culture of organism	Ampicillin 2 g 6-hourly plus Gentamicin 120 mg 12-hourly	Adjust gentamicin to renal function
Enterobacteriaceae	On culture of organism	Cefotaxime 2 g 6-hourly or Ceftriaxone 2 g 12-hourly plus Aminoglycoside, e.g. gentamicin 120 mg 12-hourly	Adjust aminoglycoside dose to renal function
Pseudomonas aeruginosa	On culture of organism	Ceftazidime 2 g 6-hourly or Tazocin 4.5 g 8-hourly or Meropenem 1 g 8-hourly plus Aminoglycoside, e.g. gentamicin 120 mg 12-hourly	Adjust aminoglycoside dose to renal function
Staphylococcus aureus	On culture of organism	Flucloxacillin 2 g 6-hourly or, if methicillin-resistant Staphylococcus aureus: Vancomycin 1 g 12-hourly	Adjust vancomycin dose to renal function

Viral encephalitis

Viral encephalitis is common in the elderly. The two main causative agents are herpes simplex and herpes zoster viruses.

Herpes simplex may cause encephalitis as a primary infection, spreading from the nasopharynx along nerves or as a reactivation of a latent infection travelling from the trigeminal ganglion. Treatment is with intravenous aciclovir at 10 mg/kg per dose every 8 hours adjusted to renal function. However mortality is about 30% even with prompt treatment and the condition carries a high rate of cognitive impairment.

Herpes zoster encephalitis is a rare complication of herpes zoster, usually starting 7–10 days after the start of skin eruption. It is usually self-limiting and treatment with aciclovir may be given by the oral route if the patient is able to tolerate medication. Alternatively, the prodrug valaciclovir, which achieves good oral absorption, may be considered.

Neurosyphilis

Neurosyphilis causes psychiatric symptoms. It may occur up to 30 years after initial exposure; the diagnosis may be missed in older patients because of a high prevalence of neurological and psychiatric disorders. However diagnosis from serology is unreliable; a positive result may be incidental to the disease process.[37] Treatment is with a prolonged course of penicillin or a cephalosporin, but it rarely results in improvement of neurological symptoms.

Cardiovascular infections

Infective endocarditis

This is a relatively uncommon but life-threatening disease, carrying substantial morbidity and mortality. In the UK there are about 2 cases per 10 000 population per year and over 50% of patients are aged over 50 years.[38] A wide range of microorganisms may be implicated.

Endocarditis usually occurs as a result of bacteraemia with opportunistic pathogens, which then attach to an underlying structural cardiac defect. Although up to 50% of patients with infective endocarditis may have no demonstrable cardiac defect, certain cardiac conditions are associated with endocarditis.[39] Rheumatic heart disease accounts for 25% of cases in the UK and congenital heart disease, especially bicuspid aortic valve, accounts for a further 25%. Mitral valve prolapse increases the risk of endocarditis by a factor of 8.

Degenerative cardiac lesions are an important predisposing factor in the elderly;[40] these include arteriosclerotic nodules, postinfarct mural thrombus and calcified mitral and aortic stenosis. Prosthetic cardiac valves become infected at the rate of 4% in the first year and 1% per year thereafter. Other intravascular devices such as intracardiac pacemakers and catheters, intravenous lines and shunts and fistulas may result in endocarditis. In hospitalised patients infection of indwelling intravenous devices and subsequent bacteraemia or fungaemia may result in endocarditis even in patients with relatively normal valves, especially if virulent microorganisms are present.

Bacteraemia may occur spontaneously or may follow from a focal infection such as UTI, pneumonia or cellulitis, which are all more common in the elderly. Procedures which breach mucosal surfaces colonised with bacteria can result in transient bacteraemia. Bacteraemia is associated with 80% of oral or dental procedures, but is less common with upper-airway, gastrointestinal, urological or obstetric procedures. Dental decay is an important risk factor for endocarditis.

Infective endocarditis may present as heart failure if untreated. There may be non-specific symptoms such as fever and chills or musculoskeletal symptoms. Other features include anorexia, weight loss, cough and dyspnoea and chest or abdominal pain. In the elderly the most common sign, pyrexia, may be absent. Heart murmurs are usually present in 85% of cases. In chronic infection, signs such as clubbing, splinter haemorrhages and splenomegaly may be present.

Untreated endocarditis may lead to necrosis of valves and ventricular septa. Refractory cardiac failure may develop. Infected vegetations may disrupt, leading to embolisation of vital organs such as the brain, kidneys and spleen, with resulting ischaemia and infective consequences. Other consequences include intracerebral or subarachnoid haemorrhage during acute infection or in later years.

Treatment of endocarditis requires identification of the infecting organism and antibiotic sensitivity testing including minimum inhibitory concentrations to ensure adequate treatment. Antibiotics selected should be bactericidal; penicillin should be the first choice if the organism is sensitive because of its superior intrinsic activity. Penetration into vegetations may be poor and therefore prolonged treatment is required to ensure eradication and prevent relapse but bacteria within the vegetations may be inactive and relatively insensitive to antibiotics. Antibiotic treatment guidelines are given in Table 8.13. If aminoglycosides or vancomycin form part of the regimen, serum level monitoring is required to ensure adequate levels and minimise toxicity.

Table 8.13 Suggested antibiotic choice for the treatment of endocarditis[38]

Organism	Associated with and approximate incidence	First-line therapy	Duration	Alternative therapy
Streptococcus viridans	Account for 50% of cases S. mutans: dental caries S. bovis: gastrointestinal lesions, e.g. cancer	Benzylpenicillin 1.2 g 6 × per day plus Gentamicin 120 mg twice daily (adjusted to renal function and levels)	4 weeks (longer if used alone for high-level aminoglycoside resistance) 2 weeks (gentamycin)	Ceftriaxone, Vancomycin (monitor) Streptomycin
Enterococci	May complicate genitourinary and obstetric procedures	Benzylpenicillin 1.2–2.4 g 6 × per day plus Gentamicin 120 mg twice daily (adjusted to renal function and levels)	Both for 4–6 weeks	Ampicillin, Vancomycin
Staphylococcus aureus	Accounts for > 20% of cases, associated with drug missuse Often no structural heart abnormality	Flucloxacillin 2 g 4 × per day plus Gentamicin 120 mg twice daily (adjusted for renal function and levels)	4–6 weeks 3–5 days (2 weeks if methicillin-resistant Staphylococcus aureus on prosthetic valve)	Vancomycin, Fusidic acid
Infective organism not identified	Native valve	Benzylpenicillin plus Gentamicin	Until organism identified	Ampicillin plus Gentamicin
	Prosthetic valve	Vancomycin plus Gentamicin		
Culture negative	Consider fungi, Chlamydia, Coxiella and Legionella	Initially Benzylpenicillin plus Gentamicin	6 weeks 2 weeks	According to serology or subsequent cultures

Once-daily dosing of aminoglycosides is commonly recommended but not adequately supported by trials. Chemotherapy is commonly ineffective for fungal infections. Dental work should be undertaken early in the course of treatment to prevent the emergence of resistant oral flora, or delayed to 4 weeks after treatment.

Surgical intervention is required in approximately 25% of cases; more in cases of prosthetic valve infections. Indications for surgery include valve dysfunction, dysrhythmias, refractory cardiac failure and antibiotic treatment failure indicated by persistent fever or other complications.

Antibiotic prophylaxis is recommended for high-risk groups (as given in Table 8.14) undergoing procedures such as dental work which may result in bacteraemia and subsequent endocarditis. Procedures for which prophylaxis is recommended are also given in Table 8.14.

Bacteraemia

Bacteraemia in the elderly has an overall fatality rate of 15%, which increases in cases of comorbidity such as renal or cardiac failure. Both nosocomial and community-acquired bacteraemias have an equal mortality rate in the elderly, in contrast to younger groups where mortality is greater in nosocomial infections. The risk of developing bacteraemia increases with increasing age and over 25% of such infections develop in the over 60 age group.

Community-acquired bacteraemia most commonly develops following UTI; the next most common source is the biliary tract and then the lungs. In long-term care facilities the urinary tract is the most frequent source, followed by skin and the respiratory tract.

Bacteraemia may progress to septic shock, hypotension, organ failure and death unless effectively treated. Mortality in septic shock is

Table 8.14 Cardiac conditions for which antibiotic prophylaxis is recommended[40]

High-risk group: prophylaxis recommended	Procedures for which prophylaxis recommended
Prosthetic heart valve	Dental procedures which involve
Septal defect	extraction or gingival procedures
Heart valve lesion	Upper respiratory tract procedures
Patent ductus	Genitourinary procedures
Previous endocarditis	Obstetric, gynaecological and
	gastrointestinal procedures

Adapted from *British National Formulary*.[40]

Table 8.15 Suggestions for the initial treatment of bacteraemia based on the suspected source of infection

Suspected source	Likely organism	Suggested first choice of treatment	Alternative choice of treatment
Community-acquired			
Urinary tract (uncomplicated)	Enterobacteriaceae especially *Escherichia coli* Enterococci	Fluoroquinolone or Ampicillin + Gentamicin	Co-amoxiclav or Second-generation cephalosporin
Biliary tract	Enterobacteriaceae Enterococci *Bacteroides* spp. *Clostridium* spp.	Piperacillin + Metronidazole or Ampicillin + Gentamicin + Metronidazole or Meropenem	Third-generation cephalosporin + Metronidazole or Aztreonam + Clindamycin
Lungs	*Streptococcus pneumoniae* *H. influenzae* *Mycoplasma* spp. *Legionella* spp.	Amoxicillin + Macrolide or Levofloxacin	Second-generation cephalosporin + Macrolide
Lungs: aspiration	Oral anaerobes	Amoxicillin + Metronidazole	Co-amoxiclav or Clindamycin
Hospital-acquired			
Urinary tract with catheter	Enterobacteriaceae *Pseudomonas aeruginosa* Enterococci	Piperacillin + Tazobactam or Ciprofloxacin + Gentamicin	Ampicillin + Gentamicin or Meropenem
Lungs	Aerobic Gram-negative bacilli: *Enterobacter* spp. *Klebsiella* spp. *Acinetobacter* spp. *Pseudomonas* spp. Also *Staphylococcus aureus* *Legionella* spp.	Third-generation cephalosporin + Gentamicin or Meropenem or Ciprofloxacin + Gentamicin If *Legionella* is suspected, add Erythromycin	Piperacillin + Gentamicin

about 60%. Clinical presentation in the elderly is frequently atypical with a lack of fever or hypothermia and a lack of leukocytosis in up to 30% of cases. Changes in mental status, lethargy or non-specific gastrointestinal symptoms may predominate. Unexplained acidosis or hypoglycaemia may help to suggest the diagnosis. Frail elderly patients often have few clinical signs of infection and their response to infection may be non-specific, with rapid decline.

Treatment of bacteraemia is usually started empirically, based on the suspected primary source of the infection. In general, broad-spectrum agents should be selected and given by the intravenous route in adequate doses. Cardiovascular and respiratory supportive measures may be required. If renal failure develops renal support will be required.

Suggestions for empirical antibiotic therapy of bacteraemia are given in Table 8.15. Treatment should be adjusted according to the results of bacterial culture and sensitivity testing. Blood cultures may often fail to detect a causative organism because bacteraemia is usually intermittent. Treatment should include removal of any devices such as intravascular lines or urinary catheters which may be colonised with the infecting organism.

Bone and joint infections

The commonest cause of osteomyelitis (inflammation of the bone marrow and surrounding bone) is bacterial infection which may be suppurative (usually in children) or indolent. Joint infections (infectious arthritis) may arise either from haematogenous spread of organisms through the highly vascularised synovial membrane or from the direct extension of a contiguous bone or soft-tissue infection.[41]

Osteomyelitis and infective arthritis will be treated as separate entities for the purpose of this section.

Osteomyelitis

Osteomyelitis is a different disease in adults to that found in children. In adults, because bone growth is complete, the epiphyses in the long bones are closed and therefore spontaneous infection in the long bones is less common. Osteomyelitis in adults is usually subacute or chronic in nature and associated with a traumatic insult to the involved area or implantation of a foreign body (e.g. orthopaedic device) or as a result of a very large infective inoculum.[42]

The incidence of osteomyelitis associated with traumatic fracture and subsequent fixation increases with the severity of the fracture and surrounding tissue damage. Prevention is dependent on adequate debridement of the damaged tissue and bone, full immobilisation of the fracture to prevent movement during healing and appropriate antibiotic cover at the time of surgery. Concomitant disease states which increase the risk of infection include diabetes mellitus and peripheral vascular insufficiency; such conditions are found more commonly in the elderly. *Staph. aureus* is most commonly associated with osteomyelitis resulting from fracture.

Osteomyelitis may occur in association with a surgical joint prosthesis and the infection may be acute (within 12 weeks of placement) or chronic. Staphylococci (both coagulase-positive and negative) account for 75% of the bacteria cultured from prosthetic joint infections.

Antibiotic prophylaxis should be given in the perioperative period to prevent infection during debridement and fixation of a traumatic fracture or during placement of prosthetic joints. The antibiotic chosen should cover skin flora and, in cases of trauma, anaerobes, Flucloxacillin with or without metronidazole or co-amoxiclav may be a suitable choice of agent and usually one perioperative dose is sufficient, but some surgeons give two doses postoperatively in addition. In institutions with high rates of MRSA or in penicillin-allergic patients, vancomycin may be substituted for the flucloxacillin or co-amoxiclav.

Elderly patients with diabetes or vascular insufficiency may develop osteomyelitis as a result of contiguous spread from either minor skin trauma or the more obvious chronic foot or leg ulcers. Infection occurs most commonly in the bones of the foot. Streptococci or anaerobic organisms are the bacteria associated with foot lesions and ulcers.

Osteomyelitis following bacteraemia occurs more commonly in elderly adults compared to younger adults. Infecting organisms are mainly *Staph. aureus* or, specifically in the elderly, Gram-negative rods. In patients with long-term urinary catheters *Pseudomonas aeruginosa* may cause infection which develops typically in the lumbar vertebrae.

The diagnosis of osteomyelitis requires recognition of the signs and symptoms of inflammation of bones and surrounding tissues. A good history of previous injury and subsequent treatment is necessary. Blood count with differential, X-ray and computed tomography scanning will aid diagnosis. Samples for microbiological culture and sensitivity should be taken from the deepest portion of the open wound or from bone biopsy to prevent contamination with non-infecting commensals.

Treatment of osteomyelitis requires early recognition and intervention to prevent extensive destruction of bone or necrosis. In acute haematogenous osteomyelitis surgery is usually unnecessary. In chronic disease or infected fracture surgical intervention to debride and remove any foreign material is required. Infected prosthetic joints should be removed. If a new joint is put into place in the same procedure then antibiotic-containing cement is frequently used. One-stage joint replacement without an intervening interval for antibiotic treatment carries a higher rate of re-infection. Osteomyelitis in vascular insufficiency may benefit from revascularisation to aid healing and prevent re-infection or ultimate amputation.

Antibiotics should be administered parenterally for at least 6 weeks to achieve an acceptable rate of cure; several months of therapy may be necessary in refractory cases. Because of the limited oral bioavailability of β-lactam antibiotics and poor gastrointestinal tolerance, it is better not to switch from intravenous to oral therapy with these drugs in adults with acute osteomyelitis. Antibiotic choice should be tailored to microbiolgical culture and sensitivity results. Suggested treatment options are given in Table 8.16.

Long-term oral therapy with quinolones can suppress the symptoms and signs of chronic refractory osteomyelitis. Nosocomial infections with MRSA or multidrug-resistant Gram-negative rods require prolonged intravenous therapy with glycopeptides such as vancomycin, or broad-spectrum antibiotics. The local use of antibiotics such as impregnated beads gives quite limited diffusion of antibiotic and this method has not undergone controlled study.

Infective arthritis

Infective arthritis most commonly involves the joints of the knee and hip, although any joint may become infected. In most cases only one joint is affected. Infection results in rapid joint destruction due to bacterial toxins and host defence products such as proteolytic enzymes. Disease states which predispose to joint infection include most commonly rheumatoid arthritis and corticosteroid use; other risk factors include diabetes mellitus, leukaemia, cirrhosis, granulomatous disease, hypogammaglobulinaemia, cytotoxic chemotherapy or intravenous substance abuse. Prosthetic joints are susceptible to infection. Underlying causative organisms in septic arthritis are influenced by the age of the patient, the source of infection and underlying disease states (Table 8.17).

Table 8.16   Recommendations for antibiotic choice for infectious osteomyelitis and septic arthritis

Infecting organism	Suggested first choice	Suggested alternative choice
Staphylococcus aureus	Flucloxacillin or Clindamycin	Vancomycin (with serum level monitoring) or Cefuroxime or Co-amoxiclav
Methicillin-resistant Staphylococcus aureus	Vancomycin (with serum level monitoring) plus Sodium fusidate or rifampicin	Teicoplanin Synercid
Streptococcus	Benzylpenicillin or Ampicillin	Clindamycin or Cefuroxime
Enterococcus	Ampicillin plus Gentamicin (with serum level monitoring)	Vancomycin (with serum level monitoring)
Escherichia coli Proteus mirabilis	Ampicillin (if sensitive) or Co-amoxiclav	Cefuroxime or Ciprofloxacin
P. vulgaris P. rettgeri Morganella morganii Serratia marcescens	Cefotaxime plus Aminoglycoside (with serum level monitoring)	Ciprofloxacin or Piperacillin or Meropenem
Pseudomonas aeruginosa	Ceftazidime or Piperacillin plus Aminoglycoside (with serum level monitoring)	Ciprofloxacin plus Aminoglycoside (with serum level monitoring)
Bacteroides fragilis Peptostreptococcus	Metronidazole	Clindamycin

Bacterial arthritis usually presents as fever, pain, warmth, swelling and decreased range of motion in the involved joint. Aspiration and culture of the joint effusion are important to determine the causative organism and guide antibiotic therapy.

The common causative organisms and their associated conditions in adults are given in Table 8.17. The most common causative organism is *Staph. aureus*, followed by *Streptococcus* spp. Infection occurs most commonly in adults via dissemination from the blood stream from abscesses or infected wounds. Other causes include spread from adjacent soft-tissue infection or from joint puncture or penetrating trauma.[43]

Treatment should be started promptly to prevent joint destruction.[44] Antibiotic treatment is usually necessary for up to 6 weeks.

Table 8.17   Some causative organisms and associated conditions in joint and bone infections

Organism	Comments and associated condition
Staphylococci	Most common in adults *Staphylococcus aureus* most common cause of primary septic arthritis *Staph. epidermidis* associated with prosthesis
Streptococci	Associated with prosthetic joint infections in adults
Gonococci	Uncommon – usually in sexually active persons May be monoarthritis or oligoarthritis in otherwise well individual
Anaerobes	Usually associated with trauma or in those with reduced host resistance or in polymicrobial infections associated with diabetic or decubitus ulcers
Enterobacteriaceae, e.g. *Escherichia coli* *Klebsiella pneumoniae* *Proteus mirabilis* *Salmonella* spp.	Haematogenous arthritis, e.g. from urinary tract infection, abscess Implicated in pathogenesis of ankylosing spondylitis and rheumatoid arthritis respectively More common in patients with sickle cell anaemia
Acid-fast bacilli e.g. *Mycobacterium tuberculosis* *M. leprae*	May be complication of respiratory or skin infection Often insidious in nature Tuberculosis of spine more commonly affects recent immigrants, those with acquired immune deficiency syndrome, homeless, alcoholics, drug abusers and those who work in prisons

Antibiotic choice should be guided by microbiological culture and sensitivity results. If a causative organism is not identified, empirical therapy to cover *Staph. aureus* and other Gram-positive cocci should be initiated. In elderly patients or those with rheumatoid arthritis, cover should be broadened to include Gram-negative organisms. Penetration of antibiotic into joints may be impaired because of raised intraosseous pressure, occluded blood vessels or oedema. In general, aminoglycoside antibiotics should be avoided because of poor joint and bone penetration. For suggested treatment choices, see Table 8.16.

The outcome in septic arthritis may be poor despite appropriate therapy, especially in the elderly when virulent organisms such as *Staph. aureus* or certain Gram-negative pathogens are involved. Physiotherapy is important to aid recovery and prevent joint deformity. Complications of septic arthritis include bacteraemia leading to endocarditis, cholecystitis or cerebral abscess.

Skin infections

The elderly are at increased risk of skin infections because of impaired local host defence mechanisms and impaired healing rates. Additionally, thinning of the epidermis and reduced sebaceous gland secretions impair the barrier to infection. Old people may also suffer from other disease states such as peripheral vascular disease, diabetes and dependent oedema which increase the rates of skin infections. Corticosteroid use may also be a factor.

Bacterial skin infections

Bacterial infections of the skin are common.[45] Infection may arise as a result of invasion of skin structures by bacteria harboured in the respiratory, digestive or genitourinary tract and transferred on to the skin causing transient colonisation. If there are breaches in the skin then bacteria can invade the skin, causing infection. Primary infection occurs on normal skin and secondary infection occurs on the background of pre-existing skin diseases. The most common pathogens are *Staphylococcus aureus* and group A β-haemolytic streptococci.

Cellulitis and erysipelas

Cellulitis is a spreading infection of subcutaneous connective tissue.[46] It usually develops from a penetrating lesion which introduces pathogens from the skin surface. In elderly patients abrasions from falls, cuts, small diabetic ulcers and intravenous cannula entry sites are common examples. Cellulitis appears as a red, tender swelling with indistinct margins which spread. In the community, the causative organism is nearly always *Staph. aureus* or *Streptococcus pyogenes*. Infection on the feet may be as a result of coliforms or enterococci or a mixture of organisms and therefore broad-spectrum treatment is required. Treatment is usually empirical, although swabs of exudate will give identification of the causative organism if there is doubt. Blood cultures are advisable if the patient has severe fever or painful lymphadenopathy. Hospital-acquired infections may be caused by resistant organisms such as MRSA, and cultures are advisable. Treatment suggestions are given in Table 8.18. If improvement does not occur within 24–48 h or the infection continues to spread or painful lymphadenopathy or fever develops, an aggressive infection is indicated, requiring hospitalisation and parenteral antibiotic treatment. Treatment regimens should be tailored to culture and sensitivity testing when available.

Table 8.18   Empirical treatment of bacterial skin infections

Site or type of infection	Common causative infective agent	Suggested choice for treatment
Cellulitis	Staphylococcus aureus	Flucloxacillin
Erysipelas	Streptococcus pyogenes Plus In lower limbs or feet: Coliforms Enterococci Anaerobes	Clindamycin Co-amoxiclav Ciprofloxacin + Metronidazole Cefuroxime + Metronidazole
Folliculitis Furunculosis	Staphylococcus aureus From hot baths or swimming pools: Pseudomonas aeruginosa	Flucloxacillin or Vancomycin (if methicillin-resistant Staphylococcus aureus) Ciprofloxacin Ceftazidime
Burns	Staphylococcus aureus Streptococcus pyogenes Plus In lower limbs: Enterococci Enterobacteria Pseudomonas aeruginosa	Flucloxacillin Ciprofloxacin + Metronidazole Ceftazidime + Metronidazole Piperacillin/Tazobactam
Ulcers	Polymicrobial: Staphylococci Enterococci Proteus mirabilis Escherichia coli Pseudomonas aeruginosa Anaerobic organisms	Co-amoxiclav Ciprofloxacin + Metronidazole Cefuroxime + Metronidazole

Erysipelas is an intradermal infection often affecting the face or leg. It may be difficult to differentiate between cellulitis and erysipelas. Erysipelas appears as well-defined hot erythematous plaques which may advance rapidly. The causative organism is commonly *Str. pyogenes* or *Staphylococcus aureus*. Erysipelas often occurs on a background of vascular disease, malignancy or diabetes mellitus in the elderly, which can lead to recurrent infection. Aggressive infection may disseminate into the blood and secondary sites and develop into streptococcal septicaemia, which carries a mortality of 25–30%. Treatment suggestions are given in Table 8.18.

Folliculitis and furunculosis

Folliculitis is a superficial infection of hair follicles with papules or pustules.[47] Common sites include the beard area, upper back, chest, buttocks and forearms. Furuncles are deep infections of the hair follicle extending to subcutaneous fat. They are inflammatory and may coalesce to form larger draining nodules called carbuncles, which are less common than furuncles, and occur mainly on the neck and the posterior thighs. Common risk factors for development of hair follicle infection include obesity, steroid use, diabetes, alcoholism and poor hygiene.

The causative organism is usually *Staph. aureus*, although *Pseudomonas aeruginosa* infections may result from hot-bath or swimming-pool folliculitis. Treatment of folliculitis may be with topical antibiotics if infection is limited, but if there is spreading infection or signs of inflammation, treatment with systemic antibiotics should be given. Furuncles may require treatment with systemic antistaphylococcal antibiotics. Carbuncles require treatment with antibiotics. The use of warm compresses and cleansing aids resolution but large nodules require drainage. In recurrent furunculosis, the staphylococcal carrier sites of the patient and close contacts may need to be treated.

Secondary bacterial infections of burns and ulcers

The elderly are prone to burns and make up about 15% of burn unit admissions. They have a tendency toward a greater depth and size of burn because of thinner skin, slower reaction times, reduced mobility, diminished sensation and impaired vision, smell and hearing.[48] Burns can arise from trivial incidents such as spilling tea or sitting too close to a fire. In the frail elderly, cellulitis or even septicaemia may develop.

To minimise the risk of infection an antiseptic cream such as 1% silver sulfadiazine should be used and any devitalised tissue debrided. If infection does occur then systemic antibiotics should be given. First-line agents against staphylococci and streptococci should be used (Table 8.18) and treatment tailored to culture and sensitivity results. Other organisms which may cause infection in burns include enterococci, enterobacteria and *Ps. aeruginosa*, especially in burns of the lower limbs.

Elderly individuals are prone to lower-limb ulceration due to dependent oedema or pressure from immobility and conditions such as diabetes or peripheral vascular disease. Wounds may become colonised by bacteria but this does not indicate active infection. Antibiotic treatment of colonised but not infected wounds is not generally indicated. Acute wounds tend to be more susceptible to bacterial occupation but a chronic ulcer may exist with large numbers of bacteria without demonstrating clinical signs of infection.[49] The use of topical antibiotics such as bacitracin and neomycin on clinically uninfected wounds is not recommended because it leads to colonisation with resistant organisms.

Infected wounds should be treated with systemic antibiotics. Signs of wound infection include a purulent discharge, tissue erythema, necrotic tissue, pain and other signs such as elevated white cell count and fever. Untreated infected wounds may lead to septicaemia or osteomyelitis of adjacent bone. Bacterial infections in chronic ulcers tend to be polymicrobial in nature and initial antibiotic treatment should include activity against aerobic and anaerobic organisms. Treatment should be tailored to the results of culture and sensitivity testing. Suggested treatment choices are given in Table 8.18.

Fungal skin infections

Fungal infections of the skin are very common.[50] Elderly individuals are at increased risk of developing fungal skin infections because of underlying conditions such as diabetes or exposure to antibiotics.

Candidal skin infections

Superficial candidal infections are usually caused by *Candida albicans*,[51] which is a commensal organism commonly found in the mouth and gastrointestinal tract in healthy individuals. Candidal infections typically develop in the presence of predisposing factors such as antibiotic use, dentures, debilitation, disease or immunosuppression. Common sites for candidal infections in the elderly include the mouth and the skin folds such as the inframammary or groin areas. Soreness and white patches (plaques) on an erythematous background are signs of oral candidiasis, but another variety can occur which does not form plaques, presenting as areas of erythema and soreness. Candidal infection in the corners of the mouth may present as chronic fissured inflammatory areas and occurs especially in people with poorly fitting dentures or who drool. Infection of skin presents as an erythematous rash and usually satellite pustules and papules outside the border of the lesion. Infection of nail folds (paronychia) may also be caused by *Candida* spp., especially in those whose hands have chronic exposure to water or in diabetics. Balanitis with erosions, exudate and pustules may occur on the glans of uncircumcised men, especially in those with poor hygiene.

Treatment of superficial candidal skin infections is usually with topical antifungals such imidazoles or terbinafine for 2–4 weeks. Recurrent or more extensive infections warrant the use of oral fluconazole for 7–10 days. Candidal intertrigo requires aeration and the use of loosely fitted clothing. Paronychia may require incision and drainage plus oral antibiotics to treat coexisting staphylococcal or *Pseudomonas* spp. infection. Treatment of cheilitis requires that dentures are properly fitted and thoroughly cleaned.

Onchomycosis

Onchomycosis is infection of the nail plate and is especially common in the toe nails of elderly individuals. The nails appear thickened, irregular and discoloured. Treatment is with systemic antifungals. Terbinafine is the treatment of choice and is given by mouth for 3 to 6 months. If griseofulvin is used, treatment for 9–12 months may be required to clear the infection and relapse is more common.

Viral skin infections

Herpes simplex

Herpes simplex skin disease presents as grouped vesicles on reddened skin which erode and crust within 4–5 days and heal within 10–14 days. Spread is by direct contact and lesions are contagious until crusting occurs. After primary infection, the virus remains dormant in the ganglion until reactivated by stress or illness such as influenza or respiratory tract infection in the elderly. Recurrence of herpes simplex represents reactivation of virus. The most common site of infection is the lips. In the frail elderly, eruptions may occur on the gums and hard palate as very painful ulceration. Primary herpes simplex may be treated with aciclovir 200 mg five times a day for 5 days or valaciclovir 1 g twice daily for 10 days, although such treatment is generally reserved for severe cases or immunocompromised patients.

Herpes zoster

Varicella-zoster virus is the cause of chickenpox (varicella) and shingles (herpes zoster). Herpes zoster occurs in the elderly as a reactivation of varicella in the root ganglion after childhood exposure to chickenpox. Frail elderly patients should avoid contact with children infected with chickenpox as secondary infection may reactivate the previously latent virus in the ganglion, leading to a modified varicella rash.

Shingles usually presents with sharp stabbing pain and malaise and fever which are followed within 3–4 days by vesicles which develop within a single sensory root dermatome. Secondary bacterial infection may occur. The rash lasts for 2–3 weeks. Involvement of the trigeminal nerve may lead to eye infection and damage to the cornea and iris. Postherpetic neuralgia may occur due to damage to sensory nerve fibres. It can be intractable in some cases.

Treatment of shingles is usually with aciclovir 800 mg five times a day for 7 days or valaciclovir 1 g three times a day for 7 days. Treatment should begin within 72 h of skin disease becoming apparent. Use of antiviral agents decreases the duration of postherpetic neuralgia. Parenteral aciclovir may be indicated for ophthalmic zoster and is necessary for disseminated disease.

References

1. Breitenbucher R B, Peterson P K. Infection in the elderly. In: Mandell G L, Douglas R G, Bennett J E, eds. *Principles and Practice of Infectious Diseases.* New York: Churchill Livingstone, 1990: 2315–2320.
2. Hirokawa K. Immunity and ageing. In: Pathy M S J, ed. *Principles and Practice of Geriatric Medicine.* Chichester: John Wiley, 1998: 35–47.
3. Falsey A R. Infectious disease. In: Pathy M S J, ed. *Principles and Practice of Geriatric Medicine.* Chichester: John Wiley, 1998: 281–288.
4. MacLennan W J, Watt B, Elder A T. *Infections in Elderly Patients.* London: Edward Arnold, 1994.
5. Yoshikawa T T, Norman D C. Treatment of infections in elderly patients. *Med Clin North Am* 1995; 79: 651–661.
6. Borrego F, Gleckman R. Principles of antibiotic prescribing in the elderly. *Drugs Aging* 1997; 11: 7–18.
7. Rian U N, Spencer R. Management of common infections in the elderly. *Prescriber* 1999: 10; 85–90.
8. Nicolle L E, Henderson E, Bjornson J *et al.* The association of bacteriuria with resident characteristics and survival in elderly institutionalized men. *Ann Intern Med* 1987; 106: 682–686.
9. Nordenstam G R, Brandber C A, Oden A S *et al.* Bacteriuria and mortality in an elderly population. *N Engl J Med* 1986; 314: 1152–1156.
10. Chaliha C, Stanton S. Guide to the management of urinary tract infections. *Prescriber* 1999; 10: 37–63.
11. Anon. Managing urinary tract infection in women. *Drug Ther Bull* 1998; 36: 30–32.

12. Gruneber R N. Changes in urinary pathogens and their antibiotic sensitivities, 1971–1992. *J Antimicrob Chemother* 1994; 33 (suppl A): 1–8.

13. Winstanley T G, Limb D I, Eggington R *et al*. A 10 year survey of anti-microbial susceptibility of urinary tract isolates in the UK: the microbe base project. *J Antimicrob Chemother* 1997; 40: 591–594.

14. Nicolle L E. Urinary tract infection in the elderly. *J Antimicrob Chemother* 1994; 33 (suppl A): 99–109.

15. Ward T T, Jones S R. Genitourinary tract infections. In: Reese R E, Betts R F, eds. *A Practical Approach to Infectious Diseases*. New York: Little, Brown, 1996: 472–518.

16. Rubin R H, Cotran R S, Tolkoff-Rubin N E. Urinary tract infection, pyelonephritis and reflux nephropathy. In: Brenner B M, ed. *The Kidney*. Philadelphia: W B Saunders, 1996: 1597–1654.

17. Edwards S. Balanitis and balanoposthitis: a review. *Genitourin Med* 1996; 72: 155–159.

18. Gupta A. Influenza, improving uptake of vaccination in older people. *Geriatr Med* 1999; 29: 11–13.

19. Department of Health. *Current Vaccine and Immunisation Issues*. London: Department of Health, 2001.

20. National Institute for Clinical Excellence. Guidance on the use of Zanamivir (Relenza) in the treatment of influenza. Technology Appraisal Guidance Number 15, November 2000.

21. Anon. Why not Zanamivir? *Drug Ther Bull*. 2001; 39: 9–10.

22. Diggory P, Fernandez C, Humphrey A *et al*. Comparison of elderly people's technique in using two dry powder inhalers to deliver zanamivir: randomised controlled trial. *BMJ* 2001; 322: 577–579

23. Woodhead M. Pneumonia. *Medicine* 1999; 27: 88–92.

24. Higson N. Pneumonia, the case for vaccination. *Geriatr Med* 1999; 29: 11–13.

25. British Thoracic Society. Guidelines for the management of community acquired pneumonia in adults admitted to hospital. *Br J Hosp Med* 1993; 49: 346–350.

26. Bonten M J M, Stobberingh E E. Diagnosis and treatment of nosocomial pneumonia. *Br J Hosp Med* 1995; 54: 335–340.

27. Anon. TB rates increase. *Pharm J* 1999; 263: 974.

28. Barnes N. Tuberculosis: a guide to diagnosis and treatment. *Prescriber* 1999; 10: 103–111.

29. Hedderwick S, Kauffman C A. Opportunistic fungal infections: superficial and systemic candidiasis. *Geriatrics* 1997; 52: 50–59.

30. Kelly C P, Pothoulakis C, LaMont J T. *Clostridium difficile* colitis. *N Engl J Med* 1994; 330: 257–262.

31. Martin M J, Griffin G E. Bacterial gastroenteritis. *Medicine* 1996; 24: 47–51.

32. Sanders T A B. Food production and food safety. *BMJ* 1999; 318: 1689–1693.

33. Miller L G, Choi C. Meningitis in older patients: how to diagnose and treat a deadly infection. *Geriatrics* 1997; 52: 43–55.

34. Quagliarello V J, Scheld W M. Treatment of bacterial meningitis. *N Engl J Med* 1997; 336: 708–716.

35. Domingo P, Barquet N, Alvarez M *et al*. Group B streptococcal meningitis in adults: report of 12 cases and review. *Clin Infect Dis* 1997; 25: 1180–1187.

36. Begg N, Cartwright K A V, Cohen J *et al*. Consensus statement on diagnosis, investigation, treatment and prevention of acute bacterial meningitis in immunocompetent adults. *J Infect* 1999; 39: 1–15.

37. Bharwani I L, Hershey C O. The elderly psychiatric patient with positive serology: the problem of neurosyphilis. *Int J Psychiatry Med* 1998; 28: 333.

38. Lewis D J M. Infective endocarditis. *Medicine* 1996; 24: 43–46.

39. Dajani A S, Taubert K A, Wilson W *et al*. Prevention of bacterial endocarditis, recommendations by the American Heart Association. *JAMA* 1997; 277: 1794–1801.

40. Anon. Summary of antibacterial prophylaxis. In: Mekta D K, ed. *British National Formulary*, vol. 38. London: British Medical Association/Royal Pharmaceutical Society of Great Britain, 1999: 243–244.

41. Dirschl D R, Almekinders L C. Osteomyelitis, common causes and treatment recommendations. *Drugs* 1993; 45: 29–43.

42. Mader J T, Mohan D, Calhoun J. A practical guide to the diagnosis and management of bone and joint infections. *Drugs* 1997; 54: 253–264.

43. Lew D P, Waldvogel F A. Osteomyelitis. *N Engl J Med* 1997; 336: 999–1007.

44. Axford J S. Joint and bone infections. *Medicine* 1998; 26: 47–53.

45. Shum K W. Primary care management of bacterial skin infections. *Prescriber* 2000; 11(2): 63–81.

46. Bannister B. Skin and soft tissue infections. *Medicine* 1996; 24: 59–63.

47. Ko W T, Adal K A, Tomecki K J. Office dermatology part 1: infectious diseases. *Med Clin North Am* 1998; 82: 1001–1031.

48. Staley M, Richard R. The elderly patient with burns: treatment considerations. *J Burn Care Rehab* 1993; 14: 559–565.

49. Orlando P L. Pressure ulcer management in the geriatric patient. *Ann Pharmacother* 1998; 32: 1221–1227.

50. Goodfield M. Diagnosis and treatment of fungal skin infections. *Prescriber* 2000; 11(7): 59–73.

51. Hay R J. Fungal infections. *Medicine* 1996; 24: 85–89.

9

Metabolic and endocrine disease in the elderly

Jayne Wood

All endocrine, but especially neuroendrocrine systems, are vulnerable to ageing. First, loss of functional reserve in many organs tends to lead to deficiency diseases, for example, hypothyroidism, diabetes mellitus and hypogonadism. This, coupled with the decreasing immune competence which is related to ageing and the autoimmune basis of many endocrine disorders, leads to an increased prevalence of hypoendocrine disease with increasing age and a tendency for more than one endocrine disease to occur simultaneously. Secondly, the elderly tend to have multiple diseases which affect the clinical and laboratory manifestations of endocrine diseases. The increased incidence of multiple disease states, together with non-specific and atypical presentation, can also result in diagnoses being missed, patients failing to seek medical assistance and difficulties in management. Thirdly, as most laboratory values have been developed from tests on young healthy people, apparently abnormal results may merely reflect the ageing process. Finally, ectopic hormone production from neoplasms can also mimic classic endocrine diseases.[1]

The two clinically most important changes in endocrine activity during ageing involve the pancreas and thyroid. The deterioration in glucose tolerance with increasing age means that the elderly tend to lose their ability to regulate plasma glucose fully, which leads to an increase in the prevalence of diabetes. This process is multifactorial in origin, but one major factor is the increased percentage of body fat that occurs in old age which is linked with a tendency towards obesity.[1] The risk of developing diabetes doubles for every 20% excess body weight.[2] Obesity is also associated with hyperinsulinaemia, marked insulin resistance and a decrease in the number of insulin receptors, although there are also genetic factors involved in the development of type 2 diabetes which are independent of body weight.[3]

Age-related thyroid dysfunction is also common. Normal ageing is accompanied by a slight decrease in pituitary thyrotrophin-stimulating hormone (TSH) release but especially by a decreased peripheral conversion of thyroxine (T_4) to tri-iodothyronine (T_3) which results in a gradual age-dependent decline in serum T_3 concentrations without a clinically important change in serum T_4 levels.

Three other hormonal systems also show decreased circulating hormone concentrations during normal ageing. The first system that gradually declines in activity is the growth hormone (GH)/insulin-like growth factor 1 (IGF-1) axis. Mean pulse amplitude, duration and fraction of GH secreted, but not the pulse frequency, gradually decrease during ageing. In parallel there is a progressive fall in circulating IGF-1 levels in both sexes. Secondly, in women aged about 50, a decrease in the release of luteinising hormone (LH) and follicle-stimulating hormone (FSH) with decreased secretion of estradiol from the ovaries initiate the menopause. Changes in the activity of the hypothalamo–pituitary–gonadal axis in males are slower and more subtle. A gradual decline in serum testosterone levels occurs as a result of decreased production by the testes and an age-related decrease in episodic and stimulated gonadotrophin secretion. Finally, circulating levels of dehydroepiandrosterone (DHEA) gradually decrease over time without clinically evident changes in adrenocorticotrophin (ACTH) and cortisol secretion.[4]

Endocrine disease tends to be easily treatable and correction of minor degrees of impaired endocrine dysfunction often leads to a dramatic improvement in the patient's quality of life. Therefore clinicians need to have a heightened awareness of the possibility of the existence of an endocrine disorder in the elderly patient.[4]

Diabetes mellitus

Aetiology

Diabetes mellitus currently affects between 2% and 3% of the population in the UK and up to 10% of those over 65 years of age. Another 23% of those aged between 65 and 70 have impaired glucose tolerance that tends to deteriorate over time, therefore the incidence of overt diabetes may be as high as 40% in those over 80 years of age.[2] This makes diabetes the most common endocrine disease in the elderly population.

Patients with diabetes are at risk of developing a range of microvascular complications, including nephropathy, retinopathy and neuropathy, and have an increased risk of developing cardiovascular disease. All these factors may cause significant morbidity and a substantial reduction in life expectancy. Patients with poorly controlled diabetes also have an increased susceptibility to infection and a tendency to poor wound healing which occurs as a result of impaired leukocyte function which is directly related to hyperglycaemia.[3] Although some clinicians may consider the risk of development of complications to be small in those who present with diabetes when they are aged 75 or over, some type 2 patients have complications at the time of diagnosis.

Published data indicate that people with diabetes account for between 5 and 6% of all hospital admissions and outpatient attendances.[5] There is also a high prevalence of diabetes amongst those who live in residential care homes and some of these patients may not be receiving consistent or adequate treatment.[6] This may be related to the position of residents who may be under the care of a number of general practitioners; this may make a uniform approach to the management of their diabetes difficult. However, the introduction of Primary Care Groups (PCGs), Primary Care Trusts (PCTs), Health Improvement Programmes (HimP), Clinical Governance and the National Service Framework (NSF) for diabetes in 2001 will set standards for the diagnosis and treatment of diabetes which should enable a uniform approach to the management of diabetes across a PCG or PCT.

The management goals for diabetes in patients of 75 and over may be different and more conservative than for the more motivated and otherwise fit younger elderly (those between 65 and 75 years of age) and younger adults. For example, some elderly patients will have poor vision and limited manual dexterity which may or may not be linked to a degree of cognitive impairment. Others have multiple pathology and take a number of other medications. Therefore the goals of therapy need to be both individual and realistic. In some patients they will involve only the optimisation of body weight, control of symptoms and avoidance of hypoglycaemia (which carries an increased risk of severe brain damage and may occur without the usual warning signs in the elderly). In others, reasonably tight control may be appropriate.[7]

Therefore, diabetes in the elderly is a major problem, in terms of consumption of National Health Service resources and in the complexity of the issues that need to be considered in management. There is a difficult balance between the use of aggressive treatment with its associated risk of hypoglycaemia and the benefits of reducing complications and maintaining an acceptable quality of life. As the proportion of elderly people in the population rises, management of diabetes in this age group will pose an increasing challenge to health care.

Presentation

The symptoms of type 1 and type 2 diabetes are similar, although they vary in intensity. Although the majority of the older population will be type 2 patients, slow-onset type 1 diabetes may mimic type 2 disease. Older type 1 patients will often be lean, have a history of weight loss and respond poorly to oral hypoglycaemic agents. Type 1 diabetes may occur even at the age of 80–90 years but this is extremely rare.[8] Therefore this chapter will concentrate on the management of type 2 diabetes.

The presentation of type 2 diabetes may occur in a number of different ways and is often atypical in the elderly. This is related to the increase in the renal threshold for glucose that occurs in old age. Patients may not complain of symptoms, or may have only one of the characteristic symptoms (polyuria, polydipsia and weight loss) and these may only become evident after careful questioning.[3] Many cases are asymptomatic and are discovered when biochemical tests are undertaken for other reasons. This is particularly common in obese individuals. Chronic skin infections, such as pruritus vulvae in women or balanitis in men, are presenting symptoms in many patients and are a direct result of glycosuria. Patients may also present with nocturia and/or incontinence or occasionally with complications, such as retinopathy, which may be discovered on a visit to the optician because of blurred vision, or foot ulceration which may be associated with neuropathy and/or peripheral vascular disease. Lastly, fatigue which may be associated with diabetes is often blamed on 'old age' by many patients.[3] Therefore one of the challenges of diabetes is to make an early and accurate diagnosis in order to ensure optimal management.

Aims of treatment

The primary aims of treatment in diabetes are to alleviate signs and symptoms. Secondary aims are, as far as possible, to prevent the development or slow the progression of long-term complications by controlling hyperglycaemia and minimising the occurrence of hypoglycaemia. In younger adults the fasting blood glucose should ideally be between 4 and 7 mmol/l preprandially[9] and less than 9 mmol/l postprandially in most patients[9, 10] provided that these levels do not cause frequent or severe hypoglycaemia. In the elderly it is often safer to aim for preprandial levels between 5.5 and 8 mmol/l and postprandial levels of less than 10 mmol/l. The glycated haemoglobin (or HbA_{1c}), which may be used to assess control during the previous 4–6 weeks, should be not more than 6.5% although in practice it may be difficult or impractical to obtain such a low value in many elderly patients. If this is the case, a level not more than 7% may be achievable. However, glycaemic goals are not absolute and must be appropriate to the patient's age, lifestyle and other factors such as the duration of diabetes, coexisting diseases, complications, intelligence, understanding, compliance and ability to recognise hypoglycaemia. Control of diabetes should be the best that can reasonably be achieved for each individual.

Treatment strategies

There are six categories of antidiabetic medication used in the UK: sulphonylureas, biguanides, thiazolidinediones, α-glucosidase inhibitors, meglitinides (or postprandial glucose regulators) and insulin. These agents may be used individually initially (according to their licence) or may be combined in a stepwise fashion to provide more ideal glycaemic control, as shown in Figure 9.1. As outlined earlier, application of the same measures of management is appropriate in older patients but these may need to be modified in the presence of coexisting disease, polypharmacy or social isolation.

Control of diabetes is achieved by diet alone in approximately 20% of patients, by diet and oral hypoglycaemics in about 60% of patients and with insulin in the remainder. The factors used to select a particular treatment include the patient's clinical characteristics such as degree of hyperglycaemia, weight, age and renal function.[11] As a guide, patients with fasting blood glucose levels between 7 and 12 mmol/l will need dietary advice which may include weight reduction. Patients with a blood glucose between 12 and 17 mmol/l will probably need an oral hypoglycaemic agent initially but may require insulin.[8, 10] Patients whose blood glucose is consistently greater than 17 mmol/l in the absence of overt stress, severe insulin deficiency and/or insulin resistance will probably need insulin, if not initially, then relatively soon after diagnosis. If it is decided that drug therapy is indicated selection is made according to the mode of action, the safety profile and the potential for adverse effects of the chosen drug in the individual.

Glucose control is not the sole criterion for effective treatment of diabetes. Coronary heart disease is the most common cause of morbidity and mortality in patients with type 2 diabetes and hypertension also has

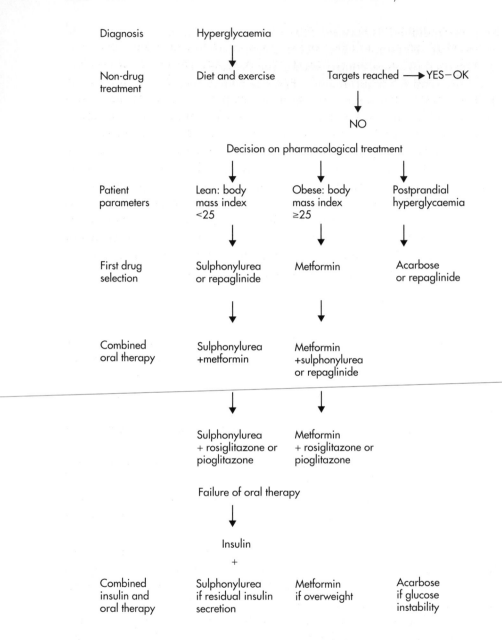

Figure 9.1 Treatment cascade for type 2 diabetes mellitus.

important implications in the development of nephropathy, stroke and myocardial infarction. Therefore advice to stop smoking and control of hypertension are extremely important. Blood pressure should be checked annually and in type 1 and type 2 patients it should ideally be 140/80 mmHg. In type 1 patients if nephropathy is present the targets are a systolic blood pressure of less than 130 mmHg and a diastolic blood pressure of < 80 mmHg or even lower if proteinuria exceeds 1 g in 24 h. Treatment of hyperlipidaemias should also be undertaken, aiming for a total cholesterol of less than 5.2 mmol/l, a high-density lipoprotein (HDL) cholesterol more than 1.1 mmol/l and a fasting triglyceride level of less than 1.7 mmol/l. However, targets for blood pressure and lipids will vary according to coexisting disease states and the patient's life expectancy as well as quality of life. Education is also an essential part of management and should include instruction about diabetes and its treatment as well as prevention of some of the complications.

Diet

The aims of diet are to reduce blood glucose and thereby to decrease symptoms and to ensure optimal weight (focusing on reduction of obesity). Diet needs to be tailored to suit the individual and habits in terms of physique, level of activity, cultural habits and religious beliefs. Elimination of simple, rapidly absorbed sugars (sucrose and glucose) is the minimum requirement for all patients with diabetes. Protein intake should usually be the same as for the general population, representing 10–15% of the total; complex carbohydrate should provide about 50% of energy intake and fat content should be reduced to less than 30%.[7] As consumption of fibre has been shown to improve blood glucose control and to lower cholesterol, patients with diabetes should also be encouraged to eat high-fibre foods.

In those elderly patients who require diet alone, initially a 3-month trial period is indicated. In the obese patient dietary advice which enables weight loss of 0.5–1 kg/week (to achieve a body mass index: BMI = weight in kg ÷ height in metres) between 20 and 25 kg/metres is desirable. However, dietary control in the elderly may be problematic when patients lack teeth, have poorly fitting dentures, cannot afford nutritious foods or fail to understand dietary instruction.[3] Depression may also lead to poor eating habits. Impaired taste perception, especially for saltiness and sweetness, is also common and may lead to oversalting or oversweetening of foods. Since the elderly are usually sedentary, calorie intake also needs to be lower than for the young adult.

Therefore early referral to the dietician is of particular benefit for the older patient.[3] Exercise may also be problematic in the elderly, especially if they have concurrent cardiac disease or arthritis. None the less 30 minutes gentle exercise every day, such as swimming or walking, can be very beneficial as long as it is approached with caution. If after 3 months of adhering to an appropriate diet fasting blood glucose is still more than 10 mmol/l, oral hypoglycaemics should be commenced (although some patients may need insulin at this stage) in conjunction with diet and exercise, where appropriate.

Oral hypoglycaemics

Sulphonylureas Sulphonylureas act chiefly by stimulating insulin release from the β cells of the pancreas together with some additional peripheral effects in lowering blood glucose. Their effect is dependent on the β-cell reserve and therefore they are only effective when there is some residual β-cell activity.[12] There are a number of different sulphonylureas. The first-generation (or older) drugs include: tolbutamide and chlorpropamide and the second-generation agents include glibenclamide, gliclazide, glipizide, gliquidone and glimepiride. Second-generation agents are used more commonly as they have equal efficacy to first-line agents but have fewer side-effects and interactions.[3, 10]

If the patient is lean (BMI less than 25) a sulphonylurea is used first-line and if obese (BMI at least 25) metformin is used first-line if there are no contraindications. This policy is used primarily because sulphonylureas stimulate weight gain and are therefore undesirable in obese patients[13] and because lean patients have profound impairment of glucose-induced insulin release.[14] However, sulphonylureas are used in combination with metformin as second-line therapy in obese patients.

Choice of sulphonylurea Maximal doses of sulphonylureas have similar efficacy; none has been shown to be better than the others or to be associated with lower failure rates in controlled trials. However, pharmacokinetic differences between different sulphonylureas have important clinical implications, particularly in relation to the risk of hypoglycaemia.[15] Choice of sulphonylurea is related to the patient's age, renal function and to a certain extent on the personal preference of the prescriber.

In patients over 65, use of shorter-acting agents such as gliclazide, glipizide, tolbutamide or gliquidone is recommended because they cause less hypoglycaemia in the elderly.[15] In patients with impaired renal function (defined as a serum creatinine more than 150 μmol/l or a creatinine clearance < 50 ml/min in practice) gliclazide is recommended because it is hepatically metabolised, but glipizide or tolbutamide would be equally suitable. However, the three-times-daily dosing schedule required for tolbutamide may make compliance a problem in some patients. It is essential to avoid longer-acting agents such as glibenclamide and chlorpropamide in the elderly because of the risk of severe hypoglycaemia, which, although uncommon, carries a high mortality.[16] Many clinicians avoid the use of sulphonylureas in patients with a serum creatinine > 200 μmol/l as they feel that insulin may be safer in these circumstances.[15]

The newest sulphonylurea, glimepiride, appears to have similar efficacy to glibenclamide, glipizide and gliclazide. It is metabolised in the liver (by P450 enzyme CYP2C9) and has one metabolite which appears to have a very minor pharmacological action, in contrast to the metabolites of glibenclamide which have significant and prolonged effects. The pharmacokinetic profile of glimepiride allows once-daily administration, which may help compliance. It also theoretically causes less hypoglycaemia than glibenclamide and appears to be well tolerated in the elderly. Therefore glimepiride may have a place in the treatment of diabetes in the elderly but any clinical differences require confirmation in wider patient use.[17, 18]

Sulphonylureas should be started at a low dose which can be increased gradually according to blood glucose measurements. In the outpatient setting this is usually undertaken at monthly intervals. In responsive patients optimal dosage of sulphonylureas will decrease the HbA_{1c} by 1–2% and fasting and postprandial blood glucose levels by 3 mmol/l.[19] However, only 60–70% of patients achieve good control with sulphonylureas. Those who are obese or have high initial fasting blood glucose levels (more than 17 mmol/l) often have a poor response and may obtain better results with metformin alone or in combination with a sulphonylurea.[11]

Metformin Metformin differs radically from the sulphonylureas in chemical structure, mode of action and side-effects. It acts by reducing hepatic gluconeogenesis, increasing peripheral uptake of glucose and, to some extent, decreasing the absorption of carbohydrates.[11] Like sulphonylureas, metformin is used in patients who have failed on diet but it is used first-line in overweight patients (BMI at least 25 or at least 120% ideal body weight) as it does not cause weight gain and it also improves insulin sensitivity and reduces hyperinsulinaemia.[14] However, these advantages may be of minor clinical significance in the very elderly who are rarely obese and may actually be underweight.[10]

Another advantage of metformin is that, unlike sulphonylureas, it does not cause clinical hypoglycaemia[10] because it lacks any stimulatory effect on insulin, it has a mild effect on decreasing gluconeogenesis and it supplies additional gluconeogenic substrate in the form of lactate from the intestine.[20] Therefore excessive falls in blood glucose are prevented because any suppression of hepatic glucose output is not sufficient to override counter-regulatory mechanisms. This is an advantage in elderly patients provided that they do not have any contraindications to its use.

The most serious side-effect of metformin is lactic acidosis. Therefore any clinical condition that is associated with a propensity to generate lactate or a decreased ability to clear lactate is a contraindication. As metformin is excreted virtually exclusively by the kidney it is contraindicated in patients with renal impairment (defined as a serum creatinine more than 150 μmol/l or a creatinine clearance less than 50 ml/min in practice), abnormal liver function tests (LFTs: usually not less than twice the upper limit of normal) or heart failure even if successfully treated. Caution should also be used in patients with peripheral vascular disease, acute or chronic pulmonary disease and in those who drink excess alcohol.[15] Although virtually all reported cases of metformin-induced lactic acidosis have occurred in patients who have had contraindications,[20] its poor prognosis and high mortality underscore the importance of its prevention. The use of metformin in the elderly remains controversial and is subject to individual clinical judgement.[21] However, provided that the patient has normal renal and hepatic function and no cardiovascular or pulmonary problems, the risks of developing lactic acidosis are probably very low.

The most troublesome side-effects of metformin include nausea, vomiting, diarrhoea and a metallic taste in the mouth. These occur in 5–20% of patients and are minimised by starting metformin at a dose of 500 mg once daily after meals and gradually increasing to a maintenance dose of 500 mg or 850 mg three times a day.[10, 11]

Use of metformin alone produces, on average, a 2–3 mmol/l reduction in fasting and postprandial blood glucose concentrations. It may also be used in combination with sulphonylureas where a further reduction of approximately 20% in blood glucose levels (or a further decrease in HbA$_{1c}$ of 1.7–1.8%) can often be achieved.[19, 20]

Acarbose   Acarbose is occasionally used as an adjunct to a sulphonylurea and/or metformin.[15] Acarbose is an α-glucosidase inhibitor which exerts a competitive dose-dependent inhibition of α-glucosidases on the brush border of the small intestine. It therefore delays the absorption of complex carbohydrates in the gut and thereby attenuates postprandial glucose peaks.[11]

The most common side-effects of acarbose are gastrointestinal and include flatulence (due to fermentation of carbohydrates in the large bowel), diarrhoea, abdominal distension and pain. They occur frequently during the first few weeks of therapy although they usually decrease with continued treatment. In order to minimise gastrointestinal problems the dose of acarbose should be increased gradually from 50 mg once daily to a maximum of 200 mg three times daily if the patient can tolerate it.[13] As there have been a few cases of raised liver transaminases with acarbose,[22] monitoring of liver function is only recommended in patients receiving 200 mg three times daily. Acarbose monotherapy does not cause hypoglycaemia, although it may potentiate the hypoglycaemic effects of other drugs, such as sulphonylureas and insulin. Acarbose also has no effect on body weight and may be beneficial in overweight patients.

Acarbose has a small effect either on its own or as an adjunct to metformin or sulphonylureas when they prove inadequate. It has been reported to reduce the HbA_{1c} by 0.5–1% and postprandial blood glucose by 2–3 mmol/l, but its effects on fasting blood glucose are weaker than with other oral hypoglycaemics.[15] Many patients either do not tolerate acarbose or do not benefit greatly from its use. However, it may be useful in patients who have modest fasting hyperglycaemia who experience postprandial glucose excursions, in elderly patients who cannot tolerate sulphonylureas or metformin, or in those in whom these agents are contraindicated.

Repaglinide Repaglinide, the first in a new class of drugs, the meglitinides, is a postprandial glucose regulator which has a distinct binding site on the β cell in addition to a common binding site with the sulphonylureas.[23] It has a novel flexible dosage regimen and is taken 30 min before a meal but only if food is eaten.[23] It is rapidly absorbed after oral administration and reaches a peak within 1 h, causing rapid release of insulin from the pancreas followed by a lowering of blood glucose concentrations. It is metabolised in the liver and excreted primarily by the bile. None of the known metabolites has any hypoglycaemic effect.[24]

The recommended starting dose of repaglinide is 500 μg for patients with an HbA_{1c} less than 8% (except for patients being transferred from other therapies or in those who have a higher HbA_{1c} where the initial dose is 1 mg). Subsequently the preprandial dose is doubled until a response is achieved or a preprandial dose of 4 mg is reached. Dose increases should be made at weekly intervals.[23] The maximum dose is 16 mg per day. Repaglinide should be used with caution in mild renal failure and is contraindicated in those with severe renal or hepatic disorders. It interacts with drugs that induce or inhibit the enzyme CYP3A4, such as erythromycin (inhibition) and rifampicin (induction).

Repaglinide is an effective first-line therapy in type 2 diabetes and may also be used in combination with metformin to produce a synergistic effect.[23] It decreases fasting and postprandial blood glucose by about 4 and 7 mmol/l respectively and HbA_{1c} by up to 2%.[23] Repaglinide may be most beneficial in patients who experience problems with postprandial glucose excursions and as single therapy in patients who eat at unpredictable times or have a tendency to miss meals. Although repaglinide has been shown to be safe and effective in patients over 65 years, it can cause hypoglycaemia and may be inappropriate for elderly patients who live alone and in those who do not experience warning signs of hypoglycaemia. It is not currently recommended for people over 75 years of age because of a lack of studies in this group. Like sulphonylureas, repaglinide also causes weight gain and therefore may not be suitable for overweight patients. Repaglinide requires wider clinical use and further comparative studies before its place in therapy can be clearly defined.

Thiazolidinediones Thiazolidinediones work by enhancing insulin action and thus promoting glucose utilisation in peripheral tissues; they reverse the defective glucose penetration into cells of the insulin resistance syndrome by an effect on the cell membrane, thereby reducing both blood glucose levels and glucose-induced insulin release from the pancreas. They have no effects on insulin secretion.[11, 24] Troglitazone was the first agent to be marketed, although it was voluntarily withdrawn in the UK at the end of 1997 and more recently in the USA due to problems with hepatic toxicity. Rosiglitazone and pioglitazone, which also belong to this class of agents, were marketed in the UK in 2000 and are currently licensed as combination therapy with either sulphonylureas or metformin. There are also a number of other thiazolidinediones currently in clinical development. Thiazolidinediones have been shown to improve glycaemic control in a range of patients, especially in those with insulin resistance. They act additively with other oral antidiabetic agents, including sulphonylureas, metformin and acarbose, as well as reducing the requirement for insulin in insulin-treated patients.[25] Either rosiglitazone or pioglitazone may be offered to patients on oral monotherapy with metformin or sulphonylureas who are unable to take metformin and sulphonylureas in combination as an alternative to transferring to insulin. The combination of a thiazolidine-dione with metformin is preferred to sulphonylureas, especially in over-weight patients. However, thiazolidinediones in combination with sulphonylureas may be useful in patients in whom metformin is contra-indicated. The future for this class of agents in the management of diabetes looks very promising.

Insulin

Indications for insulin Before starting insulin therapy it is important to ensure that patients are adhering to their diet, taking their oral hypo-glycaemics and that they are not receiving any medicines, such as corticosteroids, which might exacerbate hyperglycaemia. The level of blood glucose taken in isolation does not indicate the need for insulin (though if > 25 mmol/l the patient is likely to need it). Ketonuria (as opposed to ketoacidosis) usually but not always suggests that insulin treatment is required. If the patient's weight decreases then he or she is likely to need insulin, but if it increases the patient is probably over-eating. Insulin is likely to be needed if symptoms continue on maximum treatment, in poorly controlled overweight patients and on a temporary basis during illness.[19] Approximately 15% of patients with type 2 diabetes do not show an adequate initial response to oral agents and are termed primary failures.[19] Secondary failure to oral hypoglycaemic agents, after an initially favourable initial response, may occur in between 5% and 10% of type 2 patients on an annual basis.[26]

Starting insulin The exact procedure for starting insulin depends on the individual circumstances. The major aim initially is to reduce hyper-glycaemia without causing symptomatic hypoglycaemia. Symptoms can be alleviated with almost any insulin regimen. In some elderly patients or in those who lack motivation this is all that can be achieved. The attainment of very good control is much more difficult and quite often causes unacceptable and dangerous episodes of hypoglycaemia, espe-cially in the elderly.

The initial regimen depends on whether the patient is acutely ill, ambulant but acutely insulin-dependent, or whether the need for insulin has arisen more gradually in a type 2 patient where oral hypoglycaemics have failed. Choice of a particular regimen also depends on the patient's age, motivation and any complications present at the time the decision to start insulin is made. The main rules when starting insulin are to use small doses initially to control symptoms, to ensure that dosage changes are not normally made more than twice weekly and to limit these changes to between 10% and 20% of the total daily dose.

On the basis of glycaemic control and weight gain no preference for any treatment regimen can be discerned, although twice-daily insulin administration is the most simple and cost-effective treatment in the elderly.[19,27] With this in mind, the elderly are often started on twice-daily fixed mixtures, most commonly those that contain one-third short-acting and two-thirds intermediate-acting insulin, for example Human Mixtard 30 or Humulin M3. In a lean patient, who will probably be relatively sensitive to insulin, a reasonable starting dose is 12 units before breakfast and 8 units before tea. This will usually control symptoms adequately and can be adjusted to achieve appropriate glycaemic targets. Overweight patients are likely to be insulin-resistant, therefore their initial dose may need to be as high as 20 units before breakfast and 10 units before tea. If overnight hypoglycaemia and unacceptable morning hyperglycaemia is a problem with this regimen, improvement may be obtained by dividing the evening insulin dose so that the soluble insulin is given before tea, and the intermediate-acting insulin is given at bedtime. This three-dose regimen is very satisfactory in a number of patients; however, three injections per day may be impractical in some elderly patients. Although insulin therapy may be more difficult in the elderly than the younger adult due to limited manual dexterity and limited ability to measure doses and self-inject, there are available a variety of prefilled devices and aids to treatment.[3]

Alternatively, some lean type 2 patients who are transferred from tablets to insulin may be successfully treated with once- or twice-daily isophane insulin.[19] This approach may also be appropriate in the very elderly where symptomatic control is all that is required and where a district nurse is required to administer the insulin. However, late afternoon and evening blood glucose levels may be unacceptably high on this single daily dosing regimen[7] but this depends on the pattern of food intake of the individual. In all these cases a single daily dose of Humulin I or Human Monotard, given before breakfast, may achieve a balance between acceptable symptomatic control and convenience whilst reducing the risk of hypoglycaemia.

In patients who require temporary insulin during intercurrent illness a soluble preparation such as Humulin S or Actrapid can be given two or three times daily with a small dose of isophane insulin at bedtime to control blood glucose quickly and eliminate symptoms. The most commonly quoted regimen is 6 units of soluble insulin before each meal and 6 units of isophane insulin at bedtime. The dose is selected initially according to the patient's previous insulin requirements, if any, and adjusted according to four-times-daily blood glucose measurements.

Combination therapy

As outlined earlier, there are six categories of antidiabetic medication used in the UK: sulphonylureas, biguanides, α-glucosidase inhibitors, meglitinides (postprandial glucose regulators), thiazolidinediones and insulin. These treatments may be combined in a stepwise fashion to provide more ideal glycaemic control. If a combination of metformin and/or a sulphonylurea and/or a thiazolidinedione fails to achieve control then the patient is usually transferred to insulin. At this stage, or if insulin treatment alone fails to provide adequate control, a combination of insulin and sulphonylureas may be used, although this requires the patient to have some endogenous insulin secretion. One successful scheme is to add insulin in the evening to control basal blood glucose and to maintain the sulphonylurea to control postprandial hyperglycaemia.[7] Metformin may also be used in combination with insulin to reduce insulin requirements in obese patients and to improve glycaemic control.[28] Acarbose may also be added to insulin to reduce blood glucose variation, especially postprandial early hyperglycaemia and late hypoglycaemia. Rosiglitazone and pioglitazone have been used successfully with insulin but the combination is as yet unlicensed.

Monitoring

Several factors need to be assessed to determine whether or not treatment is adequate. Although the presence of symptoms indicates that treatment is inadequate, their absence does not necessarily indicate good control. If weight is decreasing then more intensive treatment may be required but if weight is increasing and the patient has poor control then he or she is probably overeating.

Ideally, preprandial blood glucose (before meals) should be monitored by all patients with diabetes, but especially in those with poor control and in those receiving insulin. In the initial stages of treatment and whilst hospitalised with intercurrent illness this will be measured four times daily. However, for most type 2 patients using insulin at home, who are stable, daily blood glucose measurement should suffice.

Alternatively, two to three samples per week may be acceptable in some patients.[9] If done at different times on different days the results can be used to build up an overall picture of control. Patients do not generally need to test their urine for ketones. Ketones should be measured if patients are unwell and/or their blood glucose is persistently high (e.g. more than 17 mmol/l).

Urine testing for glucose is of limited value and should be reserved for those patients who find blood testing unacceptable and some elderly patients with type 2 diabetes in whom tight control is unnecessary. It is, at best, a crude measure of glycaemic control because glycosuria appears only above the renal threshold for glucose which varies between 7 and 12 mmol/l and may be over 15 mmol/l in the elderly.[8] Urine testing also does not detect hypoglycaemia. If used, urine testing should be carried out 2 h after a meal and in most patients the aim is to abolish postprandial glycosuria.

The glycated haemoglobin (usually measured as HbA_{1c}) reflects blood glucose control over the preceding 2 months. Although the reference ranges vary amongst laboratories, an HbA_{1c} of less than 6.5% reflects good control and an HbA_{1c} of more than 7.5% reflects poor control. However in the elderly these targets may not be appropriate in every patient, especially when symptomatic control is all that is required.

During illness or infection the blood glucose concentration tends to increase and control of diabetes deteriorates. Most patients taking insulin will need larger doses and some patients on oral therapy may need insulin temporarily. When patients with diabetes become ill they should continue their normal insulin and monitor their blood glucose four times a day. If it is persistently more than 15 mmol/l the dose of soluble insulin should be increased by approximately 4 units. Additional doses of soluble insulin can be given at noon or bedtime, if needed. If hyperglycaemia is prolonged the patient should consult their diabetes specialist nurse, general practitioner or the hospital clinic.

Complications of treatment

Hypoglycaemia Hypoglycaemia (defined as a blood glucose less than 2.5 mmol/l) is the most common and serious side-effect associated with sulphonylureas and insulin as it may be complicated by stroke, myocardial infarction and even death.[3] Patients with severe hypoglycaemia should be admitted to hospital since treatment is often prolonged and relapse may occur. Approximately 5% of patients will also have permanent neurological damage.[15] Older patients are at increased risk of developing drug-induced hypoglycaemia as a result of intercurrent illness, polypharmacy and the age-related decline in hepatic oxidative enzyme activity and renal function which may interfere with the metabolism of sulphonylureas or alter insulin requirements. Counter-regulatory response to hypoglycaemia may also be attenuated with advanced age.

The symptoms of hypoglycaemia are quite variable. Whereas acute falls in plasma glucose are likely to produce sweating, palpitations and hunger, slower changes tend to lead to unusual or irrational behaviour proceeding to unsteadiness, drowsiness and coma, sometimes within a few minutes. Immediate treatment is with glucose (about 30 g or 6 teaspoonfuls) or a sugary drink. This may be repeated after a few minutes if necessary. If the patient cannot swallow, 20–50 ml of 50% glucose should be given intravenously or 1 mg of glucagon given subcutaneously.[15] When the patient is fully conscious he or she should be encouraged to take a snack containing complex carbohydrate such as a sandwich and a glass of milk. This will ensure that another hypoglycaemic episode does not occur before the next meal.

Hypoglycaemic coma The emergency treatment of severe hypoglycaemia should not be withheld to await a biochemical diagnosis. Reversal is most effectively achieved with 50 ml of 50% glucose given intravenously. On regaining consciousness the patient should be given oral carbohydrate. A continuous infusion of 5% or 10% glucose, to maintain the blood glucose between 5 and 10 mmol/l, may be necessary for several days to prevent recurrence of hypoglycaemia, which may be a particular problem if the causative agent is a long-acting insulin or long-acting sulphonylurea. Serum potassium should also be monitored and supplementation given if necessary.[15] Intramuscular glucagon (1 mg) may be of value but may be ineffective if hepatic glycogen stores are depleted after prolonged starvation or a prolonged drug-induced hypoglycaemic episode. The development of cerebral oedema should be considered in patients who fail to regain consciousness after blood glucose levels return to normal. Cerebral oedema has a high mortality and morbidity and requires urgent treatment with mannitol and/or dexamethasone, although neither agent is consistently effective.[15]

Complications of diabetes

Note: many of the following treatments are not currently licensed in the UK (see current edition of the *British National Formulary*).

Hyperosmolar non-ketotic state

This condition, which occurs only in type 2 patients, has a high mortality. Triggering factors include intercurrent illness such as a chest or urinary tract infection which may occur in a previously undiagnosed diabetic. The blood glucose is often very high (more than 40 mmol/l); however, as insulin deficiency is partial, the anticatabolic effect of insulin may be relatively well preserved while its anabolic action is not markedly accelerated. Therefore the concentration of ketone bodies in the blood remains relatively normal despite severe hyperglycaemia and dehydration due to the resultant diuretic effect.

Management is essentially the same as for diabetic ketoacidosis, with intravenous fluids and insulin. There are two main exceptions. Firstly, these patients are usually relatively sensitive to insulin and approximately half the dose of insulin recommended in diabetic keto-acidosis should be employed at least initially. Secondly, the plasma osmolality should be measured or, less accurately, calculated using the following formula based on plasma values in millimoles/l:

$$2[Na^+] + 2([K^+] + [glucose] + [urea])$$

The normal value for osmolality is 280–300 milliosmoles/l and if it is high (> 360 milliosmoles/l) 0.45% sodium chloride should be used for rehydration initially until the osmolality returns to normal, when 0.9% sodium chloride should be substituted. The overall fluid requirements also tend to be greater than for ketoacidosis but, in the frail elderly, fluid replacement should always be undertaken cautiously and replacement judged on the basis of central venous pressure and frequent plasma sodium estimations. Too rapid a fall in osmolality may be associated with the development of cerebral oedema. Use of intravenous sodium bicarbonate is never needed although subcutaneous heparin should be considered in high-risk patients to prevent thrombotic complications (stroke and/or myocardial infarction are the major causes of death).[29]

Painful sensorimotor neuropathy

Neuropathy is the most frequently encountered complication in patients with diabetes and is a diverse group of disorders. The most common form is painful diabetic polyneuropathy (DPN) which is characterised by burning, aching (dysaesthesia) or sharp stabbing pain which often lasts throughout the night and does not respond to conventional analgesia. Patients may also have an exaggerated response to painful stimulae (hyperalgesia) or to touch (hyperaesthesia).[30]

Despite continued research, treatment of DPN remains a problem. Prevention of the metabolic and vascular abnormalities implicated in the pathogenesis of DPN would be the ideal but the use of investigational drugs such as aldose reductase inhibitors (e.g. tolrestat), directed at correcting these abnormalities, has resulted in small changes in objective measures and no improvement in symptoms. Intensive treatment and tight control of diabetes, as studied in the Diabetes Control and Complications Trial (DCCT)[31] and the United Kingdom Prospective Diabetes Study (UKPDS),[32, 33] reduced the appearance and progression of microvascular complications in type 1 and type 2 patients respectively. However, this approach can only help those patients who are highly motivated and in whom tight control is appropriate. This is often not the case in the elderly. Therefore until methods of prevention are discovered we are confined to symptomatic treatment.

Drug therapy   Many of the drug trials in which the efficacy of various agents in painful diabetic neuropathy has been assessed have had insufficient statistical power. In addition, since there are no objective methods for assessing spontaneous pain, they have all used either arbitrary semiquantitative symptom scores, or visual analogue scales; these have such high variability that type 2 statistical errors (false positives) cannot be excluded with study populations of fewer than 200–300 patients. It is also important to note at this stage that the majority of these agents are unlicensed for this indication.

Tricyclic antidepressants   Tricyclic antidepressants (TCAs) are the agents of choice for symptomatic relief of painful diabetic neuropathy as their efficacy has been demonstrated in controlled trials.[34, 35] However, it remains unclear which TCA is most useful for which type of neuropathic pain. As the majority of evidence is with amitriptyline, this agent is usually the first choice, although imipramine is a popular alternative.

Imipramine or amitriptyline is started at a dose of 10–25 mg at bedtime (increased gradually to 150 or 200 mg if necessary). This regimen is often effective throughout the day and also has a nocturnal sedative effect. The dosage of imipramine may be split into three or four divided doses if patients find a single dose at night does not provide 24 h pain relief. These divided doses are generally well tolerated, even in the elderly, if imipramine is used, as it tends to be less sedating than amitriptyline.

It is postulated that TCAs mimic the actions of descending noradrenergic and possibly serotoninergic pain-modulating pathways, but this has yet to be fully elucidated. The majority of patients will get at least 50% pain relief with the median preferred dose of 75 mg at night within 2–8 days of commencing treatment.[30] The limitations of TCAs include their high rate of anticholinergic side-effects (dry mouth, drowsiness, blurred vision and confusion) which occur in about one-third of patients and most often in the elderly. Side-effects such as postural hypotension and tachyarrhythmias are also a problem. On the positive side, use of amitripyline at night is associated with an improved sleep pattern.

Antiepileptics   The clinical impression of antiepileptics is that they are useful for neuropathic pain, which is described as lancinating or burning pain. Drugs such as carbamazepine have been proposed to work by dampening down the abnormal discharge of sensory neurons. They are effective in 30–50% of patients.[36] However, carbamazepine is usually used second-line as side-effects such as nausea, ataxia, drowsiness and confusion occur in about one-third of patients and can be a particular problem in the elderly. For this reason carbamazepine should be started at a dose of 100 mg/day and the dose increased by 100–200 mg every 3 days until a response or side-effects occur. The usual maximum dose in practice is 200 mg four times daily. Sodium valproate is used occasionally and is started at a dose of 200 mg at night. This is increased by 200 mg every third day to a maximum of 1 g at night. However, side-effects, including nausea and ataxia, may also be a problem.

Interest in the use of gabapentin, an analogue of γ-aminobutyric acid (GABA), to treat painful neuropathy has increased. It is started at a dose of 300 mg at night, increasing after 3 days to 300 mg twice daily and then 300 mg three times daily. The dose may be further increased as tolerated every third day to a maximum of 3.6 g daily in divided doses. In studies it has been reported to reduce the pain score and sleep interference.[37] Side-effects include somnolence, dizziness and confusion. Therefore gabapentin should be used with care, if at all, in the elderly.

Capsaicin   Capsaicin (the active ingredient in chilli peppers) in the form of a cream (0.075%) has also been used to treat painful neuropathy.[38] Initial application of capsaicin cream to the skin or mucous membranes produces irritation and hyperaesthesia by promoting the release of substance P from the terminals of small sensory nerve fibres. Burning, stinging and erythema occur in at least 30% of patients but this reduces with repeated use. The time taken for tachyphylaxis (acute tolerance) to develop is extremely variable. It usually occurs within 72 h of repeated use but may take up to 6 or 8 weeks. Pain relief usually occurs after 14–28 days' treatment but the maximal response often does not occur until 4–6 weeks of continuous treatment.[39] Substance P is thought to be the principal transmitter of nociceptive impulses from the periphery to the central nervous system (CNS). After repeated application capsaicin depletes the neuron of substance P and it relieves pain.[40] Capsaicin may be a useful alternative in the elderly patient who is unable to tolerate therapy with a TCA or an anticonvulsant.

Mexiletine   Only two studies have been published in which the effect of mexiletine 200 mg three times daily has been assessed in DPN.[41,42] In the first it significantly reduced symptoms of pain, dysaesthesia and paraesthesia in 16 patients compared with placebo.[41] However, the bias inherent in this cross-over trial was not accounted for in the statistical analysis, which may have influenced the results. In the second study differences were not statistically significant.[42] Therefore, because of the conflicting results, the high incidence of CNS, cardiovascular and gastrointestinal side-effects, mexiletine should be reserved for patients who are unresponsive or intolerant to usual therapies, who have no evidence of heart disease and complain of sensations of burning, heat, formication or stabbing pain. Use of mexiletine in the elderly should probably be avoided.[42]

Autonomic neuropathy

The most clinically important symptoms of autonomic neuropathy include impotence in men, dizziness caused by postural hypotension as well as nausea and vomiting which occur as a consequence of gastroparesis, diabetic diarrhoea and constipation.[30] As with painful neuropathy, the majority of the agents used to treat the two former symptoms are unlicensed.

Postural hypotension   Orthostatic hypotension is a decline in blood pressure that occurs when moving from a lying to a standing position which results in symptoms of cerebral hypoperfusion, most commonly light-headedness and syncope. Although the absolute change in blood pressure to produce symptoms varies, a common definition is a decline in systolic blood pressure of more than 20 mmHg or a reduction in diastolic blood pressure of more than 10 mmHg.[43]

Non-pharmacological treatments   These include increasing sodium intake, avoiding rapid postural changes, wearing elastic garments and raising the head of the patient's bed. Patients should also be advised to avoid alcohol and large meals as these may induce vasodilatation. Orthostatic hypotension is difficult to treat pharmacologically because of varying response and adverse effects. In addition, any exacerbating drugs such as antidepressants, diuretics, antipsychotics, nitrates and any other agents which may decrease blood pressure should be stopped wherever possible. The goal of therapy is to relieve symptoms and not necessarily to return the blood pressure to normal.[43]

Fludrocortisone The mineralocorticoids are the most consistently effective agents available to treat orthostatic hypotension. The drug of choice is fludrocortisone as it has 100 times the mineralocorticoid potency of hydrocortisone, although it should be used with caution in patients with congestive cardiac failure. Starting doses of 50–100 μg once daily (usually at night) may be increased at weekly intervals to 700 μg daily (which may or may not be divided) until a response is obtained or symptoms disappear. Adverse effects such as hypokalaemia, supine hypertension and fluid retention should be closely monitored, especially in high-risk patients such as the elderly.

Although the exact mechanism by which fludrocortisone works is unclear, suggested mechanisms include expansion of plasma volume secondary to sodium retention and an increase in the sensitivity of the vasculature to noradrenaline (norepinephrine). In addition fludrocortisone may increase peripheral vascular resistance by enhancing catecholamine release and by increasing vascular reactivity as a result of elevated concentrations of sodium, potassium and water in vessel walls. However, failure of fludrocortisone therapy is common and unacceptable peripheral oedema often results before an adequate therapeutic effect is obtained.[44] This use is not currently licensed in the UK.

Non-steroidal inflammatory drugs (NSAIDs) NSAIDs such as indometacin 50 mg three times daily or flurbiprofen 50–200 mg three times daily have also been used alone and in combination with fludrocortisone to treat postural hypotension.[44] These agents inhibit the production of vasodilating prostaglandins and enhance the sensitivity of the vasculature to vasopressor substances. However, they are often of little value in clinical practice.

Midodrine Midodrine is a potent and selective peripheral α-receptor agonist which is available on a named-patient basis for refractory orthostatic hypotension (a drop in systolic blood pressure of not less than

30 mmHg when other treatments have failed or when other drugs produce intolerable side-effects). Midodrine increases standing blood pressure and improves symptoms such as weakness, syncope, blurred vision and fatigue without any associated cardiac stimulation. Dosage should start at 2.5 mg two or three times daily and be titrated weekly to a maximum of 30 mg/day according to symptomatic improvement and blood pressure measurements. Midodrine is contraindicated in patients with severe heart disease, acute renal disease, urinary retention, phaeochromocytoma and thyrotoxicosis. The most common side-effect is supine systolic hypertension. Other side-effects include hot flushes, piloerection, severe headache, dysuria, drowsiness, increasing perspiration, dry mouth, nervousness and tingling. Data from studies in over 1800 patients have shown that midodrine 2.5–10 mg/day was well tolerated and consistently raised mean supine and standing blood pressure by a maximum of 15/7 and 19/8 mmHg respectively and markedly improved orthostatic symptoms in at least 69% of patients.[45] There is little or no experience of the use of midodrine in the elderly and it should probably be avoided unless there is no alternative.

Other options β-Blockers may be helpful in managing postural hypotension in patients with impaired vasoconstriction. Agents such as propranolol and pindolol have been used[46] but should be avoided in the presence of peripheral vascular disease, congestive cardiac failure or asthma. Sympathomimetics either with or without monoamine oxidase inhibitors and ergot alkaloids should be administered only to patients with certain types of orthostatic hypotension and patients must be monitored closely. Agents such as clonidine have not been well studied and should be limited to patients with severe, refractory disease. Use of these agents may be associated with significant risks, especially in the elderly, and should probably be avoided.[43]

Gastroparesis Delayed gastric emptying or gastroparesis associated with diabetes occurs in 20–30% of patients, most often in individuals with long-standing, poorly controlled type 1 diabetes but it may also occur in type 2 patients. It may include symptoms such as postprandial nausea, epigastric pain, bloating, vomiting of undigested food eaten hours previously and early satiety. One of the consequences of gastroparesis includes unpredictable blood sugar fluctuations.[47]

Drug therapy is based on control of symptoms whilst trying to avoid fluctuations in blood glucose levels. Where gastroparesis is associated with nausea and vomiting, agents which promote gastric emptying, such as metoclopramide, domperidone or erythromycin, may be useful. However there tends to be a poor correlation between the degree of gastric stasis and the severity of symptoms; even if a powerful prokinetic agent is used, it cannot be guaranteed to relieve symptoms. In addition symptoms and gastric-emptying abnormalities are intermittent and variable and the severity of symptoms in different patients is also variable, with a few patients experiencing severe vomiting that requires admission to hospital. This makes treatment of individual patients and comparison of the efficacy of different treatments very difficult. For this reason each patient should be managed individually and a logical process of treatment selection, substitution and addition applied, according to their needs. It is also important to consider the contribution of other medications to delayed gastric emptying, e.g. anticholinergics, antidepressants and levodopa.[47] Some agents, for example, calcium channel blockers such as nifedipine, may contribute to reflux by relaxing smooth muscle in the oesophageal sphincter.[48] In patients with significant symptoms, modifying or stopping these concurrent therapies may need to be considered.

Metoclopramide Metoclopramide accelerates gastric emptying, inhibits fundal relaxation and coordinates gastric, pyloric and duodenal motility in a propulsive motion by inhibiting dopamine D_1- and D_2-receptors in the gastrointestinal tract. It is also a potent antiemetic as a result of its action on D_2-receptors in the chemoreceptor trigger zone (CTZ). Therefore it improves gastric emptying, symptoms of gastric stasis and associated nausea. Metoclopramide has been reported to produce a significant acceleration in gastric emptying after a single dose but this benefit may not be sustained on a long-term basis.[49] In addition, side-effects, including drowsiness, restlessness, lassitude, fatigue and extrapyramidal effects, are encountered in up to 10% of patients and are a particular problem in the elderly, especially in those with reduced renal function.[48] Overall, studies on the effect of metoclopramide in patients with gastroparesis have usually only evaluated small numbers of patients and so its use in practice is better governed by the response and tolerance to therapy of the individual.[47]

Domperidone Domperidone 10–20 mg four times daily orally or 30–60 mg rectally four times daily, like metoclopramide, is a potent prokinetic agent which enhances gastrointestinal smooth muscle activity by blocking inhibitory dopamine D_1-receptors and by blocking dopaminergic inhibition of neural acetylcholine release via D_2-receptors.

However, as domperidone does not cross the blood–brain barrier it is devoid of central side-effects, which is a significant advantage in the elderly. Like metoclopramide, it has been reported to lose its efficacy over time. Therefore in practice its use is governed by the response of the individual.[47]

Erythromycin   Oral or intravenous erythromycin, 250–500 mg four times daily, binds to motilin receptors and acts as a motilin agonist. In this way it accelerates gastric emptying by increasing the amplitude of antral contractions and improving antroduodenal coordination.[50] Results from a few small studies suggest that erythromycin is a promising prokinetic agent.[51] However, like metoclopramide and domperidone, it has been reported to lose its efficacy over time.[52] Combinations of metoclopramide or domperidone and erythromycin may be useful in some patients.

Surgery   In very resistant cases surgery for gastropathy may be undertaken as the last resort. However the results are not always satisfactory and in the elderly the risk of major surgery must be balanced against the potential benefits.

Diarrhoea and constipation

'Diabetic' diarrhoea is presumed to be due to autonomic nerve dysfunction. It consists of episodic, voluminous, watery diarrhoea, which is often nocturnal, and is the most common symptom attributable to small-bowel dysfunction in patients with diabetes. Although troublesome, it is not usually associated with weight loss or obvious malabsorption, but delayed small intestinal transit may predispose patients to bacterial overgrowth. Treatment relies on use of antidiarrhoeal agents such as codeine and loperamide and the use of short courses of broad-spectrum antibacterials such as tetracycline 250 mg twice daily or doxycycline 100 mg once daily for 7 days. Treatment of constipation is also symptomatic and includes the use of laxatives and stool softeners. Prokinetic drugs such as metoclopramide, domperidone or erythromycin may also be useful.

Diabetic nephropathy

Diabetic nephropathy develops in approximately 20% of people with type 2 diabetes and is usually preceded by microalbuminuria.[2] Therefore screening for microalbuminuria (urine protein excretion between 30 and 300 mg/24 h) should be undertaken in all patients with diabetes at least once each year. In patients with a confirmed diagnosis of micro-albuminuria, progression to macroalbuminuria (urine protein excretion > 300 mg/24 h) and end-stage renal failure may be prevented by the use of pharmacological agents such as angiotensin-converting enzyme (ACE) inhibitors which have been proposed to have a renoprotective effect. Initiation of ACE inhibitors is recommended in patients with established microalbuminuria and a blood pressure ⩾ 140/90 mm/Hg (and even in the absence of hypertension) provided there are no contraindications.[53] However, results from the UK Prospective Diabetes Study Group indicate that in type 2 patients tight control of blood pressure is more important than the choice of agent used for treatment and results showed no significant difference between atenolol and captopril in this context.[54, 55] However, current practice still tends towards the use of ACE inhibitors. In clinical nephropathy the same principles of treatment apply and aggressive management of blood pressure is needed to prevent or delay progression to end-stage renal failure.

Diabetic retinopathy

Diabetic retinopathy is seen in about 50% of patients who have had type 2 diabetes for more than 15 years.[2] Therefore, eye screening should be undertaken in all patients with diabetes at least once each year, and in all type 2 patients on diagnosis and yearly thereafter. In the presence of confirmed retinopathy, progression of early changes may be reduced with adequate control of blood glucose, blood pressure and serum lipids. The presence of renal impairment and autonomic neuropathy indicates that retinopathy is more likely to deteriorate rapidly. Proliferative retinopathy is treated using photocoagulation with an argon laser or xenon arc light. This allows the majority of patients to maintain their vision, although some peripheral vision may be sacrificed to maintain central vision. Vitrectomy is also beneficial in patients whose visual loss is caused by proliferative retinopathy with vitreous haemorrhage, scarring and retinal detachment.[53]

Conclusion

Diabetes mellitus affects between 2 and 3% of the population in the UK and up to 10% of those over 65 and is therefore the most common endocrine disease in the elderly. Diabetes is associated with a range of microvascular complications, including nephropathy, retinopathy, neuropathy and an increased risk of developing cardiovascular (macrovascular) disease, all of which may cause significant morbidity and a substantial reduction in life expectancy. Therefore diabetes in the elderly is a major problem, in terms of consumption of National Health Service resources and in the complexity of its management. As the proportion of elderly people in the population rises over the next few years, management of diabetes in this age group will pose an increasing challenge to health care.

Thyroid disorders

Introduction

The hormones secreted by the thyroid gland affect most tissues. Consequently, thyroid disorders can present with many symptoms. In order to understand the aetiology and treatment of thyroid disorders it is important to understand the normal secretion and functions of thyroid hormones.

The thyroid gland secretes predominantly T_4 (levothyroxine; thyroxine; tetra-iodothyronine) and only a small amount of the biologically more active T_3 (liothyronine; tri-iodothyronine) Approximately 80% of T_3 is produced from T_4 in other tissues, particularly the liver, muscle and kidney.[56] In the plasma T_4 and T_3 are almost entirely bound to proteins (albumin and thyroxine-binding globulin (TBG) but only the unbound portion of T_3 and T_4 exerts a physiological effect. Production of T_3 and T_4 is stimulated by TSH (thyrotrophin) which is produced by the anterior pituitary and this in turn is under control of the hypothalamus via thyrotrophin-releasing hormone (TRH). Thyroid hormone production is regulated predominantly by the circulating concentrations of free T_4 (FT_4) which exerts a negative feedback on TSH release.[56]

Except for diabetes and infertility, thyroid disease is by far the most common type of endocrine disease in the general population. It has an overall incidence amongst the elderly approaching 5%.[1] There seems to be a genetic element involved, with about 50% of patients having a positive family history for thyroid disease. Thyroid disease is also much more common in women than in men. All ages are affected but hyperthyroidism is more common in early adult life and hypothyroidism is more common in the elderly.

Laboratory tests of thyroid function

Thyroid function can be evaluated by various laboratory tests including total T_4 (TT_4), total T_3 (TT_3), free T_4 (FT_4), free T_3 (FT_3) and TSH but relatively few of these tests are needed in most cases.[56] TT_4 discriminates well between hyperthyroid, hypothyroid and euthyroid states but may be affected by the administration of drugs such as the phenothiazines, phenytoin and salicylates.[57] Also TT_4 reflects the level of binding proteins present and may give misleadingly high or low results.[57] Binding proteins are increased by oestrogens and decreased by androgens, anabolic steroids and corticosteroids.[57, 58] TT_3 measurements are useful in the investigation of hyperthyroidism as they are usually raised proportionately more than TT_4 levels. Measurement of TT_3 is of no value in hypothyroidism as the result is often normal. Tests that measure the concentrations of free hormones are used first-line as they provide a more reliable means of assessing thyroid status than total thyroid hormone measurements which were used a few years ago because the former avoid the interfering effects of varying TBG levels. Therefore the most useful initial tests include FT_4 and TSH. If these results are confusing then FT_3 may help interpretation. In primary hypothyroidism T_4 will be low and TSH will be high (at least twice the upper limit of normal) and in primary hyperthyroidism T_4 will be elevated and TSH will be suppressed or undetectable.[56]

Abnormal thyroid function tests are relatively common in patients aged 65 and over, but their clinical significance varies. Even when clearly abnormal, elderly patients with thyroid dysfunction may be asymptomatic or have non-specific or atypical symptoms which can easily be mistaken for the 'normal' signs of ageing or other medical conditions.[56, 59] Concurrent medical conditions and medications, which are common in the elderly, may also affect thyroid function tests, as shown in Table 9.1. For these reasons the ability to identify and correctly interpret abnormal thyroid function tests is essential to ensure that appropriate treatment is commenced in elderly patients with actual thyroid dysfunction.[56]

There is probably inadequate evidence to support biochemical screening for thyroid disease in asymptomatic older patients[57, 60–62] but there should be a low clinical threshold for their initiation. Any systemic illness, acute psychiatric disturbance or the postoperative state can modify the metabolism of T_4, T_3 and TSH, therefore screening may be prudent in elderly patients who are admitted non-electively to hospitals or nursing homes, also in those with unexplained deterioration in mental function, dementia, unexplained weight loss or lethargy, muscle weakness, tachyarrhythmias or new-onset atrial fibrillation.[1]

Table 9.1 Important effects of medication on thyroid function

Agent	Effect
Amiodarone	Multiple effects, including overt hypothyroidism or hyperthyroidism, transient elevations in TSH and decreased conversion of T_4 to T_3
Corticosteroids	Decreased TSH secretion, decreased conversion of T_4 to T_3
Lithium	Decreased T_4/T_3 synthesis and release, increased TSH secretion
Phenytoin	Multiple effects, including decreased TSH secretion, increased rate of thyroid hormone metabolism, inhibition of protein binding

Adapted from Wallace and Hofmann.[56]
TSH = Thyroid-stimulating hormone; T_4 = thyroxine; T_3 = tri-iodothyronine.

Hypothyroidism

Hypothyroidism is the clinical syndrome which results from reduced secretion of T_4 and T_3 by the thyroid gland, irrespective of the cause. The population prevalence is approximately 15 per 1000 females and 1 per 1000 males. Hypothyroidism may be caused by an intrinsic disorder of the gland (primary hypothyroidism) or may be secondary to disorders of the pituitary or hypothalamus. The most common cause of primary hypothyroidism is autoimmune (Hashimoto's) thyroiditis.[59, 63] Other relatively common causes include thyroid failure following radioiodine (iodine-131), surgery or drugs (Table 9.1). Hypothyroidism resulting from pituitary or hypothalamic disease is very rare and is usually caused by tumours or surgery.[59] In this case other hormones such as ACTH, FSH and LH are also likely to be deficient.

Clinical manifestations

The onset of hypothyroidism is often insidious in the elderly. This is because the 'classical' clinical features present in young patients are absent in up to two-thirds of the elderly population.[59, 61] Common clinical features of hypothyroidism in the elderly include a general slowing down and increasing difficulty in coping at home. Other common complaints are of weakness, sleepiness, lethargy, poor memory and concentration, weight gain and constipation. These symptoms may or may not be associated with the usual skin, hair or voice changes, but there may be facial puffiness, especially around the eyes. Hypothyroidism in the elderly may also be associated with a change in cognitive function and be responsible for treatable dementia. The clinician should also be particularly vigilant in elderly patients who have a previous history of hyperthyroidism, in those taking medicines known to cause thyroid problems and in those with a positive family history of thyroid disease.[59] Details of the presenting symptoms of hypothyroidism in the elderly and the more 'classical' symptoms found in younger adults are shown in Table 9.2. In patients with hypothyroidism the FT$_4$ index is below normal and the TSH level is increased to at least twice the upper limit of normal.[63]

Table 9.2 Clinical features of thyroid disease in old age and in the younger patient

Hyperthyroidism	*Hypothyroidism*
General	**General**
Weight loss despite good appetite	*Weight gain*
Fatigue, apathy	*Tiredness, somnolence*
Sweating and heat intolerance	*Difficulty coping at home*
Thinning of hair	Coarse hair
Goitre (diffuse[a]/nodular)	Poor memory/concentration
	Hoarse voice
	Goitre (only in primary)
	Cold intolerance
Cardiovascular	**Cardiovascular**
Atrial fibrillation	Bradycardia
~~*Angina*~~	
Heart failure	
Palpitations	
Tachycardia	
Neuromuscular	**Neuromuscular**
Generalised muscle weakness	Aches and pains
Nervousness, agitation, tremor	Muscle stiffness
Emotional lability, psychosis	Delayed relaxation of tendon reflexes
Gastrointestinal	**Gastrointestinal**
Vomiting	*Constipation*
Diarrhoea and loose stools	
Reproductive	**Reproductive**
Loss of libido, gynaecomastia	Impotence
Dermatological	**Dermatological**
Pruritus	Dry, flaky skin
Pretibial myxoedema	Myxoedema
Palmar erythema and spider naevi	Rashes
	Facial puffiness
Ocular	
Lid retraction, lid lag	

[a] Graves' disease only.
Italics: common presenting symptoms in the elderly.

Treatment

Hypothyroidism is usually treated with lifelong replacement of levothyroxine (thyroxine) which is available as 25, 50 and 100 microgram tablets in the UK. It has a long half-life which allows once-daily administration and encourages good compliance. The alternative, liothyronine, is not used routinely as it needs to be given three times a day due to its short duration of action. However, liothyronine is indicated in the initial treatment of myxoedema coma, an extreme manifestation of hypothyroidism, which is discussed later in this chapter.

Levothyroxine should be started slowly (at a dose of 25 micrograms/day in otherwise healthy patients) and gradually increased (by 25 micrograms/day) at intervals of 4–6 weeks because of the long half-life of levothyroxine (about 7 days).[61, 64] It is especially important to use a lower initial dose in elderly patients with ischaemic heart disease, as high initial doses may worsen angina and cause myocardial infarction or even death owing to the resulting increase in heart rate and cardiac work.[63] For this reason, a starting dose of 25 micrograms on alternate days, followed by very cautious increases, is recommended in patients with cardiac disease.

The maintenance dose of levothyroxine required by the elderly is lower than for younger patients and is usually between 100 and 150 micrograms/day. However, the correct dose of levothyroxine replacement is determined on the basis of clinical factors and laboratory tests. In patients who do not show an adequate clinical response, factors such as non-compliance, underlying anaemia (especially that due to vitamin B_{12} deficiency), psychiatric conditions or another autoimmune condition such as Addison's disease should be considered. If secondary hypothyroidism is suspected and there is a possibility of adrenal insufficiency, levothyroxine should be initiated after hydrocortisone replacement therapy because adrenal crisis may be precipitated if hydrocortisone is not administered first.[56]

Myxoedema coma

Myxoedema coma is an uncommon complication of hypothyroidism which is typically seen in the elderly and is often precipitated by infection, treatment with sedative drugs or inadequate heating during cold weather. Although coma does not occur in all patients, a reduced level of consciousness is common and more than 80% of patients have hypothermia. Other clinical features include hypotension, heart failure, hyponatraemia and hypoventilation with hypoxia and hypercapnia.[63]

Treatment comprises general supportive measures, including intravenous fluids, antibiotics, ventilation and slow rewarming as well as thyroid hormone replacement. Treatment is initiated with liothyronine which is given as a bolus dose of 100 micrograms intravenously. This is followed by a dose of 20 micrograms three times daily, by mouth. Levothyroxine can be substituted after 2–3 days if clinical improvement occurs.[63] If secondary hypothyroidism is suspected, and there is a possibility of adrenal insufficiency, both liothyroxine and intravenous hydrocortisone (100–200 mg three times daily) should be given as adrenal crisis may be precipitated if levothyroxine is administered before corticosteroid replacement.[56]

Response to treatment

Generally patients will begin to feel better within 2–3 weeks of starting levothyroxine but it may take 6 weeks at full dose for serum TSH levels to return to normal.[63] Reduction in weight and periorbital puffiness occur relatively quickly but restoration of skin and hair texture may take between 3 and 6 months. It is important to explain these points to patients and to emphasise the need for continued treatment. Serum T_4 and TSH are usually checked 6 weeks after treatment is commenced as the time to reach steady state with levothyroxine is prolonged due to its long half-life.[63] With effective therapy the TSH value will be within the normal range and the serum T_4 will be at the upper end of normal. Noncompliant patients who start to take their levothyroxine a few days prior to attending a clinic appointment can be detected as their thyroid function tests typically reveal a normal or even elevated T_4 and a paradoxically raised TSH.[63]

Hyperthyroidism

Introduction

Hyperthyroidism (thyrotoxicosis) is the clinical syndrome arising from exposure to excess levels of FT_4 and/or FT_3. The prevalence is between 0.5 and 2.3% depending on the criteria used for diagnosis and the population being studied.[65] Although hyperthyroidism is most common in young adulthood and middle age, 10–15% of patients with hyperthyroidism are aged over 60. The most common cause in the elderly is Graves' disease which develops as a result of the production of antibodies (thyroid stimulating immunoglobulins (TSI)) against the TSH-receptor of the thyroid cell.[59] Once bound to the receptor the antibodies stimulate thyroid hormone production in a manner similar to TSH, so leading to overproduction of hormones. TGIs which cause growth of the thyroid gland are also produced. Other relatively common causes of hyperthyroidism include toxic multinodular goitre, overtreatment with levothyroxine and iodine excess from radiographic contrast dye or amiodarone. Rare causes include TSH-secreting pituitary adenomas and other carcinomas.[56]

Clinical manifestations

The onset of symptoms of hyperthyroidism may be over a few weeks or may be insidious, especially in the elderly, and may also be obscured by coexisting illness. Although the elderly may present with symptoms and signs similar to those seen in younger people, eye signs (exophthalmos), anxiety, sweating and tremor are often absent.[61] Symptoms such as heat intolerance, frequent stools or diarrhoea are also uncommon.[59] Presentation is often termed 'apathetic thyrotoxicosis' as the patient may be tired, confused, depressed or have experienced weight loss despite a good appetite. These symptoms may be the result of physical and mental exhaustion caused by thyroid overactivity. Cardiovascular symptoms such as atrial fibrillation or high-output cardiac failure (due to increased rate of metabolism) are also common. Therefore in all these situations it is important to request thyroid function tests. In elderly hyperthyroid patients serum TSH will be undetectable and FT_4 will usually be elevated. Occasionally FT_4 may be normal and FT_3 is raised. In all situations, however, there will be no increase in TSH levels after injection of TRH and this confirms the diagnosis of thyrotoxicosis.

Treatment

Treatment of hyperthyroidism may be directed at the underlying cause, the thyroid hypersecretion or the clinical manifestations of this disease. There are three options, which include: the antithyroid drugs or thionamides (carbimazole, methimazole and propylthiouracil), surgery (subtotal thyroidectomy) and radioiodine (iodine-131). All are effective but no single method offers an absolute cure.

Antithyroid drugs There are no clinically significant differences between the three available antithyroid drugs carbimazole, methimazole and propylthiouracil. Carbimazole is a prodrug which is metabolised virtually completely to the active product methimazole, which makes the dose and effects of both drugs equivalent. Methimazole is licensed in the USA whereas carbimazole is licensed in the UK. All three antithyroid drugs act by inhibiting the uptake of iodide into organic form by the enzyme thyroid peroxidase and the coupling of iodotyrosine to form iodothyronines which in turn suppress the synthesis of thyroid hormones.[66] Carbimazole and methimazole are the preferred agents in the UK and USA respectively because they have longer half-lives than propylthiouracil and only need to be given once daily, whereas propylthiouracil needs to be taken three or four times daily. Propylthiouracil has an additional peripheral effect whereby it blocks peripheral conversion of T_4 to T_3. There is also some evidence that antithyroid drugs have immunosuppressive activity leading to a reduction of TSI levels within weeks of starting treatment.[66]

Rashes are the most common side-effect with the thionamides (affecting between 1% and 5% of patients). However, the most serious side-effect is agranulocytosis which occurs in fewer than 0.1% of patients, usually within weeks of starting treatment, and is almost always reversible following withdrawal.[66,67] Therefore patients should be advised to see their general practitioner as soon as possible if they experience a persistent sore throat, fever and malaise. Cross-sensitivity between drugs is unusual and another member of the group can usually be substituted with good effect. Other uncommon unwanted side-effects include arthralgia, myalgia, cholestatic jaundice, depigmentation of the hair, psychosis and even a lupus-like syndrome.[67]

Response to treatment The patient will feel better within 10–14 days and will be clinically and biochemically euthyroid after about 6–8 weeks.[61] The carbimazole dose can then be reduced from the initial dose of 30–60 mg/day progressively to a maintenance dose between 5 and 15 mg/day. Propylthiouracil is given initially in high doses (300–600 mg/day) in four divided doses until the patient is euthyroid. The dose is then gradually reduced every 4–8 weeks by 50–75% to a maintenance dose of between 100 and 300 mg/day in divided doses. Therapy with thionamides is usually continued for 12–18 months with a view to inducing long-term remission[66] and regular checks of FT_4 and TSH levels every 3 months.[67] FT_4 levels are usually used to guide dosage adjustment as TSH may remain suppressed in the long term.[62,66] In patients in whom antithyroid drugs are stopped after this period, about 50% will relapse within 2 years. Following treatment failure, surgery or radioiodine is usually recommended.

Subtotal thyroidectomy Subtotal thyroidectomy has a specific role to play in the treatment of hyperthyroidism. It is the treatment of choice in many patients with hyperthyroidism which recurs after a 12–18 month course of antithyroid drugs, in patients with a large goitre which does not regress significantly during antithyroid drug therapy, where poor drug compliance is suspected (resistance to drug therapy does not occur), suspected malignancy, swallowing or breathing difficulties or allergy to thionamides. During the procedure about 90% of the gland is removed, and special attention is paid to preservation of the parathyroid glands and the recurrent laryngeal nerves, leaving enough residual tissue to maintain postoperative euthyroid status.[66]

Patients must be rendered euthyroid before surgery with a thionamide or iodine. Although small amounts of iodine are required for normal thyroid hormone synthesis, large amounts inhibit thyroid function. This effect is used when patients are given iodine preparations such as Lugol's iodine (0.3 ml three times daily 24 h prior to surgery) to reduce the risk of perioperative bleeding. However its antithyroid effects do not persist as there is a reflex increase in TSH secretion. For patients taking carbimazole prior to surgery this may be stopped 2 weeks before the operation and replaced by potassium iodide 60 mg three times daily, which reduces the size and vascularity of the gland and makes surgery technically easier.

Radioactive iodine Use of radioiodine, which acts either by destroying functioning thyroid cells or by inhibiting their ability to replicate, is increasing.[66] Iodine-131 is used at a dose of 5–10 mCi orally, depending on the size of the goitre.[62] This regimen is effective within about 8–16 weeks.[61] During this lag period symptoms may be controlled by β-blockers such as propranolol, nadolol or sotalol or by carbimazole 45 mg/day for 4–6 weeks starting 48 h after radioiodine therapy. The optimal dose of radioiodine is that which partially destroys the gland, leaving sufficient functioning tissue to maintain the patient euthyroid. However, there is no reliable way of predicting the optimal dose due to the variability of response between individuals. If hyperthyroidism is still present after 12 weeks the initial dose of iodine-131 may be repeated.[62]

Radioiodine is well tolerated and is the preferred treatment for toxic nodular goitre, debilitated, cardiac or elderly patients who are poor surgical candidates, patients who fail to respond to treatment (because of non-compliance) or adverse reactions and in patients who are surgical failures. Radioiodine is more frequently being used as the primary mode of treatment for Graves' disease, especially in the elderly.[66] The disadvantage of iodine-131 therapy is the high incidence of subsequent hypothyroidism which occurs at a rate of approximately 2% per year after treatment.[59]

Role of β-adrenoceptor blockers β-Blockers block the β-adrenergic-mediated actions of thyroid hormones, producing relief from symptoms such as tremor, agitation and tachycardia. They act within 12–48 h and are useful in patients awaiting hospital consultation, the latent period before treatment is effective (10–14 days for antithyroid drugs and 8–16 weeks for iodine-131) and in combination with potassium iodide when preparing patients for surgery. However, β-blockers do not abolish all the signs and symptoms of hyperthyroidism, they do not alter thyroid hormone levels and they are therefore not indicated for long-term treatment. A non-cardioselective drug is usually used: the most widely used is propranolol as it also blocks the conversion of T_4 to T_3 in the periphery. The average dose is 160 mg of the long-acting preparation daily (Inderal LA). Alternatives are nadolol (160 mg/day) or sotalol (200 mg/day). Sotalol has additional class III antiarrhythmic activity and may be particularly valuable in thyrotoxic atrial fibrillation. Although β-blockers should be considered as adjuvant therapy in all patients with moderate or severe hyperthyroidism, they should be used with caution in the elderly as they may be more susceptible to side-effects such as peripheral vasoconstriction, bronchconstriction and bradycardia.

Conclusion

Abnormal thyroid function tests are common in the elderly, but their significance and the need for treatment vary. Even when their test results are clearly abnormal, elderly patients with thyroid dysfunction may be asymptomatic or have non-specific or atypical symptoms which can easily be mistaken for the 'normal' signs of ageing or other medical conditions. Coexisting medical conditions and concomitant medications may also affect thyroid function tests. Therefore the ability to identify and correctly interpret abnormal thyroid function tests is essential to ensure that appropriate treatment is commenced in the presence of actual thyroid dysfunction. Subclinical hypothyroidism may be a sign of early thyroid failure and requires close observation.

Pituitary disease

Pituitary tumours

Pituitary tumours account for approximately 10% of intracranial neo-plasms.[68] They are classified according to the hormones they secrete and include prolactinomas, GH-secreting tumours, ACTH-secreting tumours, TSH-secreting tumours (which are rare) and clinically inactive or 'non-functioning' tumours. Their age distribution depends princi-pally on the hormone produced. Tumours secreting prolactin and ACTH are most common in young adults whereas 'non-functioning' tumours usually present after the age of 60 years.[68]

Pituitary tumours are further divided into microadenomas, which are intrasellar adenomas up to 1 cm in diameter without sellar enlarge-ment or extrasellar extension, and macroadenomas, which are larger than 1 cm in diameter and cause focal or generalised sellar enlargement. Microadenomas usually cause symptoms or signs of hormonal excess; hypopituitarism is rare. Macroadenomas may also cause manifestations of hormonal excess, but hypopituitarism is common. Pituitary hormone deficiency tends to begin with growth hormone, followed by gonadotrophins (LH and FSH) and later by TSH and ACTH.[69] Any medication with dopamine antagonist properties, for example, metoclo-pramide, domperidone, methyldopa or a phenothiazine antipsychotic, can also cause hyperprolactinaemia.[70]

The problems created by pituitary tumours are related either to the hormones they secrete or the effects of an expanding sellar mass. For example, macroadenomas can cause visual disturbances, which range from changes in the lateral field of vision to blindness in one or both eyes. Headache is also relatively common and is described as annoying rather than disabling and often responds to analgesia. The majority of pituitary tumours are benign, although they may be invasive.[69, 71]

Treatment options for pituitary tumours

Treatment, which involves surgical resection, irradiation or drugs, aims to alleviate the symptoms and signs of hypersecretion syndromes, normalise the secretion of anterior pituitary hormones and remove or shrink large tumours to relieve pressure on vital structures. Residual anterior pituitary function should also be preserved or, if compromised, restored.[72] Whereas a single therapeutic intervention may be sufficient for microadenomas, multiple therapy may be required for large tumours and may also be less successful.[69]

Prolactinomas

Prolactin-secreting pituitary adenomas (prolactinomas) are the most common hormone-secreting adenomas and account for about 60% of primary pituitary tumours. They have different manifestations in men and women. Young women often present with galactorrhoea, amenorrhoea, oligomenorrhoea with anovulation or infertility, but prolactinomas will be silent in postmenopausal women. Men tend to experience decreased libido or impotence because serum gonadotrophin and testosterone levels are low.[71] A macroadenoma of any type may produce hypogonadism by mechanical damage to the gonadotrophin-releasing cells or by interfering with the delivery of gonadotrophin-releasing hormone (GnRH) by the hypophysial–portal system.[69, 72]

Treatment of prolactinomas   The preferred option and most effective treatment for microprolactinomas and macroprolactinomas is medical management with dopamine agonists such as bromocriptine, cabergoline or quinagolide which inhibit prolactin release and induce tumour shrinkage, although surgery is sometimes required for resistant tumours.[72] Medical therapy is also used prior to surgery to shrink large tumours to increase the likelihood of surgical cure or after failed surgery to control residual hyperprolactinaemia.[69] Radiation therapy is reserved for patients who experience persistent hyperprolactinaemia despite surgery or who cannot tolerate drug therapy. This is because there is a risk of inducing impairment of anterior pituitary function in 30–50% of patients.[69] There have also been anecdotal reports of low-grade neuronal damage, radionecrosis, vaso-occlusive disease and secondary tumours in some patients who have received radiation therapy.[71]

Bromocriptine   Bromocriptine mesylate is a semisynthetic ergot derivative of ergoline which is a dopamine D_2-receptor agonist with weak antagonist properties at D_1-receptors. Until a few years ago bromocriptine was the agent of choice for medical management of hyperprolactinaemia; however, side-effects such as nausea, vomiting, headache, dizziness and postural hypotension are common (especially in the early stages of therapy) and may be more pronounced in the elderly. Nausea and vomiting occur in up to 60% of patients and postural hypotension results in dizziness in approximately 25% of patients.[73] Side-effects may be minimised by starting with a dose of 1.25 mg taken at night.[72] The dose is then gradually increased to 7.5–15 mg/day, although some patients require 30 mg/day.[74] Side-effects often resolve after continued therapy although they necessitate permanent discontinuation of

bromocriptine in up to 12% of patients.[73] Constipation is another relatively common side-effect and occurs in up to 10% of patients but, unlike
nausea, tends to be persistent. Other side-effects, such as nasal stuffiness,
psychosis, hallucinations, nightmares, insomnia and vertigo, which are
much less common, are dose-related and can sometimes be alleviated by
dosage reduction.[73] However, since high doses may be required for
therapeutic efficacy, side-effects are often the limiting factor with
bromocriptine and make it intolerable for many elderly patients.

Another problem with bromocriptine is its short duration of action
which necessitates multiple daily dosing. In the elderly this may cause
problems with compliance since treatment needs to be lifelong in the
majority of patients. In order to overcome this problem, and to reduce
the incidence of side-effects, a long-acting parenteral formulation of
bromocriptine (Parlodel LAR) was developed which is given by intramuscular injection. However, although this formulation induced more
prolonged normalisation of prolactin no difference was shown in
tolerance. Nausea and postural hypotension were also still associated
with this formulation, usually after the first dose, although they rarely
persisted.[75] This long-acting formulation is not currently available in
the UK. Use of bromocriptine has been superseded by the use of
cabergoline.

Cabergoline   Cabergoline is an ergoline derivative with high affinity
and selectivity for dopamine D_2-receptors.[76] It has a very prolonged
duration of action and is usually given as a single daily dose either once
or twice weekly starting at 0.25 mg with dose titrations every few weeks
as required. There is a linear relationship between dose and response
between 0.25 and 1 mg twice weekly and normalisation of prolactin
levels is achieved in 95% of patients.[77] In most patients 0.5 mg twice
weekly is sufficient to normalise prolactin levels but higher doses may be
needed in some patients.[74]

The side-effects of cabergoline are similar in character to those
observed with bromocriptine and with other dopaminergic ergot derivatives but they occur less frequently than with bromocriptine.[73] The
most common problem is nausea, which occurs in up to about 10% of
patients, followed by headache, dizziness and fatigue/weakness.[78] These
adverse effects, as with bromocriptine, are generally dose-related and
can be minimised by starting at a low dosage with gradual dosage esca-
lation. Another advantage of cabergoline is that it may be effective in
patients who are resistant to bromocriptine.[79] However, whether the
dosage regimen of cabergoline is ideal in the elderly is debatable, as

difficulty may be experienced remembering to take a drug once weekly as opposed to once daily for an agent such as quinagolide.

Quinagolide Quinagolide is a non-ergot (octahydrobenzyl(g)-quinoline) dopamine D_2-agonist which has a prolonged suppressive activity on serum prolactin when given once daily.[72] The starting dose is 25 micrograms/day for 3 days, 50 micrograms/day for the next 3 days then 75 micrograms/day and the usual maintenance dose is between 75 and 150 micrograms/day. The side-effects of quinagolide are similar to bromocriptine, and include nausea, vomiting, headache, dizziness and fatigue. Again, these are usually transient and occur within the first few days of starting treatment and after dosage increments. Overall, quinagolide appears to be better tolerated than bromocriptine, although the relevant studies are smaller and the data less conclusive than for cabergoline.[80, 81]

Therefore cabergoline or quinagolide may be better tolerated in the elderly than bromocriptine. However, as quinagolide is more expensive, cabergoline has become first-line therapy in many centres and quinagolide is generally reserved for patients who do not tolerate either cabergoline or bromocriptine.

Growth hormone-secreting tumours

GH-secreting pituitary tumours account for about 20% of all primary pituitary tumours[72, 82] and are responsible for the majority of cases of acromegaly. Long-term GH excess has deleterious effects on many systems and results in serious morbidity and a shortened life expectancy. In adults acromegaly is characterised by a local overgrowth of bone, particularly of the skull and mandible, although previous fusion of the long bone epiphyses prevents linear growth. It is a slowly progressing disorder that causes cosmetic deformity which consists of a coarsening of the features with a thickened appearance to the bones of the forehead and jaw as well as broadening of the hands and feet. Associated soft-tissue swelling may cause enlarged hands, feet and tongue, the skin may appear thicker and patients may complain of increased hair growth. Acromegaly is also associated with chronic disabling degenerative arthritis as well as an increased mortality from cardiovascular atherosclerosis and respiratory diseases.[69, 83]

Treatment of acromegaly The aims of treatment of acromegaly caused by a pituitary tumour are to remove or destroy the tumour, reverse GH hypersecretion, maintain normal anterior and posterior pituitary function, relieve symptoms of GH excess and prevent long-term consequences.[84] Although the latter may seem less important in a patient who has a short life expectancy,[69] due to its insidious nature, diagnosis of acromegaly may be delayed for several years.[85]

The preferred treatment for GH-secreting microadenomas in younger patients is surgery. Selective removal of the adenoma by transsphenoidal resection has a high success rate, especially for small tumours.[85] However, as tumours in the elderly may be more sensitive to somatostatin analogues than those in younger patients, medical therapy may be used first-line, especially in those who are at high risk of surgical complications. Also, in patients with larger tumours and pronounced GH hypersecretion, more than one therapy may be required. Radiation therapy, although effective, is reserved for patients with persistent GH hypersecretion after surgery as its effects are slow and hypothyroidism, hypoadrenalism and hypogonadism may follow.[69, 72]

Bromocriptine does reduce GH levels; however, sufficient reduction is only obtained in about 10% of patients.[86] Similar results have been obtained with cabergoline whereas quinagolide appears to normalise GH and IGF-1 levels in over 45% of patients.[87] However, dopamine agonists are only used as adjunctive therapy in patients with acromegaly who have had their GH levels adequately reduced by surgery or radiation.

Octreotide acetate, a somatostatin analogue, has replaced the use of dopamine agonists as first-line medical therapy in acromegaly. It reduces GH and IGF-1 levels to normal in most patients and in some cases causes tumour shrinkage. Effective doses appear to be in the range 100–500 μg administered subcutaneously three times daily.[72] This requirement for frequent subcutaneous injections is due to the short plasma half-life of octreotide (approximately 2 h) and is inconvenient for patients.[69] For this reason a long-acting preparation has been marketed (Sandostatin LAR) which only needs to be injected once every month.[88] This preparation offers increased convenience, should improve compliance and increases acceptability of treatment.

Octreotide is well tolerated, and also normalises GH levels in 60% of patients.[85] Most side-effects are short-lived and relate to drug-induced suppression of gastrointestinal motility and secretion. These effects, which include nausea, abdominal pain, fat malabsorption, steatorrhoea and diarrhoea, usually occur in about one-third of patients and remit within 2 weeks of starting therapy. Other side-effects include cholelithiasis, mild glucose intolerance, asymptomatic bradycardia and depression as well as pain at the injection site.[72] Overall, the tolerability of the standard subcutaneous injection of GH and the depot preparation are similar.[88, 89] No dosage reduction is required in the elderly (≥ 65 years) or in those with impaired renal or hepatic function.

Corticotrophin-secreting adenomas – Cushing's disease

Corticotrophin hypersecretion by a pituitary adenoma (Cushing's disease) is now recognised as the most common cause of spontaneous hypercortisolism (Cushing's syndrome). It is much more common in women than men (8 : 1). Corticotrophin-secreting pituitary tumours are almost always benign and most are small (< 5 mm in diameter). The classic clinical manifestations include weight gain characterised by a peculiar fat distribution with truncal obesity, round face, dorsocervical fat accumulation (buffalo hump), supraclavicular fat pads and a relative sparing of the extremities. Excessive glucocorticoid action results in a catabolic state with thin skin and easy bruising as well as osteoporosis. Hyperglycaemia is also common. Adrenal androgen excess produces hirsuitism and acne.[69, 71]

The treatment of choice for corticotrophin-secreting pituitary tumours involves selective transsphenoidal resection because of its efficacy, rapid clinical response and low complication rate.[71, 72] Radiotherapy has a delayed response and only achieves a 40% cure rate.[71] Cortisol-lowering drugs have only a supportive role in Cushing's disease and are reserved for patients in whom surgery has not provided a cure and are usually given with pituitary irradiation to block peripheral (adrenal) effects of high ACTH levels.

In the USA mitotane therapy combined with irradiation is the preferred medical treatment after surgical failure; it is also used until the delayed clinical improvement induced by irradiation therapy occurs. Aminoglutethimide or metyrapone can also be combined with mitotane to improve the success rate. Combination of metyrapone with aminoglutethimide is also effective.[72] However, the usefulness of these agents is limited by their side-effects, which include nausea, oedema, somnolence and hypertension.[71] Mitotane is not currently marketed in the UK.

Thyrotrophin-secreting tumours

Thyrotrophin-secreting pituitary adenomas, which are rare and account for 0.5–1% of all pituitary adenomas,[72] are usually treated with surgery. If thyrotrophin secretion persists then ablative treatment of the thyroid with radioactive iodine (iodine-131) or surgery is necessary.[69]

Clinically endocrine inactive or 'non-functioning' pituitary tumours

Endocrine inactive or 'non-functioning' pituitary tumours are usually large at the time of diagnosis and are therefore associated with neurological manifestations, typically loss of visual acuity and/or visual fields, headache and hypopituitarism. The endocrine manifestations tend to develop over a period of years.[69] Initial management of tumours causing extrasellar pressure involves transsphenoidal surgery which is undertaken primarily to improve visual field defects and loss of visual acuity and to remove as much tumour as possible.[68] Surgical complications occur in about 8% of patients, who are principally elderly and have partially treated hypopituitarism. As the recurrence rate after surgery is between 12 and 22% after 3–5 years, postoperative external pituitary irradiation is recommended unless regular follow-up, which includes regular imaging, is available.[68] There is virtually no role for medical treatment of 'non-functioning' pituitary tumours as they respond poorly to dopamine agonist therapy with only modest tumour shrinkage in fewer than 10% of patients.

Hypopituitarism

Hypopituitarism is the partial or complete insufficiency of anterior pituitary hormone secretion and may result from pituitary or hypothalamic disease. In adults there are a number of causes of hypopituitarism, including pituitary or peripituitary tumours, surgery, irradiation, infarction, trauma and infection. The most common causes include functional and non-functional pituitary adenomas.[68] Restoration of pituitary insufficiency necessitates lifelong replacement therapy.

Clinical features

The clinical manifestations of hypopituitarism vary depending on the extent, severity and duration of the pituitary hormone deficiencies. Hypopituitarism is also often insidious in onset. In adults with large pituitary adenomas, headache and visual impairment may occur. However, in the elderly visual disturbances may be masked by glaucoma or macular degeneration. Patients may also have accompanying symptoms of corticotrophin deficiency such as chronic fatigue, sensitivity to cold, constipation and weight gain. Although in most cases mineralocorticoid secretion remains intact, corticotrophin deficiency can still be life-threatening since patients lose their ability to respond to stress, especially during infectious illness, or after trauma or surgery. In addition hypoglycaemia can result from cortisol and GH deficiency, whereas hyponatraemia commonly occurs in the elderly. Raised serum prolactin concentrations also occur with pituitary hypofunction, often in association with macroprolactinomas. Finally, hypothyroidism due to thyrotrophin deficiency is similar in clinical presentation to primary hypothyroidism, but is often less severe because some thyrotrophin activity is preserved.[90]

Cortisol deficiency

There is no universal agreement on the appropriate dose, timing and monitoring of hydrocortisone replacement therapy. Conventional treatment uses two doses of hydrocortisone per day usually 20 mg at 8 a.m. and 10 mg at 6 p.m. although thrice-daily dosing (10 mg before breakfast, 5 mg at lunchtime and 5 mg in the early evening) has been shown to mimic the normal pattern of cortisol secretion more closely than twice-daily administration.[91] However, patients on both these regimens may still complain of early-morning fatigue and headache that improve after breakfast and taking their morning dose of hydrocortisone. This may reflect overnight cortisol deficiency.[92]

As patients with cortisol deficiency are not able to respond to surgery, trauma, infections and other severe illnesses with an increase in cortisol production they should be given supplemental corticosteroids in all these situations.[93] During minor illness patients should be instructed to double their dose of oral steroids and intravenous hydrocortisone should be used to cover major illness or surgery. Patients should also be instructed to carry steroid cards with them at all times.

Thyrotrophin deficiency

Levothyroxine is the treatment of choice for secondary hypothyroidism and is used according to the same criteria outlined earlier in this chapter, starting with 25 μg/day or on alternate days in the presence of coexisting ishaemic heart disease. The dosage should be increased at 4-weekly intervals, if tolerated, according to the restoration of FT_4 into the normal range and the disappearance of signs and symptoms of hypothyroidism.[63]

Gonadotrophin deficiency

In older women a combination of estradiol valerate 2 mg or conjugated oestrogen 0.625–1.25 mg/day may be given cyclically or continuously with a progestogen in those with a uterus. There are a number of formulations of hormone replacement therapy (HRT) available, which are discussed in detail in Chapter 10.

Normal circulating androgen concentrations are essential in men of all ages to ensure normal sexual function, normal bone and muscle mass and good general health.[4] Hypogonadotrophic hypogonadism in males is shown by low serum testosterone concentrations with low or normal concentrations of FSH and LH. The results should be compared with normal values for age and hyperprolactinaemia must be excluded.[94] The choice of therapy for this indication depends on whether fertility is desired. To maintain fertility, pulse therapy with gonadotrophin-releasing hormone or gonadotrophin replacement therapy should be used. Various doses and frequencies of administration of FSH and LH have been suggested.[95] Testosterone may be administered orally as testosterone undecanoate at a dose of 40 mg two to four times daily or parenterally as the enantate or propionate at a dose of 200 mg every 2 weeks. Both these salts have clinically equivalent durations of action and effectiveness. Alternatively, transdermal testosterone patches are available, although these are currently more expensive than oral or injectable therapies. The patches each deliver 4–6 mg of testosterone when changed daily. Dosage of oral or transdermal agents and the intervals between injections (if used) should be titrated according to clinical response which is judged by improvements in sexual function, energy and mood and serum testosterone levels. Lower doses of testosterone are recommended in older men with benign prostatic hyperplasia.

Growth hormone deficiency

GH deficiency usually presents as an impaired sense of well-being which is manifested by symptoms of chronic fatigue, decreased mobility and a tendency towards social isolation. The routine use of GH replacement therapy in GH-deficient adults is not generally recommended primarily due to its high yearly costs but also because of doubts about its perceived benefit(s). The decision to start GH therapy in adults is based on alterations in body composition such as increased central obesity, low muscle mass (and strength) and lowered bone mineral density.

If it is decided to use GH in a particular individual then the recommended dose varies between patients, since the dose is dependent on body weight. A starting dose of 0.02–0.04 mg/kg (0.5–0.9 units), given as daily subcutaneous injections, is recommended to minimise initial side-effects which include oedema, paraesthesia, arthralgia and carpel tunnel syndrome. The dosage is then gradually increased, at monthly intervals, depending on side-effects. The recommended weekly maintenance dose is 0.04–0.08 mg/kg (0.01 mg/kg = 0.03 units/kg)[96] but this will vary and is optimised by measuring the serum IGF-1 according to age and sex. Other variables which can be used to judge efficacy include an increase in muscle strength and exercise capacity, increased mental energy, restoration of the ability to cope with daily life and a decrease in central obesity.[96] If the patient perceives no benefit from GH therapy after about 6 months then its withdrawal should be considered.

Vasopressin deficiency

Diabetes insipidus is characterised by the passing of large amounts of dilute urine (more than 3 l in 24 h and osmolality less than 300 mmol/kg).[97] Following diagnosis, which is usually undertaken following the water deprivation test or infusion of hypertonic saline, a therapeutic trial of desmopressin (10–20 mg intranasally or 100–300 mg orally) should be given. Patients with cranial diabetes insipidus will have an instant response. The optimum dose (generally 100–200 mg orally twice daily) varies between individuals and should be titrated to regulate thirst, polyuria and nocturia. However, particular care is needed to ensure that hyponatraemia is avoided if the patient continues to drink inappropriately despite antidiuresis. This may be a particular problem in the elderly.[97]

Conclusion

Selection of treatment for pituitary tumours, which involves surgical resection, irradiation or drugs, is related to the likely response of the tumour and associated symptoms. Medical and radiation therapy may have a greater role to play in elderly patients who are unlikely to tolerate surgery. In patients with hypopituitarism optimal replacement therapy with hydrocortisone, levothyroxine, sex steroids, GH and desmopressin is required. In cases of multiple pituitary hormone deficiencies (panhypopituitarism) cortisol should always be replaced first, followed by levothyroxine, and sex steroids once that patient's condition has stabilised. If necessary, GH can be replaced last. Replacement therapy is largely imprecise and does not quite achieve the normal physiological condition as it is often a compromise between theory, practicality and convenience to patients, as the end-points for treatment relate more to clinical judgement than precise measurement. For this reason management of these patients in specialist centres is warranted. In addition the complicated therapy and expense of a number of the available treatments warrant study of new strategies aimed at prevention of loss of pituitary function.

Disorders of the prostate

Prostatic enlargement is part of the normal ageing process and is found in approximately 80% of men between the ages of 60 and 70.[98,99] The most common cause is benign prostatic hyperplasia (BPH) which is a non-malignant enlargement of the prostate gland. Although the aetiology of BPH is not fully understood, it is well established that the condition results from proliferation of the stromal and epithelial elements of the prostate gland. BPH-related bladder outflow obstruction is believed to consist of two components: a dynamic part and a static part. The former is caused by the tone of the prostate, especially the prostate capsule smooth muscle which is innervated and regulated by the adrenergic component of the autonomic nervous system. The static component is caused by the pressure of prostatic hyperplasia which obstructs urine outflow.[100] Carcinoma of the prostate is a significant cause of morbidity and mortality. It is the third most common cause of male cancer death in the UK after cancer of the lung and of the colon.[101] Therefore the management of prostate disorders is an important consideration in the elderly male.

Presentation

The clinical manifestations of BPH range from minimal urinary symptoms such as hesitancy or poor flow with terminal dribbling and/or incomplete voiding, through nocturia, dysuria, urinary frequency or urge incontinence to urinary retention and even end-stage renal failure. However, the severity or number of symptoms does not appear to correlate with prostate size or urinary flow rate. Clinical BPH is defined as a prostate weight in excess of 20 g in association with symptomatic urinary dysfunction and/or a urinary flow of less than 15 ml/s.[102] Differential diagnosis involves a full digital rectal examination to examine the condition of the prostate, urinalysis with culture, urea and electrolytes and a serum prostatic-specific antigen (PSA). Elevated levels of the latter in the presence of a suspicious prostate indicate the need for biopsy to rule out prostatic carcinoma.[103]

Benign prostatic hyperplasia

Patients who have an enlarged prostate but no symptoms generally require no treatment. Others who have mild symptoms may be content to tolerate the inconvenience and prefer to be reviewed on an annual basis as symptoms do not necessarily become more severe over time and may even ameliorate if left untreated.[103] Treatment is only required when patients become bothered by their symptoms and their lifestyle becomes affected. However, retired men are less likely than working men to seek medical attention about symptomatic BPH as they tend to adapt their lifestyle to avoid situations where symptoms such as urgency or frequency may pose difficulties.[104] Such self-imposed restrictions can have a considerable negative impact on their quality of life.[103]

Treatment for BPH is clearly indicated in men with urinary retention, recurrent urinary tract infection, recurrent or persistent gross haematuria, bladder stones or renal insufficiency. In these situations transurethral resection of the prostate (TURP) remains the gold-standard treatment. However, surgery is not indicated for all men with BPH as, although it may provide symptomatic relief, complications such as erectile dysfunction, incontinence or retrograde ejaculation are common and the long-term outcome is not always satisfactory.[105] In addition, the risk of peri- and postoperative complications is significantly higher in men over 80 years of age.[102] In some high-risk patients who require surgery one of the minimally invasive procedures, such as transurethral incision of the prostate, prostatic stenting, microwave therapy or laser prostatectomy may be useful alternatives.[105, 106]

The problems with surgery, as well as the desire of many men to avoid it, has led to the development of medical treatments to manage all but the most severe cases of BPH. These are used in approximately 80% of patients.[98] The available pharmacological therapies include 5α-reductase inhibitors such as finasteride, and selective postsynaptic α-blockers such as alfuzosin, doxazosin, indoramin, prazosin, tamsulosin and terazosin. As many elderly men with symptomatic BPH have other age-related conditions such as atherosclerosis, diabetes mellitus, hypertension or heart failure, this has direct implications for the choice of treatment. Interactions with any concurrent drug therapy and the likelihood of compliance with medical therapy are also important factors in selecting the most appropriate treatment.[103]

α-Reductase inhibitors

Finasteride, the only currently available inhibitor of 5α-reductase, impairs prostatic growth by inhibiting the conversion of testosterone to the more active dihydrotestosterone. Dihydrotestosterone is essential for prostatic growth and therefore finasteride ameliorates symptoms of BPH by causing shrinkage of prostatic tissue.[103] It is given once daily, which encourages compliance. Finasteride has been shown to reduce the volume of the hyperplastic prostate after 3–6 months of therapy (although it may take up to 12 months to be fully effective). It is well tolerated by most patients and may be most beneficial in men with large prostates (more than 40 g) who do not require surgical intervention.[107] Its main side-effects are associated with sexual dysfunction and include erectile dysfunction, decreased libido and ejaculatory problems.[102, 108] In long-term therapy finasteride has been shown to decrease the need for prostate surgery and the risk of acute urinary retention.[109]

Finasteride appears to be of modest benefit to most patients with symptomatic BPH, with about 30–40% of patients showing signs of symptomatic improvement.[98, 103, 110] Its limited efficacy may be attributed to excessive α-adrenergic stimulation of the prostate, urethra and bladder neck; bladder decompensation due to long-standing BPH; or a lack of effect on stromal tissue.[110]

α-Adrenergic blockers

α-Blockers continue to be the predominant form of medical therapy for BPH. The rationale for their use is based on the fact that the tension of prostatic smooth muscle regulates the degree of outflow obstruction in men with prostatism and this tension is mediated by the α-adrenoceptor. Both the prostate and the prostatic capsule have predominantly α_1-receptors. Three subtypes of α_1-adrenoceptors have been identified (α_{1a}, α_{1b} and α_{1d}) and α_{1a} appears to be responsible for mediating the contraction of smooth muscle in the prostate.[99]

Use of α_1-blockers is intended to relax the smooth muscle of the prostate and the bladder neck and thereby to decrease bladder outlet resistance to urinary flow; they do not reduce prostate size.[110] The selective α_1-blockers licensed for the treatment of symptomatic BPH include alfuzosin, doxazosin, indoramin, prazosin, tamsulosin and terazosin. The use of prazosin has been superseded by the newer agents, especially in the elderly, as a result of side-effects such as postural hypotension, which is a particular problem with the first dose. Therefore prazosin will not be discussed in further detail.

The choice of α_1-blocker is based on coexisting medical conditions, concomitant medications, the likelihood of compliance and the potential risk of side-effects in the individual. The incidence of side-effects with α_1-blockers, which is about 30%, is minimised by starting with a low dose and gradually titrating upwards until clinical improvement occurs. Administration at bedtime is also encouraged. The most troublesome side-effects are dizziness and postural hypotension, which occur in about 10% of patients overall, and are more common in the elderly.[110] Most of these side-effects are explained by cross-reactivity with other α-receptor subtypes which are mainly found in the cardiovascular system and CNS.

Doxazosin, terazosin and indoramin are effective in BPH in all age groups but especially in those patients with concurrent hypertension,[111, 112] although they have no clinically significant effects on blood pressure in normotensive patients.[112] These long-acting agents can be administered once daily in the morning or evening with a similar effect,[113] as they have a gradual onset of action which decreases the risk of postural hypotension.[103] These agents do not adversely affect lipid profiles or glucose tolerance, which is important because a significant number of patients who present with BPH also have hyperlipidaemia and/or diabetes mellitus.[114]

In men with ischaemic heart disease in whom a reflex tachycardia may be detrimental or in those who have low blood pressure, use of a more 'uro-selective' agent such as tamsulosin or alfuzosin may be preferable. These agents are prostate-selective α_{1a}-antagonists which have no clinically relevant effect on blood pressure, heart rate, vasodilatation or cardiovascular side-effects.[115–117] Another major advantage of these agents is that their dosage does not require titration. Tamsulosin is given as a slow-release preparation once daily and alfuzosin three times daily, twice daily as a slow-release formulation or once daily as a very long-acting formulation. On balance, the once-daily dosage regimen of tamsulosin or long-acting alfuzosin may be preferable in men who are likely to have compliance problems. These newer agents are becoming the drugs of first choice for medical management of BPH, especially in the elderly.[110]

Symptomatic improvement in BPH is seen with α_1-blockers in about 90% of patients.[111] They have a more rapid onset of action than finasteride and are most useful in men with smaller prostates (< 40 g) who have acute and mainly irritative symptoms. The time taken for a response in most patients is between 2 and 4 weeks.[100] However, up to 6 weeks may be required for a full response in patients who require gradual dosage titration. Following each dosage adjustment a peak clinical response occurs within 2 weeks. Although there are no randomised trials which have compared the different selective α_1-blockers, there does not appear to be a clinically significant difference between the safety or efficacy of individual drugs.[106]

Combination therapy

In theory the combination of an α_1-blocker and antiandrogen therapy should provide greater efficacy than monotherapy as the symptoms of BPH are due to a combination of static and dynamic factors that may be better addressed by dual therapy. However, the results of a study in which a combination of terazosin and finasteride was compared with finasteride alone, terazosin alone and placebo showed that combination therapy was no more effective than terazosin alone.[118]

Prostatic cancer

Presentation

Prostatic cancer is often asymptomatic, and may be diagnosed during routine rectal examination or during a TURP for BPH. However, locally extensive prostate cancer may produce outflow obstruction with symptoms of hesitancy or urgency of micturition. Painful bone metastases are also common on presentation and can develop during the course of the disease. When tumours are asymptomatic and confined to the prostate gland, progression rates are slow: about 10–15% progress over 5 years to produce local symptoms or spread of disease. With metastatic disease 50% of patients will live at least $2\frac{1}{2}$ years after diagnosis.[101]

Treatment options for prostatic cancer

The choice of treatment for prostatic cancer is influenced primarily by the stage of the disease (whether it is localised or disseminated) but also by the patient's age, physical condition, acceptance of treatment and response to prior therapy. All treatments for advanced prostatic cancer are palliative. Recommendations currently range from no treatment in elderly patients with early disease and in those with asymptomatic advanced disease, through radiotherapy, medical therapy, chemotherapy to radical prostatectomy and castration or orchidectomy.[119]

For localised, clinically undetectable (stage A) disease watchful waiting is recommended in patients with low PSA levels (< 0.1 ng/ml). For patients with a PSA > 10 ng/ml radical prostatectomy or radiation therapy is recommended. In those with a PSA between 1 and 10 ng/ml either of these options is acceptable and can be discussed with the patient. In those with clinically detectable (stage B) disease, which is confined to the prostate, either radical prostatectomy or radiation is recommended. In stage C disease, where local spread has occurred, radiation is used as there are no data to support use of radical prostatectomy. Lastly, in stage D disease which has metastasised, watchful waiting may be used for patients without symptoms, as this has not been shown to affect survival rate adversely and hormonal therapy used for those with symptomatic or progressive stage D disease.[119]

Surgery   Bilateral subcapsular orchidectomy eliminates the source of 95% of serum testosterone and commonly produces a response lasting 12–18 months. Its advantages include a rapid symptomatic relief, low cost and the need for a single procedure that is very effective. Compliance with this mode of treatment is also not an issue. Its disadvantages include the psychological impact of the procedure on the patient as well as the subsequent loss of libido and impotence. Surgery may also be too risky for elderly patients with coexisting medical conditions.[101, 119]

Hormonal therapy   The use of oestrogen therapy, such as diethylstilbestrol, has been superseded by use of GnRH analogues, such as goserelin and leuprorelin, due to its feminising effects and associated cardiovascular complications. For these reasons it will not be discussed further. Other options to block the action of testosterone include androgen-blocking agents such as flutamide or cyproterone.

GnRH analogues, which are available as depot preparations given either monthly or 3-monthly, abolish testicular stimulation and lower serum levels of testosterone. They are useful agents as there are no compliance problems and no dosage adjustment is required in the elderly or in those with renal impairment. Other advantages include a lower incidence of cardiovascular side-effects and less gynaecomastia, breast tenderness, gastrointestinal upset and peripheral oedema.[119] In studies goserelin and leuprorelin have been shown to be therapeutically equivalent to orchidectomy.[120, 121] However, these agents are relatively expensive. Most side-effects associated with GnRH analogues result from their effects on the levels of sex hormones. Impotence and decreased libido occur in the majority of patients, usually within 3 months of starting a treatment.[122] Hot flushes also occur in 50–70% of patients. Since the latter does not subside with continued use, it may cause some patients to discontinue therapy.[119] Few patients achieve a complete response with GnRH analogues (usually less than 5%), although there is a partial response in up to 70% of patients.[122]

Antiandrogens such as flutamide, bicalutamide and cyproterone are useful to cover the increase in symptoms or 'tumour flare' that may occur for up to 2 weeks after starting GnRH analogue treatment.[123] Antiandrogens are administered about 1 week before and for up to 4 weeks after the initial GnRH analogue dose.[122] Due to concern over hepatic toxicity, use of cyproterone is confined to this indication and to alleviate 'hot flushes' experienced by patients after orchidectomy.[101]

Bicalutamide 50 mg once daily has shown to be at least as effective as flutamide three times daily in maximal androgen blockade and causes less diarrhoea.[124] At a dose of 150 mg daily it has also been shown to be as effective as monotherapy in patients with non-metastatic disease but patients with metastatic disease have been reported to respond better to castration.[125] As bicalutamide causes a number of side-effects, including angina, heart failure and dizziness, which may be more pronounced in the elderly, it should be used with caution in these patients, especially in those with coexisting diseases and hepatic dysfunction.

As prostatic cancer is often characterised by slow growth, chemotherapy has a minimal effect. Since chemotherapy is strictly palliative, assessments of quality of life are very important. There is no evidence that combination of agents is any more effective than single-agent therapy, although this area is still under investigation.[119]

Conclusion   As the male population ages, prostate problems are becoming more prevalent. Although intervention may be required for many men with symptomatic BPH, some patients may not require immediate treatment. Medical treatment with α-reductase inhibitors and α-blockers is clinically effective although it is difficult to predict which patients will benefit from which option. α-Blockers provide quicker, more reliable and more significant short-term symptomatic relief than finasteride but side-effects during treatment are more frequent. Prostate cancer is a significant cause of mortality; however, there is no consensus on screening. Treatment choice is decided according to whether the disease is localised or advanced and is selected according to the age of the patient. Radical prostatectomy or radiation are first-line treatments for localised disease. For more advanced disease GnRH analogues have replaced oestrogen therapy – and to some extent orchidectomy – as first-line hormonal therapy. Antiandrogens and other hormonal drugs are still being investigated as single agents and in combination regimens. Antineoplastic drugs have shown little promise and primarily remain investigational.

References

1. Morley J E. The ageing endocrine system: evaluation and treatment of age-related disorders. *Postgrad Med* 1983; 73: 107–120.
2. Miller M. Type II diabetes: a treatment approach for the older patient. *Geriatrics* 1996; 51: 43–49.
3. Bohannon N J V. Diabetes in the elderly: a unique set of management challenges. *Postgrad Med* 1988; 84: 283–295.
4. Lamberts S W J, van den Beld A W, van der Lely A J. The endocrinology of ageing. *Science* 1997; 278: 419–424.
5. Currie C J, Williams D R R, Peters J R. Patterns of in and out-patient activity for diabetes: a district survey. *Diabetic Med* 1996; 13: 273–280.
6. Benbow S J, Walsh A, Gill G V. Diabetes in institutionalised elderly people: a forgotten population? *BMJ* 1997; 314: 1868–1869.
7. Henry R R, Edelman S V. Advances in treatment of type II diabetes mellitus in the elderly. *Geriatrics* 1992; 47: 24–30.
8. De Sonnaville J J J, Heine R J. Non-insulin dependent diabetes: presentation and treatment. *Medicine* 1997; 25: 23–27.
9. Santiago J V. Monitoring diabetic control. *Medicine* 1997; 25: 27–30.
10. Mooradian A D. Drug therapy of non-insulin dependent diabetes mellitus in the elderly. *Drugs* 1996; 51: 931–941.
11. Scheen A J, Lefèbvre P J. Oral antidiabetic agents: a guide to selection. *Drugs* 1998; 55: 225–236.
12. Bailey C J. Hypoglycaemic and anti-hyperglycaemic drugs for the control of diabetes. *Proc Nutr Soc* 1991; 50: 619–630.
13. Scheen A J. Drug treatments of non-insulin dependent diabetes mellitus in the 1990s: achievements and future developments. *Drugs* 1997; 54: 355–368.
14. Meneilly G S, Elliott T, Tessier A *et al*. NIDDM in the elderly. *Diabetes Care* 1996; 19: 1320–1325.
15. Krentz A J, Ferner R E, Bailey C J. Comparative tolerability profiles of oral antidiabetic agents. *Drug Safety* 1994; 11: 223–241.
16. Shorr R I, Ray W A, Daugherty J R, Griffin M R. Individual sulphonylureas and serious hypoglycaemia in older people. *J Am Geriatr Soc* 1996; 44: 751–755.
17. Langtry H D, Balfour J A. Glimepiride: a review of its use in the management of type 2 diabetes. *Drugs* 1998; 55: 563–584.
18. Campbell R K. Glimepiride: role of a new sulphonylurea in the treatment of type 2 diabetes mellitus. *Ann Pharmacother* 1998; 32: 1044–1052.
19. Williams G. Management of non-insulin dependent diabetes mellitus. *Lancet* 1994; 343: 95–100.
20. Bailey C J. Metformin – an update. *Gen Pharmacol* 1993; 24: 1299–1309.
21. Chalmers J, McBain A M, Brown I R F *et al*. Metformin: its use and contra-indications in the elderly. *Pract Diabetes* 1992; 9: 51–53.
22. Campbell L K, White J R, Campbell R K. Acarbose: its role in the treatment of diabetes mellitus. *Ann Pharmacother* 1996; 30: 1255–1262.
23. Cheatham W W. Repaglinide: a new oral blood glucose-lowering agent. *Clin Diabetes* 1998; 16: 70–72.

24. Wolffenbuttel B H R, Graal M B. New treatments for patients with type 2 diabetes. *Postgrad Med J* 1996; 72: 657–662.
25. Day C. Thiazolidinediones: a new class of antidiabetic drugs. *Diabetic Med* 1999; 16: 179–192.
26. Groop L C, Pelkonen R, Koskimes S *et al.* Secondary failure to treatment with antidiabetic agents in non-insulin dependent diabetes. *Diabetes Care* 1986; 9: 129–133.
27. Wolffenbuttel B H R, Sels J-P J E, Rondas-Colbers G J W M *et al.* Comparison of different insulin regimens in elderly patients with NIDDM. *Diabetes Care* 1996; 19: 1326–1332.
28. Daniel J R, Hagmeyer K O. Metformin and insulin. Is there a role for combination therapy? *Ann Pharmacother* 1997; 31: 474–480.
29. Edwards C R W, Baird J D, Frier B M *et al.* (1995) Endocrine and metabolic diseases. In: Edwards C R W, Bouchier I A D, Haslett C, Chilvers C R, eds. *Davidson's Principles and Practice of Medicine*, 17th edn. Edinburgh: Churchill Livingstone, 1995: 670–774.
30. Macleod A F. Diabetic neuropathy. *Medicine* 1997; 25: 36–38.
31. Diabetes Control and Complications Trial. The effect of intensive treatment of diabetes on the development and progression of long-term complications in insulin dependent diabetes. *N Engl J Med* 1993; 329: 977–986.
32. UK Prospective Diabetes Study Group. Intensive blood-glucose control with sulphonylureas or insulin compared with conventional treatment and risk of complications in patients with type 2 diabetes (UKPDS 33). *Lancet* 1998; 352: 837–853.
33. UK Prospective Diabetes Study Group. Effect of intensive blood-glucose control with metformin in overweight patients with type 2 diabetes (UKPDS 34). *Lancet* 1998; 352: 854–865.
34. Wright J M. Review of the symptomatic treatment of diabetic neuropathy. *Pharmacotherapy* 1994; 14: 689–697.
35. Max M B, Lynch S A, Muir J A *et al.* Effects of desimipramine, amitriptyline and fluoxetine on pain in diabetic peripheral neuropathy. *N Engl J Med* 1992; 326: 1250–1256.
36. Rull J, Quibera R, Gonsalez-Millan H *et al.* Symptomatic treatment of diabetic peripheral neuropathy with carbamazepine: a double-blind cross-over study. *Diabetologica* 1969; 5: 215–220.
37. Backonya M, Baydoun A, Edwards K *et al.* Gabapentin for the symptomatic treatment of painful neuropathy in patients with diabetes mellitus – a randomised controlled trial. *JAMA* 1998; 28: 1831–1836.
38. Tandan R, Lewis A, Badger B. Topical capsaicin in painful diabetic neuropathy. *Diabetes Care* 1992; 15: 8–14.
39. Rumsfield J A, West D P. Topical capsaicin in dermatological and peripheral pain disorders. *Ann Pharmacother* 1991; 25: 381–387.
40. Fusco B M, Giacovazzo M. Peppers and pain. *Drugs* 1997; 53: 909–914.
41. Dejgard A, Petersen P, Kasting J. Mexilitene for the treatment of chronic painful diabetic peripheral neuropathy. *Lancet* 1988; 1: 9–11.
42. Wright J M, Oki J C, Graves L III. Mexiletine in the symptomatic relief of diabetic peripheral neuropathy. *Ann Pharmacother* 1997; 31: 29–34.

43. Stumpf J L, Mitrzyk B. Management of orthostatic hypotension. *Am J Hosp Pharm* 1994; 51: 648–660.
44. Watt S J, Tooke E, Perkins C M, Lee M R. The treatment of orthostatic hypertension: a combined fludrocortisone and flurbiprofen regime. *Q J Med* 1981; 198: 205–212.
45. McTavish D, Goa K L. Midrodrine – a review of its pharmacological properties and therapeutic use in orthostatic hypotension and secondary hypotensive disorders. *Drugs* 1989; 38: 757–777.
46. Rowe P C, Bou-Holaigah I, Kan J S, Calkins H. Is neurally mediated hypotension an unrecognised cause of chronic fatigue? *Lancet* 1995; 345: 623–624.
47. Nilsson P-H. Diabetic gastroparesis: a review. *J Diabetes Complications* 1996; 10: 113–122.
48. Horn J R. Use of prokinetic agents in special populations. *Am J Health-Syst Pharm* 1996; 53 (suppl 3): S27–S29.
49. Snape W J, Battle W M, Schwartz S S et al. Metoclopramide to treat gastroparesis due to diabetes mellitus. *Ann Intern Med* 1982; 96: 444–446.
50. Peeters T, Muls E, Janssens J et al. Effect of motilin on gastric emptying in patients with diabetic gastroparesis. *Gastroenterology* 1992; 102: 97–101.
51. Tack J, Janssens J, Vantrappen G et al. Effect of erythromycin on gastric motility in controls and diabetic gastroparesis. *Gastroenterology* 1992; 103: 72–79.
52. Richards R D, Davenport K, McCallum R W. The treatment of idiopathic and diabetic gastropathy with acute intravenous and oral erythromycin. *Am J Gastroenterol* 1993; 88: 203–207.
53. Clark C M, Lee A D. Prevention and treatment of the complications of diabetes mellitus. *N Engl J Med* 1995; 332: 1210–1217.
54. UK Prospective Diabetes Study Group. Tight blood pressure control and risk of macrovascular and microvascular complications in type 2 diabetes (UKPDS 38). *BMJ* 1998; 317: 703–713.
55. UK Prospective Diabetes Study Group. Efficacy of atenolol and captopril in reducing risk of macrovascular and microvascular complications in type 2 diabetes (UKPDS 39) *BMJ* 1998; 317: 713–720.
56. Wallace K, Hofmann M T. Thyroid dysfunction: how to manage overt and subclinical disease in older patients. *Geriatrics* 1998; 53: 32–41.
57. Rae P, Farrar J, Beckett G et al. Assessment of thyroid status in elderly people. *BMJ* 1993; 307: 177–180.
58. Millar J, Lee A. Drug-induced endocrine disorders. *Pharm J* 1998; 260: 17–21.
59. Mokshagundam S, Barzel U S. Thyroid disease in the elderly. *J Am Geriatr Soc* 1993; 41: 1361–1369.
60. Goldberg T H, Chavin S I. Preventive medicine and screening in older patients. *J Am Geriatr Soc* 1997; 45: 344–354.
61. Campbell A J. Thyroid disorders in the elderly: difficulties in diagnosis and treatment. *Drugs* 1986; 31: 455–461.
62. Kennedy J W, Caro J F. The ABCs of managing hyperthyroidism in the older patient. *Geriatrics* 1996; 51: 22–32.
63. Franklyn J A. Hypothyroidism. *Medicine* 1997; 25: 20–23.

64. Griffin J E. Review: hypothyroidism in the elderly. *Am J Med Sci* 1990; 299: 334–345.
65. Bagchi N, Brown T R, Parish R F. Thyroid dysfunction in adults over the age of 55 years. A study in an urban US community. *Arch Intern Med* 1990; 150: 785–787.
66. Gittoes N J L, Franklyn J A. Hyperthyroidism: current treatment guidelines. *Drugs* 1998; 56: 543–553.
67. Weetman A P. Thyrotoxicosis. *Medicine* 1997; 25: 24–28.
68. Lamberts S W. Non-functioning pituitary tumours and hypopituitarism. *Medicine* 1997; 25: 1–4.
69. Aron D C, Tyrrell J B, Wilson C B. Pituitary tumours: current concepts in diagnosis and management. *West J Med* 1995; 162: 340–352.
70. Kaye T B. Hyperprolactinaemia: causes, consequences and treatment options. *Postgrad Med* 1996; 99: 265–268.
71. Levy A, Lightman S L. Diagnosis and management of pituitary tumours. *BMJ* 1994; 308: 1087–1091.
72. Shimon I, Melmed S. Management of pituitary tumours. *Ann Intern Med* 1998; 129: 472–483.
73. Webster J, Piscitelli G, Polli A *et al.* Comparison of cabergoline and bromocriptine in the treatment of hyperprolactinaemic amenorrhoea. *N Engl J Med* 1994; 331: 904–909.
74. Webster J. A comparative review of the tolerability profiles of dopamine agonists in the treatment of hyperprolactinaemia and inhibition of lactation. *Drug Safety* 1996; 14: 228–238.
75. Ciccarelli E, Grottoli S, Miola C *et al.* Double-blind randomised study using oral or injectable bromocriptine in patients with hyperprolactiaemia. *Clin Endocrinol* 1994; 40: 193–198.
76. Rains C P, Bryson H M, Fitton A. Cabergoline: a review of its pharmacological properties and therapeutic potential in the treatment of hyperprolactinaemia and inhibition of lactation. *Drugs* 1995; 49: 255–279.
77. Webster J, Piscitelli G, Polli A *et al.* Dose-dependent suppression of serum prolactin by cabergoline in hyperprolactinaemia: a placebo controlled, double-blind, multicentre study. *Clin Endocrinol* 1992; 37: 534–541.
78. Webster J, Piscitelli G, Polli A *et al.* The efficacy and tolerability of long-term cabergoline therapy in hyperprolactinaemic disorders: an open uncontrolled, multicentre study. *Clin Endocrinol* 1993; 39: 323–329.
79. Colao A, Di Sano A, Sanacchio F *et al.* Prolactinomas resistant to standard dopamine agonists respond to chronic cabergoline therapy. *J Clin Endocrinol Metab* 1997; 82: 876–883.
80. van der Lely A J, Brownell J, Lamberts S W J. The efficacy and tolerability of CV 205–502 (a non-ergot dopaminergic drug) in macroprolactimoma patients and in prolactinoma patients intolerant to bromocriptine. *J Clin Endocrinol Metab* 1991; 72: 1136–1141.
81. van der Heijden P F M, de Witt W, Brownell J *et al.* CV 205–502, a new dopamine agonist, versus bromocriptine in the treatment of hyperprolactinaemia. *Eur J Obstet Gynaecol Reprod Biol* 1991; 40: 111–118.
82. Klibanski A, Zervas N T. Diagnosis and management of hormone-secreting pituitary adenomas. *N Engl J Med* 1991; 324: 822–831.

83. Wass J A H. Acromegaly. *Medicine* 1997; 25: 5–8.

84. Colao A, Lombardi G. Growth hormone and prolactin excess. *Lancet* 1998; 352: 1455–1461.

85. Melmed S, Jackson I, Kleinberg D *et al*. Current treatment guidelines for acromegaly. *J Clin Endocrinol Metab* 1998; 83: 2646–2652.

86. Jaffe C A, Barkan A L. Acromegaly: recognition and treatment. *Drugs* 1994; 47: 425–445.

87. Colao A, Ferone D, Marzullo P *et al*. Effect of different dopaminergic agents in the treatment of acromegaly. *J Clin Endocrinol Metab* 1997; 82: 518–523.

88. Gillis J C, Noble S, Goa K L. Octreotide long-acting release (LAR): a review of its pharmacological properties and therapeutic use in the management of acromegaly. *Drugs* 1997; 53: 681–699.

89. Davies P H, Stewart S E, Lancranjan I *et al*. Long-term therapy with long-acting octreotide (Sandostatin LAR) for the management of acromegaly. *Clin Endocrinol* 1998; 48: 311–316.

90. Lamberts S W J, de Herder W W, van der Lely A J. Pituitary insufficiency. *Lancet* 1998; 352: 127–134.

91. Howlett T A. An assessment of optimal hydrocortisone therapy. *Clin Endocrinol* 1997; 46: 263–268.

92. Al-Shoumer K A S, Beshyah S A, Niththyananthan R, Johnston D G. Effect of glucocorticoid replacement therapy on glucose tolerance and intermediary metabolites in hypopituitary adults. *Clin Endocrinol* 1995; 42: 85–90.

93. Lamberts S W J, Bruining H A, de Jong F H. Corticosteroid therapy in severe illness. *N Engl J Med* 1997; 337: 1285–1292.

94. Murray F T, Cameron D F, Ketchum C. Return of gonadal function in men with prolactin-secreting tumours. *J Clin Endocrinol Metab* 1984; 59: 79–85.

95. Burris A S, Rodbard H W, Winters S J, Sherins R J. Gonadotrophin therapy in men with isolated hypogonadotrophic hypogonadism: the response to human chorionic gonadotrophins predicted by testicular size. *J Clin Endocrinol Metab* 1988; 66: 1144–1151.

96. de Boer H, Blok G J, van der Veen A E. Clinical aspects of growth hormone deficiency in adults. *Endrocrinol Rev* 1995; 16: 63–86.

97. Bayliss P H. Diabetes insipidus. *Medicine* 1997; 25: 9–11.

98. Anderson J T. $\alpha\text{-}_1$ blockers versus 5α-reductase inhibitors in benign prostatic hyperplasia. *Drugs Aging* 1995; 6: 388–396.

99. Beduschi R, Beduschi M, Oesterling J E. Benign prostatic hyperplasia: use of drug therapy in primary care. *Geriatrics* 1998; 53: 24–40.

100. Jonler M, Riehman M, Bruskewitz R C. Benign prostatic hyperplasia: current pharmacological treatment. *Drugs* 1994; 47: 66–81.

101. Roberts T. Cancer of the prostate gland and bladder. *Medicine* 1995; 23: 475–477.

102. Cooper K L. α-adrenoreceptor antagonists in the treatment of benign prostatic hyperplasia. *Drugs* 1999; 57: 9–17.

103. Guthrie R. Benign prostatic hyperplasia in elderly men. What are the special issues in treatment? *Postgrad Med* 1997; 101: 141–162.

104. Tsang K K, Garraway W M. Prostatism and the burden of benign prostatic hyperplasia on elderly men. *Age Ageing* 1994; 23: 360–364.

105. Oesterling J E. Benign prostatic hyperplasia: medically and minimally invasive treatment options. *N Engl J Med* 1995; 332: 99–109.
106. Geller J, Kirchenbaum A, Lepor H *et al*. Therapeutic controversies: clinical treatment of benign prostatic hyperplasia. *J Clin Endocrinol Metab* 1995; 80: 745–756.
107. Boyle P, Gould A L, Roehrborn C G. Prostate volume predicts outcome of treatment of benign prostatic hyperplasia with finasteride: meta-analysis of randomised clinical trials. *Urology* 1996; 48: 398–405.
108. Gormley G J, Stoner E, Bruskewitz R C *et al*. The effect of finasteride in men with benign prostatic hyperplasia. *N Engl J Med* 1992; 327: 1185–1191.
109. McConnell J D, Bruskewitz R, Walsh P *et al*. The effect of finasteride on the risk of acute urinary retention and the need for surgical treatment among men with benign prostatic hyperplasia. *N Engl J Med* 1998; 338: 557–563.
110. Lee M, Sharifi R. Benign prostatic hyperplasia: diagnosis and treatment guideline. *Ann Pharmacother* 1997; 31: 481–486.
111. Lepor H, Auerbach S, Puras-Baez A *et al*. A randomised, placebo-controlled multicentre placebo-controlled study of the efficacy and safety of terazosin in the treatment of benign prostatic hyperplasia. *J Urol* 1992; 148: 1467–1474.
112. Kaplan S A. Doxazosin in the older male: efficacy in treating benign prostatic hyperplasia. *Eur Urol* 1996; 29 (suppl 1): 17–23.
113. Kaplan S A, Soldo K A, Olsson C A. Terazosin and doxazosin in normotensive men with symptomatic prostatism: a pilot study to determine the effect of dosing regimen on safety and efficacy. *Eur Urol* 1995; 28: 223–228.
114. Fulton B, Wagstaff A J, Sorkin E M. Doxazosin: an update of its clinical pharmacology and therapeutic applications in hypertension and benign prostatic hyperplasia. *Drugs* 1995; 49: 295–320.
115. Wilde M I, McTavish D. Tamsulosin: a review of its pharmacological properties and therapeutic potential in the management of symptomatic benign prostatic hyperplasia. *Drugs* 1996; 52: 883–898.
116. Wilde M I, Fitton A, McTavish D. Alfuzosin: a review of its pharmacodynamic and pharmacokinetic properties and therapeutic potential in benign prostatic hyperplasia. *Drugs* 1993; 45: 410–429.
117. Jardin A, Bensadou H, Delauche-Cavallier H C *et al*. The BPHalf group. Long-term treatment of benign prostatic hyperplasia with alfuzosin; a 24–30 month study. *Br J Urol* 1994; 74: 579–584.
118. Lepor H, Williford W O, Barry M J *et al*. Veterans Affairs Co-operative Studies BPH study group. The efficacy of terazosin, finasteride or both in benign prostatic hyperplasia. *N Engl J Med* 1996; 335: 533–539.
119. Cersosimo R J, Carr D. Prostate cancer: current and evolving strategies. *Am J Health-Syst Pharm* 1996; 53: 381–396.
120. Soloway M S, Chodak G, Vogelzang N J *et al*. Zoladex versus orchidectomy in treatment of advanced prostate cancer: a randomised trial. *Urology* 1991; 37: 46–51.
121. Leuprolide Study Group. Leuprolide versus diethylstilboestrol for metastatic prostate cancer. *N Engl J Med* 1984; 311: 1281–1286.
122. Plosker G L, Brogden R N. Leuprorelin: a review of its pharmacology and therapeutic use in prostatic cancer, endometriosis and other sex hormone-related disorders. *Drugs* 1994; 48: 930–967.

123. Brogden R N, Faulds D. Goserelin: a review of its pharmacodynamic and pharmacokinetic properties and therapeutic efficacy in prostate cancer. *Drugs Aging* 1995; 6: 324–343.

124. Anon. Bicalutamide in advanced prostate cancer: once daily does it. *Drugs Ther Perspect* 1998; 12: 1–5.

125. Goa K L, Spencer C M. Bicalutamide in advanced prostate cancer: a review. *Drugs Aging* 1998; 12: 401–422.

10

Osteoporosis and bone quality in the elderly

Marion Bennie, Janice Harris and Catherine Sedgeworth

Public health perspective

Osteoporosis (OP) is a major health problem, resulting in considerable morbidity, mortality and cost. The primary clinical consequence of osteoporosis is increased susceptibility to bone fracture. At age 70, 50% of women and 20% of men have OP of the spine and hip. By the age of 80, 8% of men and 25% of women will have experienced a fracture of the hip, wrist or spine. Even though spine fracture may not result in hospital admission, pain is often severe and may be associated with increased mortality. The most serious consequence of OP is hip fracture (estimated at 60 000 annually in the UK) which is associated with a 15–20% mortality rate. Hip fracture generally requires a lengthy stay in hospital. Many patients are unable to walk or pursue other routine activities independently again, producing demands on social care resources in the community.

OP currently results in over 200 000 fractures every year, in the UK. This causes severe pain and increased disability and costs the National Health Service over £940 million each year, with £250 million being attributed just to hospital care for hip fracture. Without intervention the number of fractures is set to rise in the future due to an increasing proportion of elderly people in the population. Treatments that are successful in reducing fracture rates will therefore make a valuable contribution to health care. The UK Royal College of Physicians (RCP), recognising the implications, in 1999 produced clinical guidelines for the prevention and treatment of OP[1] which have been a prime source for this chapter.

Bone physiology and pathophysiology

Bone provides both the rigid structure of the skeleton and a reservoir of ions such as calcium, phosphate and magnesium. Variations in plasma ion concentrations outside defined limits can rapidly produce serious defects in homeostatic function. If necessary, plasma ion concentrations are maintained at the expense of bone, as structural integrity is a longer-term issue.

Calcium homeostasis and vitamin D

In humans the major source of vitamin D is the conversion of a precursor in the skin to provitamin D_3, under the influence of sunlight. Dietary vitamin D is found in oily fish and dairy products. Vitamin D_3 (colecalciferol) is subsequently converted through the liver and kidney to 1,25-dihydroxycholecalciferol (calcitriol), the active form of vitamin D (Figure 10.1). Calcitonin, a hormone produced by the thyroid C cells in response to high plasma calcium, decreases plasma calcium by reducing bone resorption and increasing the renal excretion of calcium and phosphate.

The recommended reference nutrient intake (RNI) of calcium in the UK is 700 mg/day for adults aged 19 years or more. This amount is contained in 500 ml of semi-skimmed milk or 100 g of cheddar cheese. In the UK the recommended RNI of vitamin D for people of 65 years of age or over is 400 IU/day. Vitamin D is present in few foods, the best source being fish liver oils, with smaller quantities in butter, eggs, liver, fortified milks and margarines.

Calcium and vitamin D may be low in the housebound elderly due to limited exposure to sunlight; poor dietary intake; and decreased renal function leading to reduced conversion to calcitriol. It has been shown that elderly women in residential homes have low circulating levels of vitamin D and that this is accompanied by a secondary hyperparathyroidism, which worsens over time. It is believed that this may contribute to increased bone fragility in the very old.

Bone structure and remodelling

Bone is a connective tissue composed of a collagenous matrix, with non-collagenous proteins and deposited mineral crystals, mainly hydroxyapatite. The skeleton consists of two types of bone: cortical and trabecular. Cortical or compact bone has a low rate of turnover and is predominantly found in the shafts of the long bones. Trabecular or

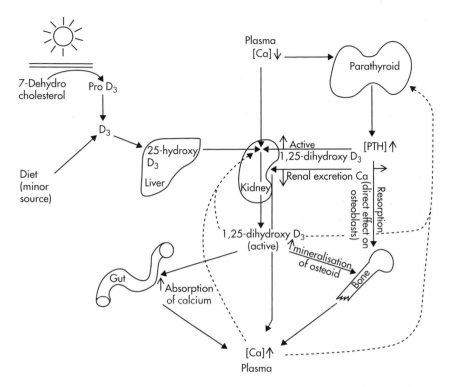

Figure 10.1   Vitamin D and calcium homeostasis. Dashed line = feedback inhibition; PTH = parathyroid hormone.

cancellous bone has a looser honeycomb-like structure and a higher rate of turnover. It is predominant in the vertebra, pelvis, distal forearm and at the end of the long bones, with the spine and distal forearm containing the highest proportion of trabecular bone. Overall, the skeleton contains 80% cortical and 20% trabecular bone.

The skeleton undergoes constant renewal with 25% of trabecular and 2–3% of cortical bone being replaced annually. This process allows for the repair and replacement of damaged bone. Bone renewal is known as remodelling and occurs in millions of discrete bone multicellular units (BMUs) on the bone surface and in cutting cones. The loose meshwork structure of trabecular bone gives it a much larger surface area, resulting in the high turnover rate and a greater sensitivity to metabolic and hormonal changes. Events in the bone remodelling sequence are shown in Figure 10.2 and described below:

1.   Osteoclasts excavate a resorption cavity from quiescent bone surface over a period of 2 weeks (resorption).

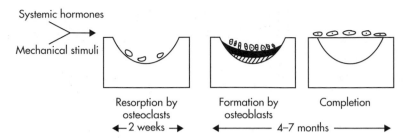

Systemic hormones

Mechanical stimuli

| Resorption by osteoclasts | Formation by osteoblasts | Completion |
| ← 2 weeks → | ← 4–7 months → | |

Figure 10.2 The bone remodelling sequence. Filled area = osteoid; cross-hatched area = calcified new bone. Adapted from Anon. Osteoporosis. *Med Intern* 1994; 22: 209–213.

2.   Osteoblasts are then attracted to the site.
3.   The osteoblasts synthesise uncalcified osteoid matrix to refill the cavity (formation).
4.   Several days later, mineralisation of the osteoid starts and may take several months to complete.

In the young adult there is a balance between bone resorption and formation, termed coupling. However, the process of formation takes longer than resorption, thus at any point in time there is an empty volume of bone representing 0.5–1% of the skeleton. The remodelling process is modified by various systemic hormones and by mechanical stress. The sex steroids oestrogen, progesterone and androgen decrease bone resorption and increase formation. Bone resorption is accelerated by thyroid hormones and parathyroid hormone (PTH). Weight bearing is associated with an increase in bone mass at the loaded site; immobilisation is associated with rapid bone loss.

After the age of 40 there is incomplete refilling of the resorption cavity and a resultant progressive loss of bone mass, accelerated by loss of oestrogen at the menopause. In age-related disease, various factors contribute to bone loss, including reduced osteoblast function (Figure 10.3).

Bone mass throughout life

Peak bone mass is achieved during the third decade of life. Age-related loss of cortical bone starts at 35–40 years and is initially lost at 0.3–0.5% per year in men and women. Cortical bone loss in women accelerates to about 2–3% per year at the menopause for a period of 10 years, before returning to the lower rate. The loss of trabecular bone starts at 30–35 years, with an annual rate of loss of 0.6–2.4% in women and 0.2–1.2% in men. The overall loss of trabecular bone in women is

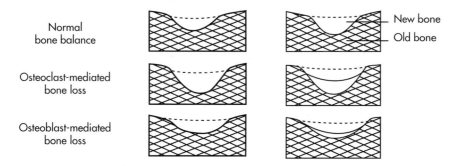

Figure 10.3 The bone-remodelling cycle at the cellular level. In normal young adults (top panels), the bone removed by the osteoclasts (left) is completely replaced by the osteoblasts (right). In osteoclast-mediated bone loss, such as that which occurs in women soon after the menopause, the osteoclasts create a deeper resorption cavity that is not refilled completely. In osteoblast-mediated bone loss, such as that which occurs with ageing, the osteoclasts create a resorption cavity of normal or decreased depth, but the osteoblasts fail to refill it. Adapted from Sagraves R, Letassy N A. Gynaecological disorders. In: Young L Y, Koda-Kimble M A, eds. *Applied Therapeutics. The Clinical Use of Drugs.* Vancouver: Applied Therapeutics, 1995: 46.27–46.38.

35–50% and of cortical bone 25–30% with advancing age, compared to 15–45% and 5–25%, respectively, in men.

Osteoporosis

Definition

In 1994 the World Health Organization described OP as 'a disease characterised by low bone mass and micro-architectural deterioration of bone tissue, leading to enhanced bone fragility and a consequent increase in fracture risk'.[1] The only measurable aspect of this definition is bone mass. Bone mass is assessed indirectly by measurement of bone mineral density (BMD), considered a good indicator of bone mass as long as bone quality is normal. A given BMD is compared to the normal distribution curve for young adult females (Figure 10.4). A T-score is assigned by comparing the measurement with standard deviation (SD) thresholds below the mean of this curve. Two thresholds are used for diagnostic purposes. Measurements between 1.0 and 2.5 SDs below the mean (T-score −1.0 to −2.49) indicate osteopenia, or low bone mass. A BMD decrease of 1.0 SD is associated with a doubling of fracture risk. A T-score of ⩽ −2.5 with documented fragility fracture indicates 'severe' or 'established' OP.

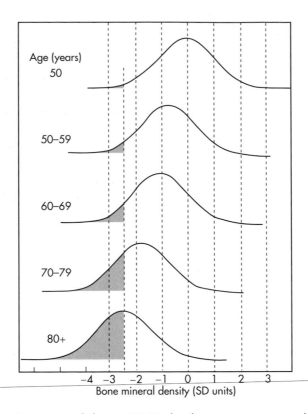

Figure 10.4   Bone mineral density (BMD) distribution in women at different ages and the prevalence of osteoporosis. BMD is normally distributed at all ages, but values decrease progressively with age. The proportion of patients with osteoporosis increases exponentially with age (SD = standard deviation shaded areas = clinical osteoporosis). Reproduced with permission of the Royal College of Physicians. *Osteoporosis: Clinical Guidelines for Prevention and Treatment.* Sudbury, Suffolk: Lavenham Press, 1999.

Diagnostic criteria for men are less well established, but it is thought to be appropriate to compare male BMD measurements to the distribution curve for women, as fracture risk is similar for any given BMD. The use of SD from the mean instead of absolute values of BMD allows direct comparison between different techniques of measurement.

Investigation

BMD can be estimated by a variety of radiographic techniques. Routine X-ray techniques are relatively insensitive, requiring loss of at least 30% of bone mass before changes are observed. They are however used to confirm fracture. More specific predictive techniques are single- and dual-energy photon and X-ray absorptiometry. BMD correlates well with fracture risk but is to some extent dependent on the site of measurement; predictive value is highest at the site of potential fracture. In the elderly, the spine is a relatively poor indicator of fracture risk. The hip is preferred because of the high risk of hip fracture in this group.

The clinical use of biochemical markers for bone formation, e.g. alkaline phosphatase, and bone resorption, e.g. hydroxyproline, has not yet been defined. Routine biochemical and haematological tests are found to be normal in OP, with the exception of alkaline phosphatase which may be raised after a fracture. A patient presenting with fracture will be investigated for other predisposing diseases, e.g. multiple myeloma, metastatic carcinoma and osteomalacia.

Classification and clinical features

OP presents with loss of height, spinal deformity or acute pain secondary to fracture, occurring after minimal trauma. OP can be subdivided into three types: primary osteoporosis type I and type II and secondary osteoporosis. The main features of type I (postmenopausal), and type II (age-related) OP are listed in Table 10.1. Secondary OP is attributed to underlying medical conditions or to drugs (Table 10.2).

Women achieve a lower peak bone mass, lose bone more rapidly than men and live longer, and therefore are much more likely than

Table 10.1 Classification of primary osteoporosis

	Type I	*Type II*
Age at presentation with fracture	51–75	> 70
Gender(female : male)	6 : 1	2 : 1
Type of bone loss	Mainly trabecular	Trabecular and cortical
Rate of bone loss	Accelerated	Not accelerated[a]
Fracture sites	Vertebrae (crush fractures)/ distal radius	Vertebrae (multiple wedge)/hip
Parathyroid function	↓	↑
Calcium absorption	↓	↓
Metabolism of 25OHD$_3$ to 1α, 25(OH)$_2$D$_3$	Secondary ↓	Primary ↓
Main causes	Factors related to the menopause	Factors related to ageing

[a] In the very old there may be accelerated bone loss, particularly at the hip.
Adapted from Riggs B L, Melton L J. The prevention and treatment of osteoporosis. *N Engl J Med* 1986; 314: 1676.

Table 10.2   Common causes of secondary osteoporosis

Medical conditions	Drugs
Cushing's syndrome	Glucocorticoids
Thyrotoxicosis	Excess levothyroxine (thyroxine)
Surgical menopause	Long-term heparin
Male hypogonadism	Antiepileptics
Diabetes mellitus	Cytotoxics
Primary hyperparathyroidism	Excessive alcohol
Liver disease	
Malabsorption	
Prolonged immobilisation	

men to experience osteoporotic fracture. Men who present with a fragility fracture are more likely to have a predisposing condition. Historically, the proportion of patients with OP has increased exponentially with age and has been paralleled by an exponential rise in hip fracture in later life.

Osteomalacia

Definition

Osteomalacia is the adult equivalent of rickets, a condition in which there is inadequate mineralisation of osteoid, leading to 'soft' bones. The common cause is insufficient vitamin D activity. Osteomalacia occurs in 4% of elderly hospitalised patients and in 20% of hip fractures.

Clinical features

Bone pain, aggravated by muscular contraction, presents commonly in the spine, shoulders, ribs and pelvis. Localised pain may be due to undisplaced fracture or pseudofractures. Muscle weakness due to myopathy, which is usually proximal (limb muscles closest to the torso), results in a waddling gait, an inability to climb stairs and to rise out of a chair. Other features include skeletal deformity with the propensity to fracture and occasionally symptoms of tetany related to hypocalcaemia.

Diagnosis

Osteomalacia can occur as a result of lack of vitamin D_3 (privational disease) or as a result of renal or metabolic disease. Here we discuss biochemical changes typical of privational disease. Plasma calcium and phosphate tend to be low and alkaline phosphatase high. Calcium is maintained at the lower end of the normal reference range by a secondary hyperparathyroidism in 50% of patients. Plasma 25-hydroxy D_3, the main circulating form of vitamin D, is low in privational disease.

Characteristic abnormalities on radiography include vertebral deformities and often the 'Looser's zone' or pseudofracture, ribbon-like zones of decalcification which occur most commonly in the thigh, pelvis and ribs. Diagnosis requires elucidation of the cause and exclusion of other diseases or drugs which inhibit mineralisation, e.g. chronic fluoride or inappropriate etidronate ingestion.

Treatment

Treatment is by supplementation with vitamin D, commonly using vitamin D_2 or D_3, except in severe renal or hepatic disease where a metabolite is indicated. Vitamin D_2 and vitamin D_3 are equipotent, while the metabolites calcitriol and 1α-hydroxycholecalciferol (alfacalcidol) are much more potent but have a much shorter duration of action. Simple deficiency is generally treated with doses up to 1000 IU vitamin D_2 or D_3 daily. Alternatively, a single intramuscular injection of 300 000 IU every 6–12 months can be used. In malabsorption syndromes up to 40 000 IU vitamin D_2 or D_3 daily may be required. Generally, the parenteral route is reserved for patients on prolonged parenteral nutrition or with complete resection of the small intestine.

Resolution of muscle weakness generally occurs within a few weeks. Bone pain takes longer, with bone structure remaining abnormal for up to 6 months and thus prone to fracture. Plasma calcium and phosphate return to normal within a few weeks, but alkaline phosphatase (possibly increasing on treatment initiation) and PTH may take several months. Vitamin D doses > 1000 IU daily require regular monitoring of plasma calcium (initially weekly) and whenever nausea and vomiting are present. The section on vitamin D treatment, below, details available types of preparation.

Prevention of osteoporosis

Strategies for prevention of OP follow two main approaches: reduction of risk factors, wherever possible, and drug therapy (principally hormone replacement therapy or HRT). Other drug treatments include bisphosphonates and the selective oestrogen receptor modulators

(SERMs), the first marketed example of which is raloxifene. These are discussed under treatment.

Risk factors

Any factor which adversely affects peak bone mass, hastens the onset of bone loss or increases the rate of bone loss predisposes to the development of OP. The following factors have been identified:

- Genetic: female gender; small body frame; positive family history; caucasian or asiatic ethnicity
- Sex hormone status: menopause (especially early); nulliparity; amenorrhoea, e.g. exercise-induced; oophorectomy (breast feeding is *protective*)
- Lifestyle: cigarette smoking; inactivity; excessive alcohol intake
- Nutritional: lifelong low daily calcium intake; high animal protein intake; caffeine; low body weight

Hormone replacement therapy (HRT)

Mechanism

The exact mechanism through which oestrogens effect a decrease in bone resorption and preserve bone is unclear. It is postulated that direct activation of oestrogen receptors on osteoblasts and osteoclasts results in a decrease in cytokines and other compounds which affect the bone-remodelling process (Figure 10.2). Oestrogens also cause an increase in calcitriol levels.

Clinical effectiveness

The evidence base relating to HRT is extensive and has been examined by the UK Royal College of Physicians (1999)[1] through a systematic review. There is good randomised control trial (RCT) evidence to demonstrate that HRT will preserve BMD, if initiated at the menopause, and the effect is sustained for the duration of therapy. However, the majority of trials are of short duration (1–2 years), prohibiting measurement of impact on clinical outcome. One small ($n = 168$) long-term (10 years) RCT has shown a reduction in frequency of vertebral fractures in women treated with cyclic oestrogen: 7 in control and 0 in HRT group.[3] This evidence is supported by several prospective cohort studies for vertebral and non-vertebral fractures. The effect of stopping HRT is unclear at the moment. Current evidence is contradictory, with some data demonstrating accelerated bone loss, while other data show a decline in bone loss similar to that in untreated patients.

Delayed initiation of HRT after the menopause can still preserve BMD compared to similarly aged controls but will not reverse existing postmenopausal loss. This positive effect on BMD has been shown in all age groups in observational studies but the extent of effect may vary at differing sites. Data on fracture rate in the elderly (type II) patient are as yet inconclusive. One study has shown that HRT in patients aged 75 years or more who commenced HRT before a diagnosis of OP is associated with a reduced forearm and hip fracture rate.[4] The effect on fracture rate in patients with past use of HRT remains contradictory. In the USA a 10-year clinical trial (1993) has commenced in women aged 50–79 which will assist in identifying the benefits of long-term HRT, commenced at and after the menopause, on fracture rate. Consequently, the optimal duration of HRT remains debatable. The UK RCP currently recommends HRT for up to 10 years, with sustained benefit after this but potentially increased risk and thus the need for individual patient assessment.

In addition to the effect on BMD and potential fracture rate, other benefits of HRT require to be recognised: reduction in vasomotor symptoms affecting about 70% of women; possible improvement in psychological and urogenital symptoms; approximate 50% reduction in coronary heart disease (CHD) in women postmenopause; possible 20–60% reduction in death secondary to stroke.

Risks of HRT are principally threefold: endometrial cancer; breast cancer; and venous thromboembolism (VTE). Unopposed cyclic oestrogen causes endometrial hyperplasia, which is negated by the addition of progestogen,[5] but data are still limited in long-cycle and continuous oestrogen use. Risk of breast cancer has undergone several meta-analyses, the most recent in 1997[6] (160 000 women); this study concluded that there was no increased risk with less 5 years' HRT use, beyond which the risk increased (5 years or more risk ratio = 1.35). The authors suggested this would translate to a cumulative risk of breast cancer from age 50 years of: 47 per 1000 (5 years' HRT), 51 per 1000 (10 years' HRT), 57 per 1000 (15 years' HRT) compared to 45 per 1000 for no treatment. Discontinuation of HRT returns the excess risk to baseline risk after 5 years. Data relating to VTE are limited but do suggest a two- to threefold increased risk, translating to 1 additional case of VTE per 3000 users of HRT per year, and the risk of VTE appears to be limited to the first year of HRT.

Patient management issues

Oestrogen preparations used in HRT are mainly 'natural' compounds (estradiol, estrone and estriol) or conjugated oestrogens, which structurally resemble natural oestrogens. The recommended daily doses are: 0.625 mg conjugated oestrogens; 2 mg estradiol; 50 μg transdermal estradiol. Tibolone, a synthetic oestrogen, is the first gonadomimetic licensed for prevention of OP in the UK and has oestrogenic, progestogenic and androgenic activity. Table 10.3 summarises the common preparation types in the UK. Women with an intact uterus must take progestogen to protect against endometrial hyperplasia. Currently, long-cycle and gonadomimetic preparations can only be used in women from 12 months after their last menstrual period. A comprehensive preassessment is essential and should include medication review, as HRT metabolism may be affected by concurrent therapy or may decrease metabolism of other drugs, e.g. corticosteroids and anticoagulants.

Evidence would suggest that there is no difference in clinical effectiveness between oral and transdermal formulations. The most important determinant is the need to select a preparation which is acceptable to the patient, since only 50% of women comply with therapy, mainly discontinuing due to vaginal bleeding (amenable to product selection) and breast tenderness (short-term 1–3 months).[7] Follow-up education/support from practitioners is key to concordance and monitoring for potential complications (at 3 months then 12–18-monthly).

Table 10.3 Types of hormone replacement therapy (HRT) available in the UK

Type[a]	Regimen	Withdrawal bleed
Cyclic	Intermittent oestrogen for 21 of each 28-day cycle	No
Sequential	Continuous oestrogen with progestogen for 10–12 days of each 28-day cycle	Yes, monthly
Long cycle	Continuous oestrogen and progestogen for 10–12 days of each 72-day cycle	Yes, 3-monthly
Continuous	Continuous oestrogen and progestogen	No
Gonadomimetic (synthetic)	Continuous	No

[a] Based on Royal College of Physicians classification.

Treatment of osteoporosis

Calcium

Mechanism

The small increase in plasma calcium produced by administration of calcium salts is thought to reduce circulating PTH and thus bone turnover.

Clinical effectiveness

A 35% reduction in vertebral fracture risk (risk ratio = 0.65; 95% confidence interval 0.48–0.87) has been demonstrated.[8] A reduction in hip fracture risk has also been shown, but is less robust as the data originate from epidemiological studies and may have been influenced by concomitant vitamin D.

The dose of calcium in studies has varied (800–1600 mg/day), with the majority using 1000–1200 mg/day.

The UK RCP recommends an intake of 1000 mg or more elemental calcium daily for treatment of OP in postmenopausal women, but indicates that calcium is not as effective as other bone-specific agents. Calcium use is primarily recommended as an adjunct to other therapy.

Patient management issues

Numerous calcium preparations are available, presently licensed for maintenance of BMD or adjunct treatment in OP, but only high-strength preparations (500–1000 mg elemental calcium) are useful. Calcium carbonate 1.25–2.5 g (chewable/non-chewable tablets and granules) provides 500–1000 mg elemental calcium. Effervescent tablets are also available in differing strengths (400–1000 mg elemental calcium); some provide calcium citrate in solution, which is more easily absorbed than calcium carbonate. Calcium carbonate absorption is dependent on gastric acid secretion, commonly reduced in the elderly, but maximised by administration with meals in divided doses.

Calcium salts are contraindicated in conditions associated with hypercalcaemia and hypercalciuria and used with caution in sarcoidosis and renal impairment (common in the elderly). Plasma calcium and urinary calcium excretion should be monitored regularly; the frequency depends on the plasma calcium level. Studies have not shown significant

Table 10.4 Evidence base for vitamin D in the treatment of osteoporosis (key studies)

Study	Patients entered Mean (SD) years	Regimen/duration	Key findings Fracture rate (%)
Chapuy et al.[9, 10]	$n = 3270$ female Age: 84 (6) years Domicile: care home/apartments for the elderly	T = vitamin D 800 IU/day and calcium 1.2 g/day plus Calcium dietary intake (mean 511 mg/day) C = calcium dietary intake (mean 514 mg/day) Duration: 18 months and 3 years	**Non-vertebral fractures 18 months** T = 11.5%; C = 15.3% Reduction 25%, $p < 0.001$ **3 years** T = 22%; C = 27% Reduction 19%, $p < 0.02$ **Hip fracture** **18 months** T = 5.8%; C = 7.8% Reduction 26%, $P < 0.004$ **3 years** T = 12%; C = 16% Reduction 25%, $P < 0.02$
Lips et al.[11]	$n = 2578$ male/female Age: 80 (6) years Domicile: own home/care home/independent	T = vitamin D 400 IU/day plus Calcium dietary intake (mean 876 mg/day) C = calcium dietary intake (mean 859 mg/day) Duration: 3.5 years	**All fractures** T = 10.5%; C = 9.5% Reduction 10.5%, $P = $ N/A **Hip fracture** T = 3.7%; C = 4.5% Reduction 17.8%, $P = 0.39$

Study	Participants	Regimen	Outcomes
Heikinheimo et al.[12]	n = 799 male/female Age: 86 (N/A) years Own home 79 (N/A) years Care home Domicile: own home/care home	T = vitamin D 150 000 IU annually (intramuscular injection) plus Calcium dietary intake: unknown C = calcium dietary intake: unknown Duration: 2–5 years	**All fractures** T = 16.4%; C = 21.8% Reduction 25%, $P = 0.034$ **Hip fracture** T = 4.4%; C = 9.4% Reduction 42%, $P = 0.18$ **Vertebral fracture** T = 2.3%; C = 1.3% Reduction N/A **Upper limb fracture** T = 2.9%; C = 6.1% Reduction 52%, $P = 0.025$
Dawson-Hughes et al.[13]	n = 389 male/female Age: 71 (N/A) years Domicile: own home	T = vitamin D 700 IU/day and calcium 500 mg/day plus Calcium dietary intake (mean 718 mg/day) C = calcium dietary intake (mean 735 mg/day) Duration: 2–5 years	**Non-vertebral fractures** T = 5.9%; C = 12.9% Reduction 54%, $P = 0.02$ **Hip fracture** T = 0%; C = 0.5% Reduction N/A **Vertebral fracture** T = 0%; C = 0% Reduction N/A
Tilyard et al.[15]	n = 622 female Age: 64 (7) years Postmenopause: 15 (8) years	T = calcitriol 0.25 mg twice daily C = calcium 1000 mg daily Duration: 3 years	**Vertebral fracture** T = 9.9/100 patient-years C = 31.5/100 patient-years Reduction 69%, $P < 0.001$ **Non-vertebral fracture** T = 5%; C = 10% Reduction 50%, $P < 0.05$

T = Treatment regimen; C = control regimen; N/A = no data available.

adverse effects with calcium, though mild gastrointestinal effects may occur.

Vitamin D

Mechanism

Lack of vitamin D, which is common in the house-bound elderly, reduces calcium absorption, producing an increase in PTH and bone loss. Prolonged vitamin D deficiency may also cause osteomalacia, which can be difficult to differentiate from OP in the elderly.

Clinical effectiveness

Calcium and vitamin D trials tend to be the only studies that have specifically examined the very old (>80 years) and the effect on hip fracture (Table 10.4). Good evidence of a 25% reduction in hip fracture rate has been provided in house-bound elderly women given a daily supplement of calcium 1.2 g and vitamin D 800 IU.[9, 10] However, this information may not be generalisable, as another study indicated no effect on hip fracture rate with vitamin D 400 IU (previously shown to reduce PTH) in an independent elderly population with adequate calcium intake.[11] This difference could be attributable to differing baseline populations: in the first studies patients had lower dietary calcium intake and 25-hydroxyD$_3$ plasma levels;[9, 10] the latter included independent patients living at home, and men.[11]

Another study[12] confirmed the effect of vitamin D in reducing fracture incidence overall, although the reduction did not achieve significance for vertebral or hip fractures: this may be due to sample size. A significant reduction in non-vertebral fracture has been reported.[13] Additionally, a large epidemiological study has shown that vitamin D is associated with a 55% reduction in hip fracture amongst elderly women with very low body mass index.[14]

Calcitriol (0.25 mg twice daily – licensed dose for OP in the UK) has been shown to be effective in reducing new vertebral fractures by 69% at 3 years compared to controls (Table 10.4).[15] No reduction in vertebral fractures at 1 year and no benefit in patients with severe OP (more than five vertebral fractures at baseline) was found. No protective effect has been shown for hip fracture to date.

The UK RCP recommends that elderly osteoporotic women should be offered treatment with calcium and vitamin D. It also states that parenteral vitamin D, with or without calcium supplements, decreases the risk of hip and other fractures in the frail elderly.

Patient management issues

At present, there are no solid oral dose preparations available in the UK which contain vitamin D alone in physiological doses, e.g. 400 IU. Calcium and ergocalciferol tablets contain a small amount of elemental calcium (97 mg/tablet) and vitamin D_2 (400 IU/tablet). Higher-strength combined calcium preparations are available: 500–600 mg of elemental calcium and 400 IU of vitamin D_3. All calcium and vitamin D tablets should be chewed or crushed before swallowing. Effervescent granules (500 mg of elemental calcium/440 IU of vitamin D_3), an oily calciferol solution and an intramuscular injection of vitamin D are available if swallowing difficulties are evident.

Patient monitoring is as for calcium therapy, with the theoretical possibility of hypercalcaemia (not observed in trials). An exception is for calcitriol, which requires serum calcium and creatinine monitoring at 4 weeks, 3 months, 6 months and thereafter 6-monthly. Other vitamin preparations containing vitamin D, e.g. multivitamins or cod-liver oil should not be taken concurrently. Vitamin D is fat-soluble, stored in adipose tissue and dependent on the presence of bile for adequate intestinal absorption. Consequently, absorption may be reduced in individuals with impaired fat absorption.

Bisphosphonates

In the UK there are currently three bisphosphonates licensed for the prevention and treatment of postmenopausal and corticosteroid-induced OP: etidronate (Didronel PMO), alendronate (Fosamax) and risedronate (Actonel). Alendronate can be given daily (10 mg) or weekly (70 mg) for the treatment of OP.

Mechanism

Bisphosphonates have a high affinity for hydroxyapatite which forms part of the mineral phase of mature bone. The bisphosphonate bone complex formed is thought to reduce osteoclast adherence to bone and when phagocytosed inhibits osteoclast activity, preventing further bone resorption. There may be slight differences between bisphosphonates but their overall effect is to reduce osteoclast activity, causing a decrease

Table 10.5 Evidence base (randomised controlled trial) for bisphosphonate in the treatment of osteoporosis (key studies)

Study	Patients entered Mean (range) years	Regimen/duration	Key findings BMD (mean values) Fracture rate (%)
Storm et al.[17] Postmenopausal women with 1–4 vertebral fractures	$n = 66$ Age: 68 (56–75) years Postmenopause: 22 (6–35) years	T = 15-week cycle: etidronate 400 mg daily for 14 days followed by calcium and vitamin D as for control C = calcium 500 mg and vitamin D 400 IU/day Duration: 150 weeks (10 cycles)	**Spine BMD (from baseline)** T = +5.3%; C = −2.7% Difference = +8% (CI 2.4%, 13.6%), $P < 0.01$ **New vertebral fracture** **Baseline to week 150** T = 18/100 patient-years; C = 43/100 patient-years Reduction 52%, $P > 0.05$ **Week 60 to week 150** T = 6/100 patient-years; C = 54/100 patient-years Reduction 89%, $P = 0.023$
Watts et al.[18] Postmenopausal women with 1–4 vertebral fractures	$n = 429$ Age: 65 years (6 > 75 years) Postmenopause: 18 (N/A) years	13-week cycle: Phosphate 1 g twice daily for 3 days, then Etidronate 400 mg daily for 14 days, then calcium 500 mg daily for remainder of cycle Four groups (all had calcium): T1 = placebo/etidronate T2 = phosphate/etidronate C1 = placebo/placebo C2 = phosphate/placebo Duration: 2 years (8 cycles)	**BMD (from baseline)** **Spine** T1 = +4.2%; T2 = +5.2%; C1 = +1.3% Difference $P < 0.01$ **Greater trochanter** T1 = +3.4%, $P < 0.017$ **New vertebral fracture (from baseline)** T1 + T2 = 29.5/1000 patient-years C1 + C2 = 62.9/1000 patient-years Reduction 53%, $P > 0.05$ **Subgroup with low bone mass at baseline** T1 + T2 = 42.3/1000 patient-years; $n = 101$ C1 + C2 = 132.7/1000 patient-years; $n = 87$ Reduction 67% ($P = 0.004$)

| Liberman et al.[22] Postmenopausal women with/without fracture and BMD ≤2.5 SD | $n = 881$ Age: 64 (45–80) years Postmenopause: 16 (N/A) years | T1 = 5 mg alendronate daily T2 = 10 mg alendronate daily T3 = 20 mg alendronate reduced to 5 mg daily in year 3 T1, T2 and T3 also received calcium 500 mg C = calcium 500 mg/day Duration: 3 years | **BMD (from baseline)** **Spine** Difference (T2 vs C) = +8.8% (SE ± 0.4%), $P < 0.001$ **Femoral neck** Difference (T2 vs C) = +5.9% (SE ± 0.5%), $P < 0.001$ **Trochanter** Difference (T2 vs C) = +7.8% (SE ± 0.6%), $P < 0.001$ **Total body** Difference (T2 vs C) = +2.2% (SE ± 0.4%), $P < 0.001$ **New vertebral fracture (from baseline)** T (pooled) = 3.2%; C = 6.2% Reduction 48%, $P = 0.03$ |
| Black et al.[23] Postmenopausal women with vertebral fracture and BMD ≤2.1 SD (Fracture Intervention Study) | $n = 2027$ Age: 71 (51–81) 539 patients 75–81 years | T = 5 mg alendronate daily for 2 years then 10 mg in year 3 C = supplement of calcium and vitamin D if required 82% of patients in each group received calcium 500 mg and vitamin D 250 IU after dietary assessment Duration: 3 years | **BMD (from baseline)** **Spine** Difference = +6.2%, $P < 0.001$ **Femoral neck** Difference = +4.1%, $P < 0.001$ **Trochanter** Difference = +6.1%, $P < 0.001$ **Total hip** Difference = +4.7%, $P < 0.001$ **Total body** Difference = +1.8%, $P < 0.001$ **New vertebral fracture (from baseline)** T = 2.3%; C = 5.0% Reduction 55%, $P < 0.001$ **New hip fracture** T = 1.1%; C = 2.2% Reduction 51%, $P = 0.047$ **New wrist fracture** T = 2.2%; C = 4.1% Reduction 48%, $P = 0.013$ |

BMD = Bone mineral density; T = treatment regimen; C = control regimen; N/A = no data available; CI = 95% confidence interval; SE = standard error of the mean.

in the number of new bone modelling units and the depth of the erosion cavities. Continuous etidronate use has been shown to have a negative effect on bone mineralisation and may induce osteomalacia.[16] It is therefore used sequentially with oral calcium, for example, as Didronel PMO: 14 days of etidronate is followed by 76 days of calcium.

Clinical effectiveness

Etidronate   Etidronate, used cyclically, has been shown to increase BMD in the spine ($P < 0.05$). The evidence at other sites is less robust but the increase in spine BMD is not at the expense of other sites. A 50% reduction in vertebral fracture rate has been demonstrated with cyclical etidronate. The two key trials[17, 18] conducted in postmenopausal women (mainly type 1 OP) with between one and four vertebral crush fractures are presented in Table 10.5. The rate of new vertebral fracture was lower[18] as the recruited patients had a higher BMD and fewer fractures at baseline. Extension to 3–5 years of these two studies has demonstrated that spine BMD continued to increase with a continued reduction in new vertebral fracture rate.[19–21] Biopsy data showed no evidence of development of osteomalacia or defective bone mineralisation. These studies however have failed to find a statistically significant reduction in non-vertebral fracture, probably due to low numbers of patients and fractures, but a postmarketing study of etidronate users ($n = 7977$) with matched controls has demonstrated a decrease of 34% in hip fracture rate with etidronate treatment ($P < 0.05$).

Alendronate   Trials have been conducted with alendronate 5–40 mg/ day but the evidence suggests that there is no advantage in using daily doses higher than 10 mg. Alendronate has been shown to increase BMD in the spine and hip ($P < 0.001$) and to reduce the incidence of new vertebral and hip fracture by 50% in women with low BMD[22, 23] (Table 10.5). A similar benefit was reported after only 1 year of therapy in women with low BMD.[24] Women with higher BMD given 4 years of alendronate did not have a reduced incidence of clinical fracture.[25]

Patient management issues

The bisphosphonates are all poorly absorbed orally and bioavailability is greatly reduced if taken with any calcium-containing substances (food, liquids or medicines). Etidronate is usually taken in the middle of a 4 hour fast and should only be swallowed with water. Alendronate is intended to be taken on rising in the morning with water and the patient informed to remain upright after swallowing to decrease the risk of oesophageal ulceration. Adherence to these directions is essential to attain patient benefit. Any underlying vitamin D deficiency should be recognised and corrected in patients commenced on etidronate. Adequate calcium intake, often from supplementation, is necessary when using alendronate. Etidronate is contraindicated in patients who have severe renal impairment, i.e. glomerular filtration rate less than 10 ml/min. Alendronate is not recommended when the glomerular filtration rate is less than 35 ml/min.

Raloxifene

Raloxifene is the first licensed SERM. It is indicated for the prevention and treatment of OP in postmenopausal women.[26]

Mechanism

Raloxifene demonstrates oestrogen agonist activity in bone, resulting in decreased bone resorption. Oestrogen antagonist activity is shown in breast and uterine tissue, with 3-year data showing no increased risk of developing endometrial cancer and a significant risk reduction for oestrogen receptor-positive invasive breast cancer.[27] Serum cholesterol is reduced but no cardioprotective effect has been demonstrated to date.[28]

Clinical effectiveness

Raloxifene 60 mg/day increases BMD of the spine and hip by 2% at 2 years.[29] Interim 2-year results from the MORE study ($n = 7705$, mean age 66 years, postmenopause mean 8 years) indicate a reduction in new vertebral fracture (34% and 42% in women with and without previous vertebral fracture) but not in non-vertebral fracture. All participants received calcium 500 mg and vitamin D 400 IU.[30]

Patient management issues

Raloxifene is associated with an increased risk of VTE compared to placebo (risk ratio = 2.49; 95% confidence intervals 1.23–5.02).[29] Treatment is associated with an increased incidence of hot flushes and leg cramps. Raloxifene is contraindicated in patients with hepatic impairment as it is metabolised primarily by the liver and plasma concentrations can multiply by up to 2.5. It is contraindicated in severe renal impairment. Supplementation is advised if dietary calcium intake is low.

Calcitonin

In the UK, calcitonin (salmon) injection (salcatonin) is licensed for short-term use in postmenopausal OP and for metastatic bone pain, although it has been used successfully for vertebral fracture bone pain. Intranasal calcitonin is licensed for treatment of OP in other countries, but only for named patients in the UK at present.

Mechanism

Calcitonin decreases bone resorption. Calcitonin (salmon) (salcatonin) is 50 times more potent than human calcitonin. Antibody formation may occur in patients on long-term therapy but is unlikely to affect efficacy.

Clinical effectiveness

Studies using injectable and, more recently, intranasal calcitonin (salmon) (salcatonin) have demonstrated a modest increase in spinal BMD. A dose–response of 1% increase has been demonstrated in spinal BMD per 100 IU calcitonin (salmon) (salcatonin) intranasal (plus 500 mg calcium), but little evidence found of preserved BMD at cortical sites, except with large doses after 2 years.[31] A reduction in vertebral fracture rate was also found in women with OP from pooled treatment data (68% reduction, $P = 0.027$).[31]

Patient management issues

Hypersensitivity reactions may occur, although they are rare, and often limited to the injection site; very occasionally there can be anaphylactic shock. Skin testing (1 : 100 dilution) is advised in patients with a history of systemic allergic reaction. Calcitonin (salmon) (salcatonin) should not reduce plasma calcium below the normal reference range. Supplementation is advised if dietary calcium and vitamin D intake is low.

Other treatments

Fluoride

There are no fluoride salts currently licensed in the UK for the management of OP. Fluoride is incorporated into bone-forming fluorapatite crystals, which are of different size and structure to hydroxyapatite crystals. Fluorapatite crystals are less soluble, thus producing reduced bone resorption. Bone density is increased but the quality and strength of the bone may depend on adequate calcium and vitamin D intake. Studies have shown an increase in bone mass and the ability to reduce vertebral fractures, but not hip fracture.

Corticosteroid-induced osteoporosis

It is estimated that 250 000 people in the UK (0.5%) take long-term oral corticosteroids. Although the incidence of corticosteroid-induced OP (CIOP) is unknown, subsequent fracture is estimated to be 30–50%, complicated by underlying disease and independent patient risk factors for OP. In one study (eight general practices) only 14% of women, aged 55 years or more and on oral corticosteroid for 3 months, received preventive treatment for CIOP. Corticosteroid therapy produces a reduction in bone mass and BMD which is more pronounced on trabecular bone. Bone loss is most rapid in the first 6–12 months of therapy, may continue at two to three times normal in older patients, and is dependent upon the dose and duration of corticosteroid. The exact threshold dose is unknown; however, oral prednisolone 7.5 mg or more, or equivalent, for more than 6 months is considered to have a clinical impact. Lower oral doses, including alternate-day dosing, and inhaled preparations do increase bone loss but the clinical impact remains unclear.

Mechanism

Corticosteroids affect bone structure through several complex mechanisms which principally alter calcium homeostasis (reduction in calcium absorption and increase in urinary calcium excretion); sex hormones (suppression of testosterone and oestrogen production); bone formation (reduction of osteoblast proliferation and activity); and muscle strength (myopathy and weakness reduce force on bone).

Clinical effectiveness

In 1998 a UK Consensus Group on the management of CIOP published a summary of the main studies.[32] In general, data are limited to small studies (20–60 patients per group), short duration (1–2 years), wide age

Table 10.6 Evidence base in primary prevention of corticosteroid-induced osteoporosis for etidronate and calcitriol (key studies)

Study	Patients entered Age: range Dose: mean	Regimen/duration	Key findings BMD (mean values) Fracture rate (%)
Adachi et al.[33] Patients with chronic inflammatory condition	n = 141 Age: 31–87 years 70 patients postmenopause Corticosteroid dose* Entry: 21–23 mg daily 1 year: 11–13 mg daily	T = 13-week cycle: etidronate 400 mg for 14 days followed by calcium 500 mg/day C = calcium 500 mg/day Duration: 1 year (three cycles)	**BMD (from baseline)** **Spine** T = +0.6%; C = −3.2% Difference = +3.8%, P = 0.02 **Trochanter** T = +1.5%; C = −2.7% Difference = +4.2%, P = 0.02 **Femoral neck and radius** Difference = P > 0.05
Roux et al.[34] Patients with chronic inflammatory condition	n = 117 Age: 18–90 years Corticosteroid dose* Entry: 17–18 mg daily 1 year: 11 mg daily	T = 13-week cycle: etidronate 400 mg for 14 days followed by calcium 500 mg/day C = calcium 500 mg/day Duration: 1 year (three cycles)	**BMD (from baseline)** **Spine** T = +0.3%; C = −2.8% Difference = +3.1%, P = 0.004 **Femoral neck** Difference = P > 0.05 **Trochanter** Difference = P > 0.05

Saag et al.[35] Patients with chronic inflammatory condition (subset of larger study)	n = 151 Age: 17–83 years Corticosteroid dose* Entry: Median 10 mg daily 48 weeks: Median 9 mg daily	T1 = 5 mg alendronate daily T2 = 10 mg alendronate daily T1 + T2 also received calcium and vitamin D as for control C = 800–1000 mg calcium and vitamin D 250–500 IU/day Duration: 48 weeks	Spine BMD (from baseline) T1 = +1.4%; T2 = +3.0%; C = −1.0% Difference = $P > 0.05$
Sambrook et al.[36] Patients with chronic inflammatory condition	n = 103 Age: 18–79 years 38 patients postmenopause Corticosteroid dose* Entry: 25 mg daily 1 year: 14 mg daily 2 years: 7.5 mg daily	T1 = calcitriol 0.5–1 µg/day + calcitonin (salmon) (salcatonin) nasal spray 400 IU + calcium 1000 mg daily T2 = calcitriol + calcium C = calcium Duration: 1 year treatment 1 year follow-up	BMD (from baseline) At 1 year Spine T1 = −0.2; T2 = −1.3; C = −4.3 Difference (T1 vs C), $P = 0.001$ Difference (T2 vs C), $P = 0.026$ Femoral neck and radius Difference = $P > 0.05$ At 2 years Spine T1 = +0.7; T2 = −3.6; C = −2.3 Difference (T1 vs C), $P = 0.17$ Difference (T2 vs C), $P = 0.94$ Femoral neck and radius Difference = $P > 0.05$

BMD = Bone mineral density; T = treatment regimen; C = control regimen.
*Corticosteroid dose = prednisolone or equivalent dose daily.

range (18–90 years) and have BMD as the clinical outcome. No studies have had the power to examine fracture rate.

Primary prevention of CIOP

The evidence is strongest – though still sparse – for an increase in spine BMD with the bisphosphonates. Most data are available on etidronate, although alendronate, pamidronate and clodronate data are emerging and expected to produce similar results (Table 10.6). Calcitriol data are limited but suggest some potential benefit. Calcium and vitamin D have not been shown to improve BMD, although calcium alone or with vitamin D is often used as adjunct therapy. Fluoride and calcitonin (salmon) (salcatonin) (intranasal and subcutaneous) in small studies have shown a variable effect on BMD and require further study. To date, no HRT studies have been conducted.

Secondary prevention or treatment

There is good evidence that etidronate, pamidronate and alendronate increase BMD in CIOP. Spine BMD has shown a 3–6% increase from baseline after 1–2 years of treatment, but the impact on femoral neck BMD remains controversial. HRT has been examined in two small studies, both demonstrating an increase in spine BMD, 4.1% and 2.2%, from baseline compared to a loss in spine BMD of 3.4% and 1.2%, respectively in control groups over a 1–2-year period. In one study testosterone use in males on long-term corticosteroids (mean 8 years) increased spine BMD by 5%, from baseline, at 1 year. Fluoride therapy has demonstrated an increase in spine BMD in small studies. A small study of intranasal calcitonin (salmon) (salcatonin) plus calcium has shown increased spine BMD, 2.7% from baseline at 1 year compared to a loss of 2.8% in a control group. Evidence for calcitriol and calcium with vitamin D is currently lacking.

Patient management issues

In 1998 the National Osteoporosis Society published guidance on the prevention and management of CIOP to be considered for all patients (excluding transplant patients) on an oral dose of 7.5 mg of prednisolone or its equivalent or more per day, or equivalent, for more than 6 months. Figure 10.5 presents a distillation of this guidance, tailored for an elderly population. Firstly, it is essential to confirm that

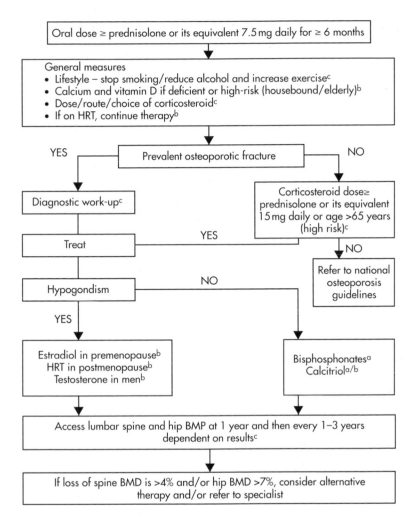

Figure 10.5 Prevention and management of corticosteroid-induced osteoporosis. Diagnostic work-up to exclude secondary causes (myeloma, endocrinologies, osteomalacia, malabsorption, hypogonadism). [a]Grade A: based on meta-analysis or at least one randomised controlled trial. [b]Grade B: based on at least one well-designed, but not necessarily controlled study, including case control and comparative studies. [c]Grade C: based on expert reports or opinion. HRT = Hormone replacement therapy; BMD = bone mineral density.

a corticosteroid is required and, if so, at the lowest effective dose. Deflazacort and budesonide may have less effect on BMD, but this requires confirmation in further studies. Calcitriol is not licensed and requires regular calcium monitoring. It must always be remembered that corticosteroid use is only one factor in the risk assessment for OP

Case study 10.1 A 66-year-old Caucasian woman (55 kg) presents to the community pharmacy seeking advice on use of calcium to prevent osteoporosis (OP)

Family history	Mother had hip fracture
Past medical history	Ischaemic heart disease (myocardial infarction 2 years ago); menopause aged 55 years
Drug history	HRT: used 10 years ago for 6 months but did not tolerate withdrawal bleeds and unclear about cancer risk; aspirin 150 mg/day; atenolol 50 mg/day
Social history	Independent, living alone; smoker; no children

Risk assessment for OP	Additional data required
PMH (mother: hip fracture)	(liaison with general practitioner)
Smoker	Renal function: 70 ml/min (GFR)
Postmenopause (11 years)	No reduced stature or kyphosis
No children	No disease/drugs predisposing to OP
	BMD measurement (desirable)

Pharmaceutical care issues
- Advice on smoking cessation
- Promote regular exercise and avoidance of excessive alcohol intake
- Ensure adequate dietary calcium intake (700 mg/day) and vitamin D (400 IU/day)
- Discuss with patient and general practitioner osteoporosis prevention drug therapy (see below): HRT considered first-line unless patient has concerns
- If BMD establishes OP therapeutic options are:
    — Calcium (> 1 g/day)
    — Bisphosphonate
    — Raloxifene

Drug therapy choice	Cautions	Compliance issues	Benefits[a]
HRT: continuous	Cancer: endometrial/ breast VTE	Possible bleeds	Cardioprotective (50% reduction in coronary heart disease) Possible stroke prevention
Bisphosphonate	Osteomalacia	Complex regimen Gastrointestinal side-effects	
Raloxifene	VTE		Possible reduced cholesterol Risk reduction in invasive breast cancer

[a] All three choices have similar effectiveness data on BMD.
HRT = Hormone replacement therapy; PMH = past medical history; BMD = bone mineral density; VTE = venous thromboembolism.

Case study 10.2   An 80-year-old woman (45 kg) is admitted to hospital after a fall at home. A stroke is diagnosed, aspirin 75 mg/day prescribed and rehabilitation initiated. She is to be discharged home but has restricted mobility, which is likely to result in her being primarily house-bound

Family history	Nil
Past medical history	Menopause aged 53 years; polymyalgia rheumatica (7 years); wrist fracture (3 years ago); kyphosis
Drug history (at discharge)	Prednisolone 2 mg daily (5 years); aspirin 75 mg daily
Social history	Lives alone; home help twice weekly

Risk assessment for osteoporosis (OP)	Additional data required (from medical notes)
• PMH (fracture/kyphosis)	• Vitamin D level: 15 nmol/l (reference range: 15–100 nmol/l)
• Steroid long-term (low dose)	• Renal function: GFR = 45 ml/min
• Reduced mobility (partially housebound)	• No other disease/drugs predisposing to OP (except steroid)
• Low body weight	

Pharmaceutical care issues
- Advice on avoidance of falls (liaise with occupational therapist)
- Review need for steroid for polymyalgia rheumatica
- Discuss with patient (and general practitioner) OP prevention drug therapy (see below) – calcium (> 1 g/day) and vitamin D (800 IU/day) first-line

Drug therapy choice	Cautions	Compliance issues	Benefits[a]
Calcium and vitamin D		Unpleasant taste with some formulations Possible gastrointestinal upset	Reduced fracture rate (25%)
Calcitriol	Hypercalcaemia Impaired renal function		Reduced vertebral fracture rate (50%) in younger population (no information on hip)
Bisphosphonate	Osteomalacia	Complex regimen Gastrointestinal side-effects	Some studies in elderly show effective increase in BMD (power too small to demonstrate fracture effect)

[a] All three choices have similar effectiveness data on BMD.
PMH = Past medical history; GFR = glomerular filtration rate; BMD = bone mineral density.

prevention and treatment. The elderly will commonly have other risk factors that trigger management.

Osteoporosis in men

OP is less common in men (about 1 in 12), possibly due to higher peak bone mass, reduced loss during ageing and shorter life expectancy. However, men still account for 15% of symptomatic vertebral and 20% of hip fractures. The pathophysiology is similar to postmenopausal OP. Decreased testosterone levels are associated with increased fracture risk, though the mechanism is not clearly defined. Relatively few studies specifically examine the prevention and treatment of male idiopathic OP. Consequently, men should initially be investigated for secondary causes (more prevalent in men) and subsequently managed similarly to women, with the exception of hypogonadism. Treatment options include bisphosphonates, testosterone, fluoride, calcium and vitamin D. Cyclical etidronate has been shown to increase spine BMD but the impact on fracture rate remains unclear. Studies are ongoing with the other bisphosphonates. Testosterone increases spine BMD in hypogonadal men and may also have a beneficial effect on eugonadism. The effect of testosterone on cardiovascular risk appears to be neutral in the short term but longer-term studies are needed. Testosterone should not be used in prostatic cancer. Preliminary results of intermittent fluoride (15 mg/day for 3 months out of 4) and calcium (1000 mg/day) appear promising. Treatment effect with calcium and vitamin D remains unclear (there is a modest effect on BMD with or without change in fracture rate), possibly due to a variable dose of vitamin D and calcium supplementation.

Acknowledgement

We wish to thank Dr Elizabeth MacDonald, Consultant Physician, Care of the Elderly, Lothian University Hospitals NHS Trust, for advice and clinical review of the chapter.

References

1. Royal College of Physicians. *Osteoporosis – Clinical Guidelines for Prevention and Treatment*. Sudbury, Suffolk: Lavenham Press, 1999.
2. Kanis J A. *Textbook of Osteoporosis*. Oxford: Blackwell Science, 1996.

3. Nachtigall L E, Nachtigall R H, Nachtigall R D *et al*. Estrogen replacement therapy I: a 10-year prospective study in the relationship to osteoporosis. *Obstet Gynecol* 1979; 53: 277–281.

4. Cauley J A, Seley D G, Ensrud K *et al*. Estrogen replacement therapy and fractures in older women. *Ann Intern Med* 1995; 122: 9–16.

5. Grady D, Gebretsadik T, Kerlikowska K *et al*. Hormone replacement therapy and endometrial cancer risk: a meta-analysis. *Obstet Gynecol* 1995; 85: 304–313.

6. Collaborative group on hormonal factors in breast cancer. Breast cancer and hormone replacement therapy: collaborative reanalysis of data from 51 epidemiological studies of 52 705 women with breast cancer and 108 411 women without breast cancer. *Lancet* 1997; 350: 1047–1059.

7. Anon. Fracture prevention in elderly women. *Prescriber Int* 1998; 7: 155–159.

8. Kanis J A. The use of calcium in the management of osteoporosis. *Bone* 1999; 24: 279–290.

9. Chapuy M C, Arlot M E, Duboeuf F *et al*. Vitamin D_3 and calcium to prevent hip fractures in elderly women. *N Engl J Med* 1992; 327: 1637–1642.

10. Chapuy M C, Arlot M E, Delmas P D *et al*. Effect of calcium and cholecalciferol treatment for three years on hip fractures in elderly women. *BMJ* 1994; 308: 1081–1082.

11. Lips P, Wilco C G, Ooms M *et al*. Vitamin D supplementation and fracture in elderly persons. *Ann Intern Med* 1996; 124: 400–406.

12. Heikinheimo R J, Inkovaara J A, Harju E J *et al*. Annual injection of vitamin D and fractures of aged bones. *Calcif Tissue Int* 1992; 51: 105–110.

13. Dawson-Hughes B, Harris S S, Krall E A *et al*. Effect of calcium and vitamin D supplementation on bone density in men and women 65years of age or older. *N Engl J Med* 1997; 337: 670–676.

14. Ramstam J, Kanis J A. Influence of age and body mass on the effect of vitamin D on hip fracture risk. *Osteoporosis Int* 1995; 5: 450–454.

15. Tilyard M W, Spears G F S, Thomson J *et al*. Treatment of postmenopausal osteoporosis with calcitriol or calcium. *N Engl J Med* 1992; 326: 357–362.

16. Adami S, Zamberlan N. Adverse effects of bisphosphonates: a comparative review. *Drug Safety* 1996; 14: 158–170.

17. Storm T, Thamsburg G, Steiniche T *et al*. Effect of intermittent cyclical etidronate therapy on bone mass and fracture rate in women with postmenopausal osteoporosis. *N Engl J Med* 1990; 322: 1265–1271.

18. Watts N B, Harris S T, Genant H K *et al*. Intermittent cyclical etidronate treatment of postmenopausal osteoporosis. *N Engl J Med* 1990; 323: 73–79.

19. Storm T, Kollerup G, Thamsborg G *et al*. Five year clinical experience with intermittent cyclical etidronate for postmenopausal osteoporosis. *J Rheumatol* 1996; 23: 1560–1564.

20. Harris S T, Watt N B, Jackson R D *et al*. Four-year study of intermittent cyclic etidronate treatment of postmenopausal osteoporosis: three years of blinded therapy followed by one year of open therapy. *Am J Med* 1993; 95: 557–567.

21. Watts N B, Miller P D, Licata A A *et al*. Seven years of cyclical etidronate: continued improvement in spine BMD and progressive decline in vertebral fracture incidence. *Bone* 1995; 17: 617.

22. Liberman U A, Weiss S R, Broll J et al. Effect of oral alendronate on bone mineral density and the incidence of fractures in postmenopausal osteoporosis. *N Engl J Med* 1995; 333: 1437–1443.

23. Black D M, Cummings S R, Karpf D B. Randomised trial of effect of alendronate on risk of fracture in women with existing vertebral fractures. *Lancet* 1996; 348: 1535–1541.

24. Pols H A P, Felsenberg D, Hanley D A et al. Multinational, placebo controlled, randomized trial of the effects of alendronate on bone density and fracture risk in postmenopausal women with low bone mass: results of the FOSIT study. *Osteoporosis Int* 1999; 9: 461–468.

25. Cummings S R, Black D M, Thompson D E et al. Effect of alendronate on risk of fracture in women with low bone density but without vertebral fractures. *JAMA* 1998; 280: 2077–2082.

26. Anon. Raloxifene to prevent postmenopausal osteoporosis. *Drug Ther Bull* 1999; 37: 33–40.

27. Cummings S R, Eckert S, Krueger K A et al. The effect of raloxifene on risk of breast cancer in post-menopausal women: results from the MORE randomised trial. Multiple Outcomes of Raloxifene Evaluation. *JAMA* 1999; 281: 2189–2197.

28. Walsh B W, Kuller L H, Wild R A et al. Effects of raloxifene on serum lipids and coagulation factors in healthy post-menopausal women. *JAMA* 1998; 279: 1445–1451.

29. *Raloxifene. ABPI Compendium of Data Sheets and Summaries of Product Characteristics*. London. Datapharm, 1999–2000.

30. Ettinger B, Black D M, Knickerbocker R K et al. Reduction of vertebral fracture risk in postmenopausal women with osteoporosis treated with raloxifene: results from a 3-year randomized clinical trial. Multiple Outcomes of Raloxifene Evaluation (MORE) investigators. *JAMA* 1999; 282: 637–645.

31. Overgaard K, Hansen M A, Jensen S B, Christiansen C. Effect of salcatonin given intranasally on bone mass and fracture rates in established osteoporosis: a dose–response study. *BMJ* 1992; 305: 556–561.

32. National Osteoporosis Society (NOS). *Guidance on the Prevention and Management of Corticosteroid Induced Osteoporosis*. Bath: NOS, 1998.

33. Adachi J D, Bensen W G, Brown J. Intermittent etidronate therapy to prevent corticosteroid-induced osteoporosis. *N Engl J Med* 1997; 337: 382–387.

34. Roux C, Oriente P, Laan R. Randomized trial of effect of cyclical etidronate in the prevention of corticosteroid-induced bone loss. *J Clin Endocrinol Metab* 1998; 83: 1128–1133.

35. Saag K, Emkey R, Schnitzer T J et al. Alendronate for the prevention and treatment of glucocorticoid-induced osteoporosis. *N Engl J Med* 1998; 339: 292–299.

36. Sambrook P, Birmingham J, Kelly R N et al. Prevention of corticosteroid osteoporosis: a comparison of calcium, calcitriol and calcitonin. *N Engl J Med* 1993; 328: 1747–1752.

Further reading

Anon. Osteoporosis. *Med Int* 1994; 22: 209–212.

Brocklehurst J C, Tallis R C, Fillit H M, eds. *Textbook of Gerontology*. London: Churchill Livingstone, 1992.

Eastell R. Treatment of postmenopausal osteoporosis. *N Engl J Med* 1998; 338: 736–746.

Eastell R, Reid D M, Compston J. A UK consensus group on management of gluco-corticoid-induced osteoporosis: an update. *J Intern Med* 1998; 244: 271–292.

Hallworth R B. Prevention and treatment of postmenopausal osteoporosis. *Pharm World Sci* 1998; 20: 198–205.

Johnson S, Johnson F N, eds. *Reviews in Contemporary Pharmacotherapy: Etidronate in Osteoporosis*. Carnforth: Maurius Press, 1998.

O'Connell M B, Bauwens S F. Osteoporosis and osteomalacia. In: Dipiro J T, Talbert R L, Yee G C *et al.*, eds. *Pharmacotherapy. A Pathophysiologic Approach*. Connecticut: Appleton and Lange, 1997: 1689–1716.

Riggs B L, Melton L J. The prevention and treatment of osteoporosis. *N Engl J Med* 1986; 314: 1676.

Sagraves R, Letassy N A. Gynaecological disorders. In: Young L Y, Koda-Kimble M A, eds. *Applied Therapeutics. The Clinical Use of Drugs*. Vancouver: Applied Therapeutics, 1995: 46.27–46.38.

11

Musculoskeletal and joint problems in the elderly

Anne M Watson, Fiona C Thomson and Aileen Muir

Musculoskeletal disorders are the most common cause of disability in the developed world. Outpatient referrals for rheumatology in England and Wales for males and females increase with age, reaching a peak rate at 55–74 years and then declining after 85 years.[1] The increasing prevalence of osteoarthritis (OA) with age is a major cause of disability in the elderly. While rheumatoid arthritis (RA) may develop in younger age groups, it is often a cause of disability, morbidity and mortality in the elderly population. Old age causes diagnostic difficulties because of one condition superimposed on another (e.g. OA and RA) and also because normal ageing may mimic disease (e.g. ulnar deviation in old age may be normal).

The use of drugs to treat musculoskeletal disorders is common but not without problems in the elderly population. Coexisting medical conditions and their treatments also complicate the management of these disorders in this patient group.

Effect of age on the immune system

Immune system abnormalities may contribute to the aetiology of many rheumatic diseases, for example autoantibodies such as rheumatoid factors are present in a number of rheumatic illnesses.

However the immune system changes with increasing age, showing decreased T-cell activity, increased incidence of monoclonal antibody and autoantibody production and an increase in erythrocyte sedimentation rate (ESR). This therefore needs to be considered when interpreting immunochemical tests. ESR, for example, can be adjusted for age using a simple formula. Caution is needed in interpreting rheumatoid factor tests in the elderly as the prevalence of positive tests increases after the age of 70 years.

Rheumatoid arthritis

RA is a chronic systemic inflammatory disease causing pain, joint destruction and loss of joint mobility. It is an autoimmune disorder characterised by symmetric erosive synovitis and sometimes multisystem involvement.[2] RA is a progressive but variable disease which has difficulties in clear diagnosis and determination of prognosis.

Epidemiology

It is estimated that 30–40% of patients with RA attending rheumatology centres are over the age of 65.[3] Increased longevity will ultimately increase the burden of RA on National Health Service resources. The overall prevalence of RA in the UK is estimated at 1% but is 3.4% in the 68–75-year age group and 1.8% in those aged 75 years and over.[3] There is a 3 : 1 preponderance of females over males; however this ratio decreases with increasing age.[4] There is no age limit on the onset of RA but the average age at onset of RA in the UK is about 55 years.[5]

Aetiology

The exact cause of RA is as yet unknown but it seems to be multifactorial. It appears that some environmental trigger factor is responsible for initiating the disease in a genetically predisposed individual. Like other forms of inflammatory arthritis, the disease tends to cluster in families. Most patients with RA have human lymphocyte antigen (HLA) serotypes HLA-DR1 or HLA-DR4 present. HLA-DR4 has been associated with severe forms of the disease. Other factors, however, are associated with the occurrence and expression of RA, including the patient's educational level, lifestyle and hormonal status (remission in pregnancy is well known). Socioeconomic status is associated with disease outcome in RA, but there is little evidence for its involvement in disease onset. A meta-analysis of the role of oral contraceptives (OC) in RA concluded that OCs have no effect on RA risk; however, overall they may postpone the disease. The Epstein–Barr virus, parvoviruses and mycobacteria have been linked to RA but there is no clear evidence as yet. Other associated risks include infection, stress, trauma, climate, metabolic and endocrine factors.[6]

Pathophysiology

Pathologically, RA is immune-mediated. Immune complexes (antigen/antibody) form within the joint and activate the complement system. There is infiltration of the synovium with lymphoid cells, formation of new blood vessels, synovial proliferation and joint destruction. T lymphocytes are attracted into the synovial fluid where they phago-cytose the immune complexes. This results in release of lysosomal enzymes and other chemical mediators of inflammation, which then play an important role in synovitis.[7]

Continued inflammation then results in proliferation of the synovium over the joint surface. The thickened synovium, or pannus, releases enzymes which erode both cartilage and bone, causing perma-nent damage. This process leads to increased laxity of ligaments around the joints, subluxation of tendons and eventually joints, and inflam-mation of many other tissues of the body.

Clinical features and diagnosis

The diagnosis of RA is made on the presenting signs and symptoms and specific investigations. The most commonly used criteria is the classifi-cation of the revised American Rheumatism Association (ARA) criteria (Table 11.1). At least four of the seven criteria must be present. The first four criteria must be present for at least 6 weeks for the diagnosis of RA to be made.[8]

RA presents as symmetrical polyarthritis which can develop over a few days or, more commonly, over weeks to months. Diagnosis of RA may be more difficult in the elderly due to the increased incidence of other misleading factors such as gout, polymyalgia and neoplastic disease. Symmetric features such as fatigue and diffuse musculoskeletal pain are not uncommon prior to 'joint' swelling. The disease commonly presents in the metacarpophalangeal joints or the metatarsophalangeal joints and wrists, although the picture may vary with age.[9] It can also affect the elbow, shoulder, knee, ankles, toes and jaw. Large joints are

Table 11.1 1987 American Rheumatism Association revised criteria for classi-fication of rheumatoid arthritis[8]

Morning stiffness of at least 1 h
Arthritis of three or more joint areas (left or right proximal interphalangeal, metacarpophalangeal, wrist, elbow, knee, ankle and metatarsophalangeal joints)
Symmetrical arthritis (50% or more of the above affected joint areas affected symmetrically)
Rheumatoid nodules
Serum rheumatoid factor-positive
Typical radiographic changes in the hand and wrist

Adapted from Arnett *et al.*[8]

more often affected at presentation in the elderly than in younger patients; this is particularly evident in the pelvic girdle and the shoulder joint, whereas younger patients have more metatarsophalangeal joint involvement. There is also a tendency for older patients to have a higher frequency of acute onset and weight loss.[9]

Morning stiffness present for more than 30 min is a common early feature which may be relieved by modest activity. Various extra features can exist with RA and these include fatigue, weight loss, dry eye (Sjögren's syndrome), cardiopulmonary diseases, haematological complications, rheumatoid nodules and vasculitis. Subcutaneous nodules are less prevalent in older patients.

In the elderly RA patient there is an excess prevalence of male gender, acute onset, systemic onset, shoulder involvement, persistently active disease and rapid functional decline.[9] The more rapid functional deterioration evident in older patients suggests that they should be treated with at least equally potent therapy to their younger counterparts.

Various investigations are undertaken in addition to the clinical examination. These are not specific diagnostic tests but may aid the diagnosis and help monitor disease progression and response to treatment. The non-specific tests, ESR and C-reactive protein (CRP), give an indication of disease activity since they are both dependent on acute-phase proteins and raised during an inflammatory response. Immunological tests are also performed to look for the presence of rheumatoid factor. Only 70–80% of patients with RA and 5% of normal patients have immunoglobulin M rheumatoid factor present. Haematological tests may also show normochromic, normocytic anaemia of chronic disease (related to disease activity) and an increase in alkaline phosphatase.

Another non-specific immunological test is that for antinuclear antibodies. X-rays, mainly of the hands and feet, are used to assist in the diagnosis of RA and to monitor progress. Erosions of joint margins and losses of joint space can be detected by X-rays. The presence of early erosive changes is a poor prognostic sign. When diagnosed, RA can progress in a variety of ways, although various factors, such as older age at onset, have been associated with poor prognosis.

Treatment

The management of RA aims to minimise pain, reduce inflammation, prevent or minimise joint destruction and suppress disease progression.

There is no known cure or prophylaxis for RA. Optimal management requires early diagnosis and the timely introduction of agents that reduce the probability of irreversible joint damage. Periodic assessment of disease activity, drug efficacy and toxicity, and effectiveness of non-pharmacological intervention by the multidisciplinary team is required.

In the UK, the Royal College of Physicians has published guidelines on RA (1992)[10] and the American College of Rheumatology issued their guidelines on RA in 1996.[2] The Scottish Intercollegiate Guideline Network (SIGN) guideline for the 'Management of Early Rheumatoid Arthritis' recommends early treatment with DMARDs to control symptoms and delay disease progression.[11] However, they still include the traditional 'pyramid' approach to drug therapy, and have not yet been revised to reflect the current move to earlier use of disease-modifying antirheumatic drugs (DMARDs). There is evidence that the rationale for earlier referral and initiation of DMARD therapy is being implemented into clinical practice.[12]

Self-management is an important feature of RA and patients are encouraged to make an informed decision on choice of management.[13] Patient education may influence disease outcome. This has particular implications for the elderly who may require written and verbal information tailored to their specific requirements.[13]

Non-pharmacological measures

The multidisciplinary team are involved in various aspects of the RA patient's management and can cooperate and provide education and support for RA patients to improve morbidity and mortality (Table 11.2).

Exercise is important, since much of the pain and stiffness in RA comes from periarticular tissues (muscles and tendons). Patients should be encouraged to perform a gentle exercise programme regularly to improve and maintain fitness and muscle bulk around the joints. This is particularly important in elderly patients to help minimise the need for pharmacological treatment, with its attendant risks.[9]

End-stage disease may result in joint deformities requiring surgical intervention and/or joint replacement. In severe and disabling disease this may provide dramatic relief from pain and improve functional ability. Age is not a contraindication but comorbid states should be taken into consideration when an elderly patient is considered for surgery.

Drug treatment

The mainstay of management of RA is the variety of very effective but also potentially toxic drugs available, hence the pharmacist has a key

Table 11.2   The multidisciplinary team approach for rheumatology patients

Doctors	Diagnosis
	Disease management
	Emotional support
Pharmacists	Advice on pharmaceutical care
	Patient education
	Emotional support
Physiotherapists	Assess needs for exercise, mechanical aids
	Electrical, heat, cold therapy
	Emotional support
Dieticians	Advice on weight reduction
	Advice on trigger foods
Occupational therapists	Advise on home/lifestyle adaptations
	Emotional support
Specialist nurses	Outpatient and patient follow-up in the community
	Emotional support
Podiatrists	Assessing foot-joint abnormalities

role within the multidisciplinary team in the delivery of pharmaceutical care.[14] Elderly patients should be treated similarly to their younger counterparts, although comorbidity, multiple medications and age-related changes in pharmacodynamics and pharmacokinetics must be taken into account.[15]

The pharmacological approach has changed in recent years, with a challenge to the traditional 'pyramid' approach. Drugs which retard the progression of the disease (i.e. the DMARDs) are now commenced much earlier in the disease, since functional damage is irreversible.

Simple analgesics   Simple analgesics such as paracetamol, dihydro-codeine or combination products such as co-proxamol provide limited benefit for the inflammatory pain of RA. These are given as adjunctive therapy and used on a regular basis if pain is persistently present. There is an increased risk of side-effects (constipation, drowsiness and liver damage) in the elderly.[16]

Non-steroidal anti-inflammatory drugs (NSAIDs)   NSAIDs constitute 5% of the National Health Service prescriptions in the UK, with ibuprofen, naproxen and diclofenac being the most commonly prescribed in general practice. Awareness of the consequences of overconsumption and rates of toxicity should minimise the problems associated with these drugs.[17] Patients should be advised to avoid additional over-the-counter

NSAIDs. Instead, patients should be advised to add regular paracetamol, if possible, to minimise any NSAID dose required.[9] NSAIDs have an analgesic and anti-inflammatory effect when taken in regular doses. NSAIDs suppress inflammation by preventing the production of prostaglandins through inhibition of the cyclo-oxygenase enzyme which has two isoforms, COX-1 and COX-2. Present research has indicated that the anti-inflammatory action of NSAIDs is due to COX-2 inhibition, whereas the side-effects, gastrointestinal and renal toxicity, may be due to COX-1 inhibition.

Recent work has focused on developments of COX-2-preferential agents (meloxicam, etodolac and nabumetone) and COX-2-selective agents (rofecoxib, celecoxib), which may have an improved safety profile without loss of anti-inflammatory effect. This may prove to be a particular benefit in elderly patients. Celecoxib is now licensed in the UK for use in RA and OA. Rofecoxib is also licensed in the UK but only for OA, although potential benefits in RA are being investigated.

Table 11.3 outlines some of the considerations in NSAID prescribing in elderly patients.[18]

The most important adverse effect of NSAIDs is gastrointestinal bleeding and/or perforation, and this clearly increases with age. Patients who are taking NSAIDs have a three- to fivefold increase in risk of gastrointestinal complications compared to non-users, and prophylaxis may be required (see Chapter 3). Gastrointestinal toxicity is dose-related and so the lowest effective dose should be used. The reduced incidence of gastrointestinal complications with the highly selective COX-2 inhibitors requires further evaluation in the long term in clinical practice, particularly in the elderly population. NSAIDs may also cause renal toxicity due to inhibition of renal prostaglandins, especially in elderly patients with limited renal capacity. The extent to which COX-2 inhibitors share the effects of non-selective NSAIDs on renal function needs to be established since the former drugs are largely eliminated in the kidney.

Morbidity and mortality due to cardiac side-effects have also been attributed to NSAIDs. They may cause fluid retention and may interfere with antihypertensive treatment, especially in the elderly who require closer monitoring.

There are a large number of NSAIDs on the market with few differences in efficacy, although there is variability in individual patient response. The choice of NSAID should be based on the Committee on Safety of Medicines advice on relative safety profiles, as referred to in Table 11.3.[19]

Table 11.3 Prescribing non-steroidal anti-inflammatory drugs (NSAIDs) in elderly patients

Choice of drugs	Special considerations in elderly	Common adverse effects	Contraindications/precautions
NSAIDs	**Choice of drug**	Gastrointestinal bleeding/	Congestive cardiac failure
Lowest risk	Use safest drug	perforation[a]	Renal impairment
Ibuprofen		(consider prophylaxis if	Peptic ulcer disease
Intermediate risk,	**Dose of drug**	other risk factors are present)	Hypertension
possibly higher	Use lowest effective dose		
for piroxicam	May need reduced dose if	Hypersensitivity reactions	
Piroxicam	renal impairment	Skin reactions	
Ketoprofen			
Indometacin	**Cautions/contraindications/drug**	Fluid retention	
Naproxen	**interactions**	Central nervous system	
Diclofenac	Concomitant disease states/	reaction	
Highest risk[19]	interacting drugs more common	Hepatotoxicity	
Azapropazone	in elderly	Blood dyscrasias	
	Monitoring		
COX-2 inhibitors	For efficacy/adverse effects	Insomnia, pharyngitis	Renal impairment
Rofecoxib			Inflammatory bowel disease
Celecoxib	**Patient education**		Severe congestive cardiac failure
			Celecoxib-sulphonamide sensitivity

[a] Age-related risks.
COX-2 = Cyclo-oxygenase-2.
Adapted from Suarez-Almzo.[18]

DMARDs There is now good evidence that both inflammation and rate of appearance of radiological erosions can be decreased by DMARDs. A more aggressive approach is now recommended using DMARD therapy, as soon as diagnosis is made, to suppress symptoms, delay joint damage and potentially delay deformity.[20] There is a delicate balance between benefit and risk of drug toxicity in terms of choice of DMARD, particularly in the elderly with their inherent problems, discussed earlier. The relative toxicities of DMARDs and NSAIDs are however similar. The precise mechanisms of action of most of the DMARDs are unknown and hence choice of therapy is difficult. Although over 50% of patients remain on methotrexate for 5 years or more, about half of the rest stop other DMARDs within 1–2.5 years because of inefficacy, loss of clinical benefit or unwanted side-effects. A recent study found better results, in terms of effectiveness and toxicity, with sulfasalazine or methotrexate than with oral gold (less effective) or intramuscular gold or oral penicillamine (more toxic).[21]

Some of the toxicities that appear to be more prevalent in elderly patients include skin rash and taste disturbances with penicillamine, retinopathy with antimalarials (regular monitoring is required, as this may be mistaken for normal macular degeneration in ageing), serious liver disease with methotrexate, blood dyscrasias or nephrotic syndrome with parenteral gold, and gastrointestinal symptoms with sulfasalazine.[9] However, this tendency to increased toxicity may be due to longer disease duration rather than age itself.

Systematic reviews of randomised controlled trials have found no evidence of a difference in effectiveness between most DMARDs, although oral gold (auranofin) seems to be the least effective. Assessments by meta-analysis have suggested that methotrexate and hydroxychloroquine have the highest efficacy : toxicity ratio. Sulfasalazine, intramuscular gold, penicillamine and methotrexate are thought to be equally effective and more effective than hydroxychloroquine or oral gold.[22] The immunosuppressive drugs azathioprine, ciclosporin, cyclophosphamide and chlorambucil are the most effective but also the most toxic DMARDs and hence are reserved for more severe, unresponsive RA, particularly where there is extra-articular involvement.

Table 11.4 includes information on DMARD use in the elderly.

New DMARD developments

Combination DMARDs This development aims to use the synergistic effect of two or more drugs in combinations to provide greater efficacy.

Table 11.4 Use of disease-modifying antirheumatic drugs (DMARDs) in the elderly

Drug	Evidence base/use in practice	Monitoring
Hydroxychloroquine	Meta-analysis demonstrates a relatively high efficacy : toxicity ratio compared with other DMARDs.[21,22] Its use is usually restricted to patients with mild non-erosive disease or where patients have comorbidities such as renal impairment, where a more powerful DMARD is deemed unsuitable	Antimalarials are the least toxic of the DMARDs, with retinopathy being the adverse effect of concern, despite the incidence being extremely rare and related to cumulative dose. Baseline assessment is recommended for all patients, with yearly checks. Twice-yearly assessments are advised in the elderly population since age-related degeneration may mimic antimalarial-induced retinopathy.
Auranofin	Oral gold is significantly less effective than any of the other DMARDs and hence is reserved for patients with mild disease[22]	Diarrhoea limits the use of oral gold
Sulfasalazine	Sulfasalazine is as effective as injectable gold, penicillamine and methotrexate and better than oral gold and hydroxychloroquine. No age-related differences in toxicity or efficacy of sulfasalazine have been found[23,24] The enteric-coated preparation of sulfasalazine should be used. The dose is 500 mg/day increased weekly to a target dose of 40 mg/kg per day	It has been suggested that older patients withdraw from treatment more often from nausea and vomiting. Adverse effects include gastrointestinal or central nervous system complications, neutropenia, skin rashes and hepatotoxicity. Full blood counts are recommended every 2–4 weeks for the first 3 months and then every 3 months thereafter. Liver function tests should be checked monthly for the first 3 months and then every 3–6 months thereafter
Parenteral gold	Parenteral gold has no difference in toxicity or efficacy in elderly and younger rheumatoid arthritis patients.[3] Treatment should start with a 10 mg test dose by deep intramuscular injection followed by 50 mg intramuscularly weekly injections until a sustained regimen is achieved. Thereafter less frequent injections should be introduced	Compliance and monitoring are ensured, which may be beneficial in the elderly.[3] Haematological, renal and pulmonary side-effects can occur hence a full blood count and proteinuria should be checked prior to each injection. Liver function tests and plasma creatinine should be checked every 3 months

Penicillamine	Penicillamine again shows no age-related differences in efficacy. There is, however, a higher incidence of taste disturbances, gastrointestinal upset and rashes among elderly users[3]	Side-effects are dose-dependent and haemoglobin, full blood count and proteinuria should be tested every 2 weeks until the dosage is stable, and then every 1–3 months. Oral iron, antacids and zinc can impair absorption and should not be given within 2 h of the penicillamine dose
Methotrexate	Methotrexate is probably the most effective and most rapidly acting DMARD.[21–23, 25, 26] In the UK 80% of newly diagnosed patients with rheumatoid arthritis receive this drug in the first year. Methotrexate is given on a once-weekly dosing schedule with a rapid onset of action, usually within 1 month.[27] Methotrexate is principally excreted by the kidneys and hence caution should be used in patients with impaired renal function; this is particularly important in the elderly population	Methotrexate is usually given in doses of 5–15 mg once weekly followed 4 days later by folic acid to reduce stomatitis and gastrointestinal toxicity. Caution is required in co-prescribing non-steroidal anti-inflammatory drugs with methotrexate due to gastrointestinal toxicity and reduced renal elimination of methotrexate. The commonest toxicities associated with methotrexate are nausea and vomiting and hepatic and pulmonary toxicity which appear to be more common in elderly patients. Concomitant alcohol is not recommended due to the increased risk of hepatic toxicity
Corticosteroids	Meta-analysis of studies of oral prednisolone 2.5–15.5 mg/day confirms effectiveness in symptomatic control.[27, 28] Intra-articular administration of steroids (methylprednisolone or triamcinolone) is an effective way of restoring functional ability and relieving pain in synovitic joints. This route of administration minimises the risk of systemic corticosteroid effects and may be the preferred route as 'bridge' therapy in patients experiencing a flare of rheumatoid arthritis. It has a short-term effect (lasting up to 8 weeks) and only three injections should be administered to any one joint in a year	Check glucose and blood pressure every 3–6 months. Long-term adverse effects such as osteoporosis and the comorbidities which the elderly are more likely to have may limit their use in this population

Although there is increasing interest in this approach, there is still not enough evidence to support its widespread use in any age group. Several drugs may be used in combination to induce remission in RA with a subsequent 'step-down' approach in which drugs are revised from the regimen or lower doses of the individual drugs may be used (the 'sawtooth' approach). Table 11.5 shows some combinations which have been used in small-scale studies.

Leflunomide Leflunomide is newly licensed in the UK as a DMARD with a rapid onset of effect (within 4 weeks). Side-effects include skin disorders, diarrhoea, abdominal pain, alopecia, dizziness and hypertension. Liver function should be monitored during therapy. Some studies have looked at its combination with methotrexate, which appears more effective than methotrexate alone, although there is increased risk of liver toxicity. There is little specific information on use in elderly patients, but caution should be exercised in patients with renal dysfunction.[29]

Minocycline Minocycline may be useful in RA, particularly in controlling disease activity in seropositive RA within the first year of disease. However, randomised controlled trials (conducted in patients with seropositive RA) are limited so its place in therapy is not yet clear. The main side-effect is hyperpigmentation.[30]

Use of other drugs in the elderly Ciclosporin is not usually used in the elderly population as these patients are at increased risk from ciclosporin renal toxicity, perhaps due to underlying arteriosclerotic

Table 11.5 Some disease-modifying antirheumatic drug (DMARD) combinations that have been studied

Triple therapy with hydroxychloroquine, sulfasalazine and methotrexate is more effective than either hydroxychloroquine/sulfasalazine or methotrexate alone[27]

Triple combinations of sulfasalazine, corticosteroid and methotrexate are more effective than sulfasalazine alone[25]

Combination of corticosteroids increases the effectiveness of oral or intramuscular gold[22, 23]

Combinations of methotrexate with ciclosporin and with sulfasalazine and hydroxychloroquine show better clinical outcomes than methotrexate alone[26, 27]

Combined penicillamine and oral gold shows improved outcomes over penicillamine alone[21, 22]

Addition of prednisolone 7.5 mg to other DMARD regimens show short-term rather than long-term effects[22]

Table 11.6 Key points in the management of rheumatoid arthritis

• Aims of management are to reduce pain and disability and to limit joint damage
• Analgesics/non-steroidal anti-inflammatory drugs are useful for symptomatic treatment
• DMARDs should be used early in treatment to delay joint damage and improve long-term disability and may be used singly or in combination
• Changes to DMARD therapy should be carried out systematically

cardiovascular disease, and have reduced ability to metabolise the drug through decreased cytochrome P450 enzyme activity. Studies of other cytotoxics in elderly patients have not been carried out.

Biological agents   Various biological products are under investigation in RA. These include vaccination, modulation of T cells and modulation of cytokines, inflammatory mediators, such as tumour necrosis factor-α (TNF-α) and interleukin-1 (IL-1). Alteration of cytokines may be achieved by local or systemic monoclonal antibodies (e.g. infliximab), soluble cytokine receptors (e.g. etanercept), cytokine receptor antagonists and administration of competing cytokines. Both infliximab and etanercept have the advantage of a rapid onset of action. Etanercept may have more potential for use as monotherapy than infliximab, which causes antibody formation, and may need to be given with methotrexate. Initially these agents may be useful for short-term therapy of aggressive disease. It is not yet known whether these agents can reduce the need for NSAIDs, DMARDs and corticosteroids, with consequent benefits in terms of drug-related morbidity, or the extent of any effect on progression of joint damage.[31]

Table 11.6 summarises the key points in the management of RA.

Osteoarthritis

Osteoarthritis (OA) is the most common rheumatic disease, the single most important cause of locomotor disability and a major challenge to health care. It is the most common chronic disease in the elderly, affecting up to 25% of the world's elderly population and it is one of the most common causes of musculoskeletal pain in the elderly.

OA is confined to the joints and is characterised by destruction of the articular cartilage and subchondral bone demonstrating inflammatory, erosive and reparative features. Radiographic changes in OA occur later in the disease and include joint space narrowing from the eroded cartilage (Figure 11.1) and osteophyte formation (bony outgrowths that occur as a result of bone destruction and reformation). It is the main indication for joint replacement surgery.

Epidemiology

Overall, OA affects 2.5% of the UK population, with this figure increasing with advancing age.[32] Approximately 12% of the population aged 65 years and over in the UK are affected by OA.[32] OA is becoming the fourth highest impact condition in women and the eighth in men.[33]

Aetiology

OA can be classified as primary or secondary. Primary OA has no known cause, although recent research indicates that there may be a genetic link which may result from an immune-mediated insult in genetically predisposed individuals. This is often referred to as nodal generalised OA or menopausal OA (due to symptoms commonly starting around the

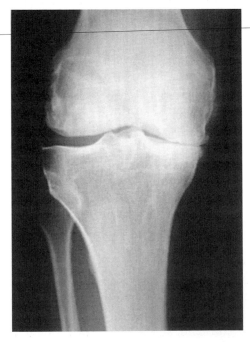

Figure 11.1 Osteoarthritis of the knee joint. Reproduced with the permission of Dr P Marazzi/SPL.

menopause). A suggested protective effect of hormone replacement therapy against OA has not, however, been established.[34]

Secondary OA occurs in response to other mechanisms, including injury, infection and metabolic disorders.

The incidence of OA is strongly related to age: it is uncommon in people aged under 45 years.[35] The prevalence increases up to the age of 65, when at least 50% of people have radiographic evidence of OA in at least one joint; however, the evidence for increases in prevalence over the age of 65 are less clear.[36] OA was previously considered as a degenerative disease which was an inevitable consequence of ageing and trauma, which led to negative approaches to research and treatment.[37] Research now indicates that it is a metabolically active disease which is increasingly amenable to treatment. Severe radiographic grades of OA and particular joint involvement are more common in females.[36] Oestrogen use has been suggested as a contributing factor to OA but no clear relationship has been shown.[39]

Cohort studies have shown a clear association with obesity, particularly for knee OA and more weakly linked to hip OA. It has also been shown that weight reduction can provide mild-to-moderate pain relief for knee OA. Occupation-related repetitive injury and physical trauma to particular joints may be a contributing factor.[36]

Long-term outcomes thus rely on integration of drug treatment with exercise, lifestyle adjustment and physiotherapy.

Diagnosis

OA is diagnosed by a triad of typical symptoms, physical findings and radiographic changes.

The best diagnostic tool for recognising OA is simply X-ray imaging, with different diagnostic X-ray signs for each joint. For example, the most sensitive and specific indicator for OA of the knee is the presence of a definite osteophyte, accompanied by joint space narrowing in hip OA and sclerosis of subchondral bone in hand OA. Arthroscopy can be used to image articular structures directly.

Although clinical signs and symptoms, such as pain, stiffness and restriction of movements, may contribute to the diagnosis, 40% of radiologically detectable OA is asymptomatic.[38] In contrast, there is a group of clinically positive but radiologically negative cases with a quickly progressing disease. Laboratory markers do not play a role in the diagnosis of OA since there is no systemic inflammatory component of the condition.

Clinical features

The most frequently reported symptom of OA is pain.[39] Although there is no nerve supply in cartilage, the pain arises from different structures. Characteristically it is worsened by loading and movement but eased by rest, though patients with severe disease may even have pain at rest. It is often worst at the end of the day.

Morning stiffness and stiffness following inactivity (gel phenomena) rarely exceed 30 min.[39] Physical findings in OA joints include bony prominences, crepitus and deficits in range of motion. Progressive cartilage destruction, malalignment, joint effusions and subchondral bone collapse contribute to irreversible deformity.

Treatment

There is no cure for OA. The main management goals are to reduce pain, stiffness and disability, and to limit the risk of progressive joint damage, while minimising adverse effects. Various outcome measures have been used to evaluate treatment, including frequency and severity of joint pain (particularly activity-related and night pain); stiffness; functional impairment and disability, and quality-of-life measures.

Features of OA include variability in disease presentation, periods of remission and relapse for individual patients and poor correlation of radiographic changes with patients' symptoms. These factors, coupled with altered pharmacokinetics and pharmacodynamics in the elderly population, require therapy to be tailored to the individual patient's needs. It is also important to consider whether the patient has anxiety or depression as this may further aggravate arthritic pain.

Most patients have only moderate pain and disability and can often be controlled without systemic drug treatments, which is useful in the elderly population who may have a variety of comorbid states. Patients and their carers should be given a full explanation of the disease and treatments.

Drug treatment

Drug treatment is largely aimed at relieving pain and reducing inflammation, if present. Options include local therapy (topical applications, intra-articular corticosteroids) and systemic drugs such as analgesics, NSAIDs and low-dose antidepressants.

Local treatment Since OA is not a systemic disease, targeting treatment to a local area, especially if only a few joints are involved, may be beneficial in reducing systemic toxicity in the elderly.

Rubefacients and counter-irritants These produce vasodilatation and/or mild irritation in tissues around joints. This warming effect may relieve joint symptoms. Counter-irritants distract the patient's attention from the arthritic pain. There is no evidence base for these commonly used products.

NSAID creams and gels Although it has been suggested that topical NSAIDs may help to limit unwanted systemic side-effects of oral NSAIDs in this patient group, side-effects such as renal impairment have been reported rarely,[40] and long-term safety studies or comparisons with safety or efficacy of oral NSAIDs or paracetamol are lacking. In this context, despite a systematic review of randomised controlled trials finding that topical NSAIDs are effective compared with placebo in acute and chronic pain conditions, they cannot be recommended as an evidence-based treatment at present.[41, 42]

Capsaicin cream The analgesic properties of capsaicin are as a result of its ability to stimulate nociceptive neurons, resulting in the release of neuropeptides, including substance P. Although this can result in an initial inflammatory response, this tends to settle with continued application (two to four times daily), due to depletion of neuropeptides from the nerve fibres.

Although several small studies have shown the benefits on pain with capsaicin cream compared to placebo, there is not enough evidence to indicate whether topical capsaicin or NSAID is superior to simple rubefacients.[43] Patients may experience some mild temporary localised burning but there are no systemic side-effects from topical capsaicin.

Intra-articular corticosteroid injections OA was traditionally thought of as a non-inflammatory disease but there is growing evidence that there may be an inflammatory component involved in some phases of the disease.

Intra-articular steroids have been used as a common therapeutic alternative in OA, especially during an inflammatory phase of the condition, when patients present with pain and synovitis. There are few clinical trials on their efficacy or the optimal frequency of their administration, but they are thought to be particularly effective for OA of the knee joint and the thumb base joint.[43]

Long-term effects are unknown so they should be reserved as adjunctive therapy and their use should be restricted to patients with clinical evidence of synovitis and no more than three or four injections given in 1 year. Injections of triamcinolone or methylprednisolone have been shown to have a positive, although short-acting effect (up to 8 weeks). Their use in the elderly may be beneficial due to the limitation of side-effects, although they may affect glycaemic control in diabetics.

Viscosupplementation with hyaluronic acid (HA)   HA is the major constituent of both synovial fluid and the surface layer of the articular cartilage. Intra-articular hyaluronan (Hyalgan) and its derivative (Synvisc) are licensed for use in the UK for the treatment of knee OA, as a series of 3–5-weekly injections, with benefits on pain over placebo. Their efficacy appears similar to intra-articular corticosteroids and continuous NSAID treatment but data are limited, there is no evidence to substantiate repeat courses and they are expensive. Local adverse effects and synovitis have been reported. The place of these agents in the overall management of OA is uncertain and should be reserved for patients where other measures have failed or are contraindicated and where surgical intervention is inappropriate.[43, 44]

Systemic treatment   Patients may require oral analgesia or NSAID treatment if physical and/or topical therapy does not control symptoms.

Analgesics   Management should commence with simple analgesics, e.g. paracetamol, adjusted according to the patient's requirements, which controls symptoms in 50% of patients.[45] Liver function, other drug therapies and comorbid conditions must be taken into consideration, particularly in the elderly. If pain still remains, combination products of paracetamol with opioid derivatives such as codeine or dextropropoxyphene may be beneficial. These should be used with caution in the elderly due to increased likelihood of drowsiness and constipation. Analgesics should be taken regularly rather than 'as required' during periods of pain, and may be taken prophylactically when the patient is about to undertake an activity which normally causes pain.

Non-steroidal anti-inflammatory drugs   There is no good evidence that NSAIDs are superior to simple analgesics such as paracetamol.[42] These are only indicated when other therapy options have failed and during an inflammatory phase of the disease.[46] The 25% of OA patients who may benefit from NSAIDs cannot be identified in advance.[45] Further, there is some evidence to support transfer of elderly patients taking regular NSAIDs to paracetamol alone, which is of particular importance in minimising morbidity and mortality in this group. Table 11.3 outlines some factors to be considered when prescribing NSAIDs in elderly patients.

Antidepressants Low-dose antidepressants (commonly amitriptyline) are sometimes used as adjunctive treatment for arthritic pain associated with sleep disturbance. There are no controlled trial data as yet on their effectiveness.[42]

Alternative medicines Many patients with OA try alternative treatments such as green-lipped mussel and animal cartilage extracts. There has been much interest in glucosamine and the limited evidence available appears to suggest potential benefits, but long-term studies have not been carried out.[47,48]

Physical and functional interventions Health professionals should encourage physical activity and reassure patients that, rather than cause further joint damage, this may help ease symptoms by increasing general fitness, muscle strength around affected joints and the range of joint movement. Emotional support, stress management and other coping strategies may help older patients, who often become depressed because of chronic pain, reduced mobility and increasing disability.[33] Surgery, including arthroscopy, osteotomy or arthroplasty, may be indicated in patients with persistent pain at rest and during the night accompanied by significant disability, where response to drug therapy is inadequate, or for severe knee and hip OA. The functional status, particularly the cardiovascular system, must be taken into account when considering surgical intervention for elderly patients.[32]

Future therapeutic options Protection of the cartilage is a central aim of the management of OA. NSAIDs have different *in vitro* actions on cartilage metabolism. There is speculation that some may be protective or even anabolic – termed as a chondroprotective action. Various agents are under investigation and include glycosaminoglycans, tetracyclines, superoxide dismutase, bone-resorptive agents, certain cytokines and growth factors. The nutritional supplement, high-dose glucosamine, has been reported in the press to 'cure' OA but long-term trials are required.

The key points in the management of osteoarthritis are summarised in Table 11.7.

Table 11.7 Key points in the management of osteoarthritis

- Main management goals are to reduce pain, stiffness and disability and limit progressive joint damage
- Local treatment may be adequate in patients with moderate pain in single joints
- Systemic treatment should commence with simple analgesia i.e. paracetamol
- Non-steroidal anti-inflammatory drugs may also be used and may provide additional symptomatic relief in some patients. However, they are usually no more effective than simple analgesics and there is a risk of adverse effects in the elderly
- Adverse effects of drug treatments are more likely in elderly patients
- Other illnesses, such as depression, which may make pain worse, should be treated promptly

Gout

Clinical features

Gout is characterised by acute onset (within 1 day) with monoarticular arthritis, commonly occurring in the toe but possibly affecting other joints. The joint will be extremely painful, red and swollen and the patient often experiences fever. Gout is sometimes difficult to recognise in elderly patients as it may mimic rheumatoid arthritis,[49] but is increasingly diagnosed in this patient group.

Aetiology

Gout occurs due to deposition of urate crystals in joints, causing an acute inflammatory response. The presence of urate crystals in the joint fluid is diagnostic of acute gout, as is the development of tophi (chalky deposits in tissues near affected joints).[50] Hyperuricaemia alone is not the only factor involved in the development of gout but the risk increases as plasma urate concentrations rise above $600 \, \mu mol/l$.[51]

Gout in the elderly tends to be more equally distributed between males and females, involves polyarticular joints and has fewer acute episodes but more likelihood of tophi developing.[52]

Pseudogout is a term used to describe calcium pyrophosphate arthropathy, which has similar features to gout. It tends to be less acute but runs a more prolonged course.

Treatment

Treatment and prophylaxis of gout in the elderly are complicated by coexisting medical conditions such as congestive cardiac failure and renal impairment. This leads to a higher risk of drug adverse effects, and should be considered when choosing treatment.

If hyperuricaemia is asymptomatic, drug treatment is not required, although causes should be investigated and removed or reduced.

Treatment of acute gout

NSAIDs   The usual preferred option in treating acute gout is NSAIDs which reduce the pain and inflammation of acute gout and should be initiated soon after the onset of the attack. However these should be used with extreme caution in the elderly, at the lowest effective dose, for the shortest possible duration, with close monitoring of renal function.[51] Prophylaxis against gastrointestinal damage may be required (see Chapter 3). They are not recommended in elderly patients with congestive heart failure or pre-existing renal impairment. Many NSAIDs have been shown to be effective, but those with a long half-life or high incidence of toxicity should be avoided. They should be given initially at high doses, reducing after 1–3 days. Indometacin 50 mg four times a day is effective but poorly tolerated in the elderly. Less toxic alternatives include diclofenac 50 mg three times a day, naproxen 500 mg twice a day, flurbiprofen 100 mg three times a day and sulindac 200 mg twice a day.[53] It should be noted that salicylates, including aspirin, are not effective in treating gout.

Colchicine   Colchicine is an alternative to NSAIDs for acute gout. It has a slower onset of action and is associated with vomiting and diarrhoea. It is poorly tolerated by the elderly and significant toxicity often occurs before clinical improvement is seen[54] so it is not generally recommended in this patient group. However, it does not cause fluid retention and is an option in patients with heart failure who may be at risk from the fluid-retaining effects of NSAIDs or those taking oral anti-coagulants, where NSAIDs may interact. The recommended dose is 1 mg initially, followed by 500 micrograms every 2–3 h until pain relief is obtained or vomiting or diarrhoea occurs (up to a total of 6 mg). The course should not be repeated for at least 3 days. Lower doses (500 μg four times a day) have been recommended; these carry less likelihood of toxicity but are still effective.[54]

Corticosteroids Short courses of oral, intravenous or intra-articular (where a single joint is affected) corticosteroids have been used infrequently where other treatment is unsuitable or ineffective.[49] Short courses may minimise side-effects such as hypertension and fluid retention but carry a risk of joint infection[52] or rebound phenomenon if withdrawn too quickly.

Other measures Precipitating factors should be considered and addressed. Use of diuretics in the elderly is common. Change to an alternative antihypertensive may help reduce urate levels, especially since hypertension control is a factor in gout. Low-dose aspirin may also precipitate gout and may necessitate consideration of alternative antiplatelet agents. The patient should be encouraged to make lifestyle changes, such as weight loss and reduced purine and alcohol consumption, to reduce the risk of a recurrence.[53] Further supplies of medicines, to enable the patient to initiate treatment rapidly if recurrence does occur, have been advocated.

Prevention of gout

Prophylactic drug treatment may not be necessary if precipitating factors are addressed. Initiation of prophylaxis should be considered carefully as this is likely to be lifelong treatment. Where pharmacological prophylaxis is indicated urate-lowering agents can be used.[50]

Allopurinol Allopurinol is the drug of choice. It can be given as a once-daily dose and is usually started at a low dose (50–100 mg), with adequate fluid intake, and increased weekly until the serum urate is below 300 μmol/l. Maintenance doses can vary from 50 to 800 mg/day. Lower doses are recommended in elderly patients due to possible renal impairment that reduces the ability to excrete allopurinol, and increases the risk of serious rash,[55] requiring discontinuation of the drug. If a rash occurs, slow reintroduction of allopurinol is possible with close monitoring for recurrence.

Uricosurics The place of uricosuric drugs (probenecid, sulfinpyrazone) in the prevention of gout episodes in the elderly is limited to patients with good renal function; they are generally ineffective in moderate or severe renal failure (glomerular filtration rates < 50 ml/min). If renal function is normal they can be used, sometimes in combination with allopurinol, to prevent attacks of gout,[52] by increasing the renal

Table 11.8   Key points in the management of gout

• The mainstay of treatment for acute gout is high-dose NSAIDs but these are unsuitable for many elderly patients
• Colchicine is an alternative that does not cause fluid retention but vomiting and diarrhoea limit its use
• Short-term corticosteroids may be an alternative option for acute management if NSAIDs or colchicine is unsuitable
• Precipitating factors should be removed and lifestyle changes made
• Allopurinol may be used for the prevention of gout, but the dose may need to be reduced in renal impairment, and should not be initiated during an acute attack

NSAIDs = Non-steroidal anti-inflammatory drugs.

secretion of urate. This can lead to deposition of uric acid crystals in the renal tubules, resulting in renal colic or impaired renal function. The possibility can be minimised by starting at low doses, increased over 2–4 weeks until serum urate levels are normal, and ensuring that the urine is kept alkaline.

Introduction of urate-lowering drugs can initially produce a worsening of gout symptoms or bring on an attack. It is therefore useful to wait for an acute attack to have settled and to use a NSAID or colchicine at low doses as prophylaxis until serum urate falls to normal levels.[51]

The key points in the management of gout are summarised in Table 11.8.

Polymyalgia rheumatica and cranial (giant cell) arteritis

These diseases usually occur in middle-aged and elderly patients and are rare in patients under 50 years, with a mean age at onset of about 70 years. Women are affected about twice as often as men. The two diseases are closely related and may occur separately or together. Polymyalgia rheumatica and cranial arteritis may have a genetic link, possibly linked to the immune system.

Features of polymyalgia rheumatica include pain and stiffness in the neck, shoulder and pelvic girdles, low-grade fever, fatigue and weight loss. The condition mainly affects muscles; however, there may also be an association between synovitis and muscle symptoms. In cranial arteritis (other terms used include temporal arteritis, giant cell arteritis and granulomatous arteritis), features may differ depending on affected arteries. Symptoms may include fatigue, headaches, joint pain and tenderness of the scalp around the temporal and occipital arteries, visual symptoms (amaurosis fugax, diplopia and partial or complete loss of vision). The onset of these symptoms may occur abruptly or insidiously over weeks or months.

The ESR and CRP concentrations are usually, but not always, raised in these conditions.

Drug treatment

The aim of treatment is to relieve symptoms and minimise vascular complications, particularly blindness, the most serious and irreversible feature (which may occur with both polymyalgia rheumatica and, especially, giant cell arteritis). Early diagnosis is essential to prevent consequences such as blindness, stroke or dissection of the aorta.[56]

The mainstay of treatment is corticosteroid treatment, as oral prednisolone, to control the disease process. Corticosteroids are used in high doses initially then reduced gradually over a period of several months. Initial response is often rapid, with clear improvement within days contributing to the diagnosis. Treatment may need to be continued for 3–4 years, although an attempt at withdrawal after 2 years is reasonable.[57] NSAIDs are sometimes used to alleviate symptoms, but do not modify the disease process.

Recommended doses vary between 10 and 100 mg oral prednisolone daily. Intravenous corticosteroids are occasionally used if visual complications are already present. There is insufficient evidence to recommend any particular starting dose, though some small studies to assess optimal doses have been carried out[58] and others have suggested risk factors to aid in decisions about doses.[59,60] Many clinicians use doses at the higher end of the scale initially, particularly where ocular involvement is demonstrated. Lower doses of 10–20 mg prednisolone daily to treat polymyalgia and 40–60 mg daily for cranial arteritis (where there is a higher risk of developing the complications of arteritis) may be used. There is some evidence that clinical and biochemical parameters indicating the presence of a strong acute-phase response may define a subgroup of patients at low risk of developing cranial ischaemic complications and this may suggest a rationale for using less aggressive treatment schedules in these patients.[61] The potential benefits of higher doses need to be balanced against the risk of adverse effects in elderly patients. Serious side-effects are related to high initial doses, maintenance doses, cumulative doses and increased duration of treatment.

Prolonged treatment using corticosteroids may result in the usual spectrum of side-effects. These can be minimised by using the lowest dose

Table 11.9 Key points in the management of polymyalgia rheumatica and cranial arteritis

- Use an adequate dose of prednisolone for the first month to achieve good symptomatic control and prevent complications
- Use a higher dose if visual disturbances are already present
- Aim to reduce dose gradually, with trial of withdrawal after 2 years
- Monitor for relapse and increase steroid dose accordingly
- Consider other methods of minimising steroid side-effects (e.g. use of prophylaxis against steroid-induced osteoporosis)
- Reassure the patient that the condition responds well to treatment, and treatment can usually be discontinued after 2–3 years. Advise to report signs of relapse

of prednisolone possible, and coadministering prophylactic treatment against steroid-induced osteoporosis (see Chapter 10). Addition of steroid-sparing agents (e.g. azathioprine, methotrexate) may be considered, although the benefits of these have not been established.[62]

Return of clinical features may indicate a relapse, despite normal ESR and CRP measurements. Relapses are unpredictable and may occur either during treatment or at any time after corticosteroids have been discontinued. Monitoring for relapse should continue for 6–12 months and patients advised to report urgently any recurrence of symptoms at any stage.

Key points in the management of polymyalgia rheumatica and cranial arteritis are summarised in Table 11.9.

References

1. Office for National Statistics. *Key Health Statistics from General Practice 1996*. London: HMSO, 1996.
2. American College of Rheumatology Ad Hoc Committee on Clinical Guidelines. Guidelines for the management of rheumatoid arthritis. *Arthritis Rheum* 1996; 39: 713–722.
3. Hamilton J, Capell H. Treatment of rheumatoid arthritis in the elderly. *Prescriber* 1998; 9: 121–132.
4. Akil M, Amos R S. Rheumatoid arthritis – clinical features and diagnosis. *BMJ* 1995; 310: 587–590.
5. Symmons D P M, Barrett E M, Bankhead C *et al*. The incidence of rheumatoid arthritis in the United Kingdom: results from the Norfolk Arthritis Register. *Br J Rheumatol* 1994; 33: 735–739.
6. Brooks P M. Rheumatoid arthritis: aetiology and clinical features. *Medicine* 1998; 26: 28–31.

7. Kaye E. Rheumatoid arthritis and osteoarthritis. *Pharm J* 1988; 241: 296–299.

8. Arnett F C, Edworthy S M, Block D A *et al*. The American Rheumatism Association 1987 revised criteria for the classification of rheumatoid arthritis. *Arthritis Rheum* 1988; 31: 315–324.

9. Van Schardenburg D. Rheumatoid arthritis in the elderly – prevalence and optimal management. *Drugs Aging* 1985; 7: 30–37.

10. Report of a joint working group of the British Society for Rheumatology and the research unit of the Royal College of Physicians. Guidelines and audit measures for the specialist supervision of patients with rheumatoid arthritis. *J R Coll Physicians Lond* 1992; 26: 76–81.

11. Scottish Intercollegiate Guideline Network. Management of Early Rheumatoid Arthritis. Edinburgh: SIGN, 2000, No 48.

12. Irvine S, Munro R, Porter D. Early referral, diagnosis and treatment of rheumatoid arthritis: evidence for changing medical practice. *Ann Rheum Dis* 1999; 58: 510–513.

13. Bendtsen P, Akerlind I, Hornquist J O. Pharmacological intervention in older patients with rheumatoid arthritis. Quality of life aspects. *Drugs Aging* 1995; 7: 338–346.

14. Bayraktar A, Hudson S, Watson A, Fraser S. Pharmaceutical care (7): arthritis. *Pharm J* 1998; 264: 57–67.

15. Watson M. Rheumatoid arthritis. *Pharm J* 1998; 260: 310–311.

16. Brooks P M. Management of rheumatoid arthritis. *Medicine* 1998; 26: 32–35.

17. Brooks P M, Day R O. Nonsteroidal anti-inflammatory drugs – differences and similarities. *N Engl J Med* 1991; 324: 1716–1725.

18. Suarez-Almzo M E. Rheumatoid arthritis. In: Barton S, ed. *Clinical Evidence*. London: BMJ Publishing Group, 1999: 225–237.

19. Committee on Safety of Medicines. Relative safety of oral non-aspirin NSAIDs. *Curr Probl Pharmacovigilance* 1994; 20: 9–11.

20. Van Jaarsfeld C H M, Jacobs J W G, van der Veen M J *et al*. Aggressive treatment in early rheumatoid arthritis: a randomised controlled trial. *Ann Rheum Dis* 2000; 59: 468–477.

21. Felson D T, Anderson J J, Meenan R F. The comparative efficacy and toxicity of second line drugs in rheumatoid arthritis. Two meta-analyses. *Arthritis Rheum* 1990; 33: 1449–1461.

22. Felson D T, Anderson J J, Meenan R F. Use of short term efficacy/toxicity trade-offs to select second-line drugs in rheumatoid arthritis. A meta-analysis of published clinical trials. *Arthritis Rheum* 1992; 35: 1117–1125.

23. Verhoeven A C, Boers M, Tugwell P. Combination therapy in rheumatoid arthritis: updated systematic review. *Br J Rheumatol* 1998; 37: 612–619.

24. Boers M, Verhoeven A C, Markusse H M *et al*. Randomised comparison of combined step-down prednisolone, methotrexate and sulphasalazine with sulphasalazine alone in early in rheumatoid arthritis. *Lancet* 1997; 350: 309–318.

25. Tugwell P, Pincas T, Yocum D *et al*. Combination therapy with cyclosporin and methotrexate in severe rheumatoid arthritis. *N Engl J Med* 1995; 333: 137–141.

26. O'Dell J R, Haire C E, Erikson N *et al*. Treatment of rheumatoid arthritis with methotrexate alone, sulfasalazine and hydroxychloroquine or a combination of all three medications. *N Engl J Med* 1995; 334: 1287–1291.

27. Gotzche P C, Johansen K H. Meta-analysis of short-term low-dose prednisolone versus placebo and non-steroidal anti-inflammatory drugs in rheumatoid arthritis. *BMJ* 1998; 316: 811–818.

28. Kirwan J R. The effect of glucocorticoids on joint destruction in rheumatoid arthritis. *N Engl J Med* 1995; 333: 142–146.

29. Anon. Leflunomide is an effective new DMARD for active rheumatoid arthritis. *Drugs Ther Perspect* 2000; 16: 1–5.

30. O'Dell J R, Paulsen G, Haire C E *et al*. Treatment of early seropositive rheumatoid arthritis with minocycline: four year followup of a double-blind, placebo-controlled trial. *Arthritis Rheum* 1999; 42: 1691–1695.

31. Anon. Intercepting TNF-alpha with etanercept to treat rheumatoid arthritis. *Drugs Ther Perspect* 1999; 14: 1–5.

32. Watson M. Management of patients with osteoarthritis. *Pharm J* 1997; 259: 296–297.

33. Ling S M, Bathon J M. Osteoarthritis in older adults. *J Am Geriatr Soc* 1998; 46: 216–225.

34. Erb A, Brenner H, Gunther K-P, Sturmer T. Hormone replacement therapy and patterns of osteoarthritis: baseline data from the Ulm osteoarthritis study. *Ann Rheum Dis* 2000; 59: 105–109.

35. Cicuttini F M, Spector T D. Osteoarthritis in the aged: epidemiological issues and optimal management. *Drugs Aging* 1995; 6: 409–420.

36. Jones A, Docherty M. *Osteoarthritis. ABC of Rheumatology*. London: BMJ Publishing Group, 1997: 28–31.

37. Dieppe P. Osteoarthritis; time to shift the paradigm. *BMJ* 1999; 318: 1299–1300.

38. Anon. Osteoarthritis and its treatment. *MeRec Bull* 1994; 5: 13–16.

39. Scott D L, Shipley M, Dawson A *et al*. The clinical management of rheumatoid arthritis and osteoarthritis; strategies for improving clinical effectiveness. *Br J Rheum* 1998; 37: 546–554.

40. Krummel T, Dimitrov Y, Moulin B, Hannedouche T. Acute renal failure induced by topical ketoprofen. *BMJ* 2000; 320: 93.

41. Anon. Topical NSAIDs for joint disease. *Drugs Ther Bull* 1999; 27: 87–88.

42. Dieppe P, Chard J. Osteoarthritis. In: Barton S, ed. *Clinical Evidence*. London: BMJ Publishing Group, 1999: 219–223.

43. Hamilton J, Sturrock R. Osteoarthritis; current management approaches. *Prescriber* 1999; 10: 48–58.

44. Anon. Hyaluronan or hyalans for knee osteoarthritis? *Drugs Ther Bull* 1999; 37: 71–72.

45. Wynne H A. Osteoarthritis. *Prescribers' J* 1998; 38: 211–216.

46. Eccles M, Freemantle N, Mason J. North of England evidence-based guideline development proposed; summary guidelines for non-steroidal anti-inflammatory drugs versus basic analgesia in treating the pain of degenerative arthritis. *BMJ* 1998; 317: 526–530.

47. Rapport L, Lockwood B. Glucosamine. *Pharm J* 2000; 265: 134–135.

48. McAlindon T E, LaValley M P, Gulinn J P, Felson D T. Glucosamine and chondroitin for treatment of osteoarthritis. *JAMA* 2000; 283: 1469–1475.
49. Anon. Diagnosis and treatment of gout in the elderly is not always easy. *Drugs Ther Perpect* 1999; 14: 8–11.
50. Emerson B T. Drug therapy: the management of gout. *N Engl J Med* 1996; 334: 445–451.
51. Snaith M L. Gout, hyperuricaemia and crystal arthritis. *BMJ* 1995; 310: 521–524.
52. Fam A G. Gout in the elderly. Clinical presentation and treatment. *Drugs Aging* 1998; 13: 229–243.
53. Star V L, Hochberg M C. Prevention and management of gout. *Drugs* 1993; 45: 212–222.
54. Jolobe O. Treating gout in the presence of cardiac failure. *Practitioner* 1994; 238: 489–490.
55. Parfitt K, ed. *Martindale, The complete drug reference*, 32nd edn. London: Pharmaceutical Press, 1999: 390–391.
56. Dwolatzky T, Sonnenblick M, Nesher G. Giant cell arteritis and polymyalgia rheumatica: clues to early diagnosis. *Geriatrics* 1997; 52: 38–44.
57. Kyle V, Hazelman B L. Stopping steroids in polymalgia rheumatica and giant cell arthritis. *BMJ* 1990; 300: 344–345.
58. Nesher G, Rubinow A, Sonneblick M. Efficacy and adverse effects of different corticosteroid regimens in temporal arthritis: a retrospective study. *Clin Exp Rheumatol* 1997; 15: 303–306.
59. Seriolo B, Cutolo M, Garnero A, Accardo S. Risk factors for thrombotic events in giant cell arteritis and polymyalgia rheumatica. *Br J Rheumatol* 1998; 37: 1251–1253.
60. Gonzalez-Gay M A, Blanco R, Rodriguez-Valverde V *et al*. Permanent visual loss and cerebrovascular accidents in giant cell arteritis: predictors and response to treatment. *Arthritis Rheum* 1998; 41: 1497–1504.
61. Cid M C, Font C, Oristrell J *et al*. Association between strong inflammatory response and low risk of developing visual loss and other cranial ischaemic complications in giant cell (temporal) arthritis. *Arthritis Rheum* 1998; 41: 26–32.
62. van der Veen M J, Dinant HJ, van Booma-Frankfort C *et al*. Can methotrexate be used as a steroid-sparing agent in the treatment of polymyalgia rheumatica and giant cell arteritis? *Ann Rheum Dis* 1996; 55: 218–223.

12

Eye, ear and mouth problems in the elderly

Duncan Livingstone

Eye

Visual degeneration can be regarded as an inevitable consequence of ageing. Of people in the UK registered blind or partially sighted, more than three-quarters are aged 65 years and over. Conservative estimates suggest that glaucoma and cataracts are at least eight times more common in people over 65 years compared with the general population. Given the increasing longevity of the UK population, the number of patients with degenerative eye disease will undoubtedly continue to grow.

Between the ages of about 40 and 65 years, there is a gradual loss of elasticity of the lens, leading to a progressive inability of the ciliary muscles to focus the lens on near objects. The resultant short-sightedness is usually corrected in people with otherwise healthy eyes by the use of appropriate reading glasses. Ageing also causes a decrease in the diameter of the pupil, allowing less light into the eye; furthermore, the rate at which the pupil reacts to light and dark by constriction and dilatation is retarded. The consequences of these changes may be particularly significant at night for elderly car drivers and those with poorly lit homes. As these degenerative changes are insidious, there are undoubtedly many elderly people who are unaware of their visual impairment and hence their increased risk of accident and injury.

Dry eye

Dry eye is a problem which commonly occurs in the elderly due to progressive diminution of tear secretion with advancing age. Sufferers of rheumatoid arthritis and some other systemic diseases are particularly prone to dry eye. Symptoms vary from minimal to severe discomfort with sensations of grittiness and burning (keratoconjunctivitis sicca). If left untreated, corneal ulceration may arise. The ideal solution to dry eye would be controlled stimulation of tear secretion, but as yet this remains impractical. A wide range of artificial tear solutions have been developed incorporating polyvinyl alcohol, cellulose derivatives and sodium hyaluronate. The artificial tear solutions based on hypromellose (hydroxypropylmethylcellulose) are most widely used and inexpensive. Although usually effective, hypromellose eye drops require frequent instillation and patients should be advised to use them as often as required to eliminate discomfort. Patients who regularly need to use their artificial tears more than eight times each day will require further investigation.

A more recent innovation are the gel artificial tear drops (GelTears, Viscotears) which contain carbomer 980 (polyacrylic acid). These preparations have the advantage of a longer duration of action than hypromellose and therefore require less frequent instillation. Hydrophobic, liquid paraffin-based eye ointments (Lacri-Lube, Lubri-Tears) can also be used to treat dry-eye conditions and are useful when applied at night due to their resistance to evaporation and drainage.

Hypersensitivity (usually to the preservative, benzalkonium chloride) may develop after artificial tear solutions have been used for some time. This is usually manifest as local irritation, conjunctivitis and sometimes periorbital eczematous changes. The addition of a topical anti-inflammatory or antihistamine is rarely appropriate; substitution with a preservative-free formulation is preferable. The widespread use of benzalkonium chloride in ocular lubricants appears somewhat paradoxical because it is directly irritant to the cornea and, being a surfactant, facilitates the break-up of the tear film! Benzalkonium chloride-preserved eye drops should also be avoided by wearers of soft contact lenses as the preservative is absorbed by the lenses which become cloudy. Preservative-free formulations exist for many, although not all, eye drop preparations. Whilst allergy/irritation is reduced by such products, their relatively high cost, difficulty in manipulation and the requirement to use a fresh container after each dose has been administered tend to prevent their widespread adoption.

Glaucoma

Glaucoma is the term applied to a number of eye conditions which are characterised by an increase in the intraocular pressure (IOP). Raised IOP may be due to obstructed outflow or increased secretion of aqueous humour. These result in a progressive loss of visual field which may ultimately lead to blindness if untreated. Glaucoma tends to run in families and is more common in Afro-Caribbeans than Caucasians. The incidence of glaucoma increases with age; about 1% of people aged 40 years and over exhibit glaucoma, rising to 10% in those aged 70 years and over.

Glaucoma can be subclassified into two major types: closed-angle (acute) and open-angle (chronic). Closed-angle glaucoma, the less common of the two, is usually unilateral and occurs four times more frequently in females than males. Characteristically, it is a disease of rapid onset with sudden pain in and around the eye, blurring of vision, nausea and vomiting. Closed-angle glaucoma should be regarded as a medical emergency and requires urgent treatment if blindness is not to ensue. Drug therapy is generally an interim measure pending surgical or laser treatment to facilitate drainage of aqueous humour. Closed-angle glaucoma may be precipitated or exacerbated by many drugs (including over-the-counter medicines) which are given for unrelated disorders. Elderly patients with multiple pathologies are particularly at risk of adverse effects and care should be taken when prescribing drugs with significant anticholinergic effects. Such drugs include tricyclic anti-depressants, antihistamines, antispasmodics and phenothiazines.

Open-angle glaucoma is usually a bilateral eye condition which progresses slowly and insidiously. Long-term treatment with topically and occasionally systemically administered drugs is required to control the IOP and prevent loss of vision. The preferred initial therapy for the majority of patients is a topical β-adrenoceptor antagonist (betaxolol, carteolol, levobunolol, timolol). β-Adrenoceptor antagonists are absorbed systemically and may be contraindicated for patients with asthma, chronic obstructive pulmonary disease (COPD), congestive cardiac failure, sick sinus syndrome and second- or third-degree heart block. Due to the risk of bronchospasm, the Committee on Safety of Medicines (CSM) has advised that asthmatic patients and those with COPD should not be prescribed a β-adrenoceptor antagonist, including the apparently cardioselective betaxolol, unless no alternative treatment is available.

If a β-adrenoceptor antagonist fails to produce an adequate response, is contraindicated or side-effects are unacceptable, topical adrenaline (epinephrine) can be added or substituted. Dipivefrine which is a prodrug of adrenaline, may be preferred for some of those in whom adrenaline is poorly tolerated. Acute hypertensive crisis is a rare but serious side-effect of adrenaline and dipivefrine. These drugs must therefore be used with caution in patients with hypertension and other cardiovascular disorders. Brimonidine is a recently introduced selective α_2-adrenoceptor agonist which has been shown to have efficacy comparable to timolol but fewer serious adverse effects. In addition, brimonidine does not cause mydriasis (dilatation of the pupil) in contrast to non-selective α-adrenoceptor agonists and consequently brimonidine has displaced adrenaline and dipivefrine as the α-adrenoceptor agonist of choice.

Pilocarpine eye drops, which were formerly the mainstay of open-angle glaucoma treatment, now tend to be reserved as third-line therapy due to undesirable side-effects. Pilocarpine, particularly in higher concentrations, causes ocular pain and a loss of visual acuity and such problems may be less tolerable to the patient than the symptoms of glaucoma.

The last decade has also seen a dramatic decline of systemic treatment of open-angle glaucoma with the carbonic anhydrase inhibitor acetazolamide as the previously mentioned topical agents alone or in combination usually produce a therapeutically adequate response. In addition the elderly are more prone to the systemic side-effects of acetazolamide, including increased frequency of urination, drowsiness, nausea, hypokalaemia and paraesthesia. Acetazolamide should be used with particular care in patients with a history of renal impairment. Dorzolamide and brinzolamide, more recently introduced topical carbonic anhydrase inhibitors, exhibit systemic adverse effects rather less commonly than acetazolamide but may nevertheless cause local problems, including blurred vision and conjunctival irritation which require discontinuation of the drug.

The prostaglandin $F_{2\alpha}$ analogue latanoprost effectively reduces IOP and may be useful for patients with open-angle glaucoma which is resistant to other drugs or when other drugs are contraindicated. Latanoprost has the somewhat bizarre side-effect of increasing the brown pigmentation of the iris. This may be a particular problem for susceptible blue-eyed individuals who are receiving treatment to one eye only and patients should be alerted to this effect accordingly. The widespread use of latanoprost is further inhibited by its relatively high cost when compared with β-adrenoceptor antagonists and α-adrenoceptor agonists.

Cataract

Cataracts are a common condition in the elderly; indeed, it is likely that some degree of cataract formation is present in all those over 70 years of age. Cataract is a condition where the lens becomes progressively less clear causing a gradual loss of vision and ultimately blindness. Ageing appears to be the leading cause of cataract formation, but the process may be accelerated by a hereditary factor, trauma, poorly controlled diabetes mellitus and the chronic use of topical or systemic corticosteroids and high-dose phenothiazines. In cases of iatrogenic and diabetes-related cataracts appropriate medical intervention may slow down the rate of degeneration; however, the treatment of cataract is essentially surgical. Treatment is usually delayed until visual impairment is sufficient to impair normal activity significantly; the affected lens is removed and replaced with an artificial intraocular substitute. Postoperatively the eye is usually inflamed and treatment for a few weeks is common with a topical preparation containing a steroid and antibacterial, e.g. Maxitrol, Neo-Cortef.

Macular degeneration

Macular degeneration is a leading cause of blindness in the elderly. The macula is the central 10% of the retina and is responsible for sharp and near vision. The remainder of the eye is principally responsible for peripheral vision. The macula slowly deteriorates from middle age onwards, although this process appears to accelerate significantly in the elderly. Total blindness is unlikely with macular degeneration, but normal activity is severely impaired. The exact causes of macular degeneration remain unclear, although ultraviolet light and free radicals may be implicated. Consequently, wearing of ultraviolet-blocking sunglasses and taking antioxidant vitamins (A, C, E) and zinc have been advocated, although evidence of their clinical value is very sparse. Recent innovations using photodynamic (laser) treatment have dramatically improved the outlook for 30% of sufferers of macular degeneration, but cost is currently high and availability limited.

Entropion and ectropion

Entropion is an eye problem usually associated with ageing. Most commonly, the lower eyelid turns inward due to muscle spasm or as a response to trauma and scarring of the eyelid. These result in damage to the eye with irritation and pain, often requiring remedial surgery. Ectropion is when the lower lid margin is turned outward and is no longer in contact with the surface of the eye (usually due to loss of muscle tone). This causes the eye to dry excessively with resultant soreness and tearing. Sufferers of ectropion tend to rub their eyes and this increases the vulnerability of the eye to infection. Regular use of an ocular lubricant and/or a topical antimicrobial, e.g. chloramphenicol eye ointment, may be required pending surgery.

Miscellaneous iatrogenic eye disease

It is well recognised that the elderly are more prone to the adverse effects of drugs than younger adults. Many drugs prescribed for systemic diseases in the elderly are associated with ocular adverse effects. Derivatives of chloroquine used in the treatment of rheumatoid arthritis have been demonstrated to cause retinal damage, although wide variations of incidence are reported. Long-term systemic use of corticosteroids may exacerbate the development of cataracts in susceptible individuals. The antiarrhythmic drugs digoxin and amiodarone may cause visual disturbances even at therapeutic doses, although such effects usually reverse following withdrawal of treatment.

Use of eye drops by the elderly

The overwhelming majority of elderly patients who are prescribed drugs for an eye condition will be treated with an eye drop formulation. Patients will frequently need comprehensive counselling about their treatments and appropriate administration techniques. Ideally, new patients should be asked to self-administer in the presence of the pharmacist to assess administration technique. Some patients, e.g. those with rheumatoid arthritis or Parkinson's disease, may have particular difficulties with eye drops due to their inability to squeeze the bottle or dropper, difficulty in keeping the eye open or an inability to direct the drops into the eye. In such cases, training of a carer to administer the eye drops may be more appropriate. Alternatively, compliance aids such as Autodrop may help patients to direct their eye drops correctly whilst keeping the eye open during administration. An alternative approach for patients who experience difficulty in self-administering eye drops may be the use of an eye ointment containing the same or similar active moiety. Unfortunately, the greasy bases used in most eye ointments may produce a sight-blurring film across the eye.

Ear disorders

Hearing impairment in the elderly (presbycusis) is very common and may be regarded as a normal trait of the ageing process. It has been conservatively estimated that 30% of people over the age of 65 years have a degree of hearing loss great enough to impair normal everyday communication. Poor hearing may put elderly patients at risk whilst undertaking routine tasks such as crossing the road. In addition, patients may misunderstand information given to them or questions asked of them – the author has experience of an elderly patient who achieved a mental score of 2/10 and was diagnosed as suffering from dementia; when a hearing aid was tried, the patient's condition apparently improved dramatically, meriting a score of 7/10! Because hearing loss is usually insidious, many elderly people are unaware of a problem and do not volunteer any such information.

Loss of hearing has been reported with a number of drugs, notably furosemide (frusemide), quinine-based antimalarials, some cytotoxics (particularly cisplatin) and the aminoglycoside antibiotics. Most cases of ototoxicity have arisen from rapid high-dose intravenous administration of these compounds, but rare instances of permanent hearing impairment have been reported with orally administered formulations. Damage to hearing may be prevented or reduced if patients are alerted to report early signs of aural toxicity such as vertigo and tinnitus, thus allowing opportune modification of therapy.

Ear wax

Wax (cerumen) is a normal secretion produced by the outer ear and is believed to have a physiological role in maintaining the integrity of the aural canal. Total or partial blockage of the outer ear canal by wax is common in the elderly. Although it might appear that ear wax production is increased in the elderly, evidence would suggest that it is the drier nature of the wax secreted in old age and inability to remove it readily which allow blockage of the outer ear canal to occur. Males are somewhat more prone to blockage than females due to subtle differences in the aural anatomy. The degree of occlusion of the ear will dictate the degree of hearing impairment.

Removal of impacted earwax can give a dramatic improvement in hearing and consequently the quality of life of an affected individual. Syringing the ear with warm water can provide rapid relief from impacted earwax, but carries a small risk of damage to the ear drum and the possibility of permanent deafness. It is not recommended for individuals with a perforated ear drum or recent history of ear surgery. Syringing should also be avoided if there is a history of recurrent otitis externa. Expulsion of earwax may be facilitated by the application of warm olive or almond oil to the affected ear for several days prior to syringing. A number of inexpensive proprietary ear drop solutions are marketed for the removal of earwax but evidence for their efficacy when used without subsequent syringing is lacking. In addition, some of the ingredients of the proprietary earwax removal solutions may irritate the outer ear canal and ear drum.

Tinnitus

Tinnitus is a condition experienced by up to a quarter of those over 65 years. It is characterised by unpleasant, intermittent or unceasing noises in the ears, typically hissing, buzzing, ringing or whistling. In a small proportion of those affected, symptoms may be very debilitating with a marked reduction in quality of life. The causes of tinnitus are diverse, but are usually associated with some degree of pathological change to the middle and inner ear. Some drugs, particularly aspirin, have been implicated as causes of tinnitus although usually when given in excess of the normal therapeutic doses. There is however wide interindividual variation of sensitivity to salicylate-induced tinnitus and some individuals may suffer this effect when taking 'normal' doses of aspirin. Tinnitus, together with vertigo and deafness, are common symptoms of Ménière's disease. This disease is rare below the age of 30 and appears to increase in incidence with age. Antihistamines such as cinnarizine and cyclizine and phenothiazines such as prochlorperazine may reduce vertigo and associated nausea, but tinnitus rarely responds to drug therapy. Betahistine, although specifically indicated for the treatment of Ménière's disease, appears to offer little or no advantage over the antihistamines and phenothiazines apart from avoiding antimuscarinic and antidopaminergic adverse effects.

The use of a hearing aid can be an effective method of managing tinnitus; the resultant increase in perception of extrinsic sound helps to mask the disturbing intrinsic tinnitus sounds. Sufferers of tinnitus often find the problem to be worse in bed at night due to lack of normal daytime background noise and other sensory distraction and some individuals gain benefit from employment of an extrinsic sound source, e.g. radio, to act as a so-called 'pillow masker'. Fatigue and stress are recognised to be aggravating factors for tinnitus. Anxiolytic drugs may cause more problems than they solve and are unlikely to be advantageous in the long term, but alteration of lifestyle and learning of relaxation techniques may aid some sufferers.

The mouth

Mouth care of the elderly is a very important but frequently neglected practice. In the past the loss of teeth with advancing age was accepted as part of the normal ageing process. As general health, education and prosperity have improved over the last half-century, so the likelihood of retaining natural teeth into old age has increased. In common with many other disease states, there is a significant correlation between socio-economic class and dental health. The reasons why the elderly fail to exercise good dental care are many, but include difficulty in attending a dental surgery, apathy, fear of cost and fear of radical treatment.

It can be demonstrated that good dental care with preservation of natural teeth can reduce general ill health and help to attenuate the visible signs of aging. Loss of teeth and mandibular bone decreases support of the overlying tissue and consequently the face takes on a sunken, wrinkled and weak appearance. Well-fitted dentures can help to restore fuller contours to the face but it should be emphasised that natural teeth, whether undecayed or correctly restored, are usually preferable to dentures.

Many individuals with no remaining natural teeth either do not possess or fail to use their dentures. These problems can lead to difficulty in eating certain foods as well as giving the face a sunken or haggard appearance. Old, worn and ill-fitting dentures are commonly encountered and may cause pain, oral disease and lead to malnutrition. Oral thrush (candidiasis) due to the yeast *Candida albicans* is frequently encountered in the elderly and is especially common and persistent in patients with poor dental hygiene and/or ill-fitting dentures. Certain drugs, including corticosteroids and other immunosuppressants, may also predispose to this condition. Rigorous cleaning and sterilising of the dentures with a chlorine-based disinfectant such as Milton plus regular application of a topical antifungal containing miconazole (Daktarin Oral Gel, Dumicoat) to the surface of the dentures may overcome problems of persistent or recurrent thrush. Care should be exercised when using such miconazole-based preparations as significant systemic absorption of miconazole may occur, allowing the possibility of interaction with other drugs, including oral anticoagulants, antiepileptics and hypoglycaemics if taken concurrently.

Dry mouth

Dry mouth (xerostomia) is a common condition affecting approximately 20% of the population aged 65 years and over. Dry mouth may

cause discomfort, eating difficulties and dental decay and allow opportunistic infection to occur. Normal ageing itself is not believed to cause
a significant reduction of saliva secretion. Sjögren's syndrome, dehydration, diabetes and radiotherapy may all reduce saliva secretion. Drugs
are perhaps the most frequent extrinsic cause of dry mouth in the
elderly; antihistamines, antispasmodics, tricyclic antidepressants,
phenothiazines, atenolol and diuretics are common culprits. Dry mouth
due to drug therapy can often be managed by instructing patients to
increase their fluid intake or by removal or substitution of the offending
drug. Artificial saliva products (Glandosane, Saliva Orthana) may
provide some relief for dry mouth, but require frequent administration
(usually every 2 h). Pilocarpine, which exerts parasympathomimetic
activity similar to acetylcholine, has been used successfully to treat
severe dry mouth arising from radiotherapy for head and neck cancer.
Side-effects are common and include abdominal pain, nausea, vomiting
and diarrhoea and limit the general utility of pilocarpine. In addition,
pilocarpine is contraindicated for patients with asthma or COPD –
common problems in the elderly.

Mouth ulcers

Mouth ulcers (aphthous ulcers) can occur at any age, but frequently
occur in the elderly. Many cases of ulceration are idiopathic, but it is
recognised that some disease states, nutritional deficiencies and drugs
may increase the incidence and/or severity of mouth ulcers. Many
different drug treatments for mouth ulceration have been advocated,
although success has varied widely and no single drug has been shown
to be beneficial in all cases. Most ulcers will heal without intervention in
less than 10 days, although warm salt-water mouthwashes may reduce
the pain and inflammation. Antiseptic mouthwashes are widely
employed to treat mouth ulcers but evidence that they reduce the
duration and rate of recurrence of ulceration is lacking. Pain relief may
be otherwise obtained by the application of a salicylate-based gel or the
use of a topical local anaesthetic. Care must be taken with the latter, as
significant anaesthesia of the mouth and tongue may allow inadvertent
scalding to occur when hot beverages are consumed. Topical corticosteroids in lozenges or pellet form have been demonstrated to provide
worthwhile relief from mouth ulcers, although some patients may find
application to the immediate area of ulceration difficult. Patients with
very large and/or persistent mouth ulcers (over 2 weeks' duration)

should be referred to their dentist or doctor due to the risk of underlying oral malignancy.

Lichen planus

Lichen planus is a condition which can appear at any age, but is somewhat more prevalent in the elderly. It is estimated that approximately 1% of the UK population suffer from lichen planus, with a slightly higher incidence in females than males. The underlying cause has never been fully established, but an autoimmune factor is generally believed to be implicated. It is recognised that it may be precipitated or exacerbated by certain drugs, including 5-aminosalicylic acid derivatives, gold salts, penicillamine and spironolactone, and also by stress.

The disease is characterised by bilateral lesions of the oral mucosa. These may vary in appearance, but most cases are exhibited as white patches or striae (lines). The name is derived from the superficial resemblance of the lesions to lichen growing on rock. Pain and discomfort are uncommon and the lesions may be present for months or even years before detection. Most subjects with asymptomatic lichen planus do not require treatment, but less common erosive forms of the condition may necessitate therapeutic intervention. It has been suggested that the condition may be a precursor to oral cancer in a small number of patients, although this theory remains unproven. Topical corticosteroids – hydrocortisone, betamethasone, beclometasone and triamcinolone – administered as lozenges, mouthwashes, gels or sprays, two to four times daily are the mainstays of treatment; intralesional triamcinolone has also been used with some success. The concurrent use of a topical antifungal such as miconazole or nystatin has been advocated to prevent development of oral thrush. Systemic prednisolone has been shown to produce complete remission in over 70% of cases of lichen planus, but carries the risk of systemic adverse effects and, paradoxically, oral thrush. Tetracycline and chlorhexidine mouthwashes were formerly used, but in the absence of a topical corticosteroid they appear to exert little beneficial effect in their own right.

The autoimmune nature of lichen planus has attracted much research interest; treatment with a ciclosporin mouthwash has been investigated, but no clinical benefit has been identified. Where a drug has been identified as a precipitating or exacerbating factor, withdrawal of the offending substance can be beneficial, but lesions may remain for many months. The administration of anxiolytics has been promoted for cases where stress is believed to be a significant contributor, but their use is equivocal.

Further reading

Exton-Smith A N, Weksler M E. *Practical Geriatric Medicine*. Edinburgh: Churchill Livingstone, 1985.

Khaw P T, Elkington A R. *ABC of Eyes*, 2nd edn. London: BMJ Publishing Group, 1994.

Lewis M A O, Lamey P-J. *Clinical Oral Medicine*. Oxford: Butterworth-Heinemann, 1995.

Matteson M A, McConnell E S, Linton A D. *Gerontological Nursing*, 2nd edn. Philadelphia: Sunders, 1997.

Perry J P, Tullo A B, eds. *Care of the Ophthalmic Patient*, 2nd edn. London: Chapman & Hall, 1995.

Walker R, Edwards C, eds. *Clinical Pharmacy and Therapeutics*, 2nd edn. Edinburgh: Churchill Livingstone, 1999.

13

The skin in the elderly

Virginia A Hill

The skin in old age is a neglected subject, despite the fact that society places such a high value on youthful appearance. In no other organ are the signs of ageing so apparent as in the skin.[1] Ageing in the skin is a complex interplay between intrinsic processes and environmental damage, in particular photodamage.

The classical changes in ageing skin are wrinkling and roughness.[2] The epidermal thickness is reduced; the dermis undergoes atrophy with a reduction in connective tissue elements as well as blood vessels, nerve endings, sweat and sebaceous glands. In addition the hair loses colour and becomes thinner. Drying of the skin becomes a particular problem. The ageing appearance of the skin and hair loss can be a major cause of psychological problems.[3,4]

Particular considerations in the skin of the elderly are the effects of internal organ pathology as well as multiple drug therapy, as a result of which drug eruptions appear to be common. Infirmity may impair understanding and ability to comply with treatment, as can poverty and isolation.

The following sections discuss some of the common dermatological problems seen in the elderly and their treatment.

Eczema

Eczema is an inflammatory skin condition characterised by itching, redness and scaling, which may be induced by a wide range of factors. These factors may be endogenous, mediated by processes within the body, including alterations in the skin immune system, i.e. atopy. Exogenous factors include contact allergens, inhaled and ingested allergens, ambient temperature, humidity and sunlight, and psychosocial stress. There is an increased familial tendency.

The skin becomes drier with age and it is not unusual for women to develop eczema for the first time after the menopause. There are many types of eczema, the incidence of which varies with age. Alterations in immunity may contribute to atopic eczema and contact dermatitis being less common in the elderly, although they still occur, while asteatotic eczema, seborrhoeic dermatitis, discoid eczema and venous eczema are more common.[5,6] There have been few studies of the incidence and prevalence of eczema, but it appears to be the most common dermatological problem in general practice and one of the most common in hospital dermatology. An American study showed that the prevalence of all forms of eczema was 18 per 1000; asteatotic eczema and discoid eczema each accounts for 2 per 1000.[7]

Asteatotic eczema

The skin develops a mosaic, scaly, dry appearance, particularly on the shins. This problem is more common in the winter, particularly in hospitalised and nursing-home patients, due to the excessive dehydration of the skin by low ambient humidity. This form of eczema is thought to be endogenous, so there may be a past history of skin problems.

The most important aspect of treatment is liberal use of moisturisers including replacement of soaps with moisturisers and emollients in the bath. Topical steroids may be needed if the skin is inflamed.

Seborrhoeic dermatitis

Erythematous, slightly moist, scaly patches develop on the central part of the face, behind the ears and in the flexures of the trunk. The scalp may also be involved. The yeast *Pityrosporum ovale* is implicated, as well as other microorganisms. There is an endogenous component in this condition, so again there may be a relevant past history of eczema. Many patients mention that it is stress-related.

Treatment again includes the use of moisturisers, replacement of soap with an emollient and weak or moderately potent topical steroids combined with antifungal agents. Scalp involvement can be treated with a tar-based, salicylic acid-based or antimicrobial shampoo.

Discoid eczema

Discoid eczema is an endogenous form of eczema which is uncommon in young people, but is seen more in the elderly. Lesions are red, scaly, well demarcated and resemble a disc. They occur most commonly on the limbs and are typically persistent and itchy.

Treatments include moisturisers, emollients as cleansers and in the bath, as well as potent topical steroids. Antihistamines may be useful if itching is a feature, and systemic treatments may be necessary as it is often resistant to treatment.

Venous eczema

This is a condition that is only seen in patients with venous disease and therefore occurs on the lower legs. It is common in the elderly. If it becomes severe it may trigger a widespread eczematous eruption. There may also be an allergic component if the patient has received topical treatment for venous ulcers or bandaging.

Treatment is much the same as for other forms of eczema, but compression bandaging and long-term compression hosiery are also required to reverse the effects of venous disease. Walking regularly and elevation of the legs while resting are also helpful. If contact sensitivity is suspected and particularly if the eczema is slow to respond to treatment, patch testing is necessary.

Systemic treatment in eczema

Severe, persistent widespread eczema in the elderly requires investigation to exclude underlying causes such as malignancy, drug reactions, contact sensitivity and exclusion of infestations such as scabies.

If topical therapy is ineffective, systemic treatment may be required. The most commonly used drugs in the elderly include prednisolone, azathioprine and ciclosporin. The lowest dose possible should be used to minimise the risk of side-effects, which are more common in the elderly. Light therapy, including ultraviolet B (UVB) and psoralen-ultraviolet A may be useful options, particularly if pruritus is a major symptom.

Psoriasis

Psoriasis is a common inflammatory skin condition which has a prevalence of 2% of the population in western Europe and Scandinavia, and a lower prevalence in other countries.[8] There are no studies of incidence. It is chronic, and in some cases can be severe, causing significant psychological and physical disability. There are two peaks of onset: the first in the late teens and early 20s, the second in late middle age. There is a definite association with high alcohol intake and a less well-known association with cigarette smoking. A family history of psoriasis is present in about a quarter of patients,[9] but there is a controversy over the mode of inheritance. There is a strong human lymphocyte antigen (HLA) association with HLA-Cw6.[8] The basic underlying molecular genetic defect has yet to be elucidated but is likely to be an abnormality of the interaction between T lymphocytes and keratinocytes.

Triggering factors include trauma, infections, hormonal changes, drugs (e.g. lithium, β-blockers, antimalarials, steroid withdrawal) and psychosocial stress.[8]

It is important to assess patients' understanding of their skin condition, and the effect it has on their life as a primary part of their treatment; even mild psoriasis may cause significant distress.

The following patterns of psoriasis are seen.

Classical or chronic plaque psoriasis

Salmon-pink, scaly, well demarcated plaques are typically seen on the elbows, knees, shins and sacrum. The scalp and nails may also be involved and plaques can appear on any other part of the body. This is the most common form of psoriasis, and lesions tend to be stable and chronic. Pruritus is not usually a feature. The appearance of the lesions and the persistent shedding of scale are the major problems.

Scalp psoriasis

The scalp is often involved in psoriasis but occasionally may be the only area affected.

Nail psoriasis

Pitting, onycholysis (lifting up) and thickening of the nails are common in psoriasis. Again, this may be seen as an isolated problem. Fungal infection of the nail may need to be excluded.

Guttate psoriasis

Usually a problem of teenagers and young adults, this form of psoriasis is typically acute and follows an infection. The lesions are small and profuse, and it tends to be self-limiting.

Flexural psoriasis

This form of psoriasis is more common in the elderly and may be difficult to differentiate from seborrhoeic eczema. Anogenital involvement may be persistent, distressing and resistant to treatment. In addition, elderly patients may be reluctant to admit involvement of this area.

Erythrodermic psoriasis

The whole skin is involved with pink, unstable psoriasis, resulting in excessive heat and water loss. In the elderly this may be life-threatening. Systemic or very potent topical steroids can precipitate it.

Acute generalised pustular psoriasis

This is also a life-threatening but rare condition, particularly in the elderly as the patient is unable to conserve heat or water and becomes systemically unwell. It can occur spontaneously or can be triggered by withdrawal or use of systemic steroids.

Palmoplantar pustular psoriasis

This is a more chronic form of pustular psoriasis involving only the palms and soles. The condition may be quite disabling. It is seen more often in late middle age and old age than in younger people. A severe nail dystrophy may also be associated with it.

Psoriatic arthopathy

A specific form of arthritis may accompany psoriasis in a minority of cases. Rarely this can cause gross deformity. It may occur in isolation.

Treatment

Topical treatment

Topical treatments are often adequate for limited forms of psoriasis, including emollients, tar-based products, salicylic acid, topical steroids (which may be combined with tar and/or salicylic acid) and calcipotriol. Dithranol has been used for decades, and can be used as proprietary preparations at home, or in Lassar's paste for inpatient treatment of widespread psoriasis, classically combined with UVB light therapy. Care must be taken to start at low strengths and increase gradually as it is easy to burn the skin with dithranol, which can lead to worsening psoriasis and even erythroderma.

The use of topical treatment requires careful explanation, and adequate compliance with regular application is important for success. This may not be possible for elderly patients who may be unable to hear properly, have poor vision, short-term memory loss, physical disabilities, and may be living on their own. Enlisting the help of a district nurse may be invaluable.

Light therapy

Light therapy may be a useful adjunct to topical therapy and can be used with systemic therapy, as psoriasis often responds well to sunlight. UVB therapy is typically given three to five times weekly. Narrow-band UVB (TL01) has been found to be more effective and only needs to be used twice weekly. UVA therapy is also used, usually combined with oral methoxypsoralen, which sensitises the skin to light. It is more effective than UVB or TL01 therapy but increased sensitivity of the eyes to sunlight, as well as a long-term risk of skin cancer, are potential disadvantages. Light therapy is always hospital-based, which may be a cause of difficulty if transport is a problem, or if the patient is unable to stand upright in the machine.

Systemic treatment

Systemic treatment is appropriate for severe psoriasis, though may be used in milder forms if the patient is distressed by the condition or unable to comply with topical treatment. Although there is a greater risk of side-effects in the elderly, teratogenicity and long-term side-effects are less of a concern. Systemic treatments are therefore used more often than in younger patients.

Methotrexate   Methotrexate is a very useful drug which also helps nail dystrophy and psoriatic arthropathy. It is an antimetabolite, which can cause bone marrow suppression, immunosuppression and hepatic toxicity. It is usually given as a once-weekly oral dose, although it can be given by intramuscular injection if the tablets cause nausea or if the patient has acute, severe psoriasis. Regular monitoring of blood count, renal and liver function tests is required as well as liver ultrasound or biopsy, but it is usually well tolerated by patients, including the elderly.

Acitretin   Acitretin is a synthetic retinoid which reduces skin turnover and at least flattens psoriatic plaques. It has little effect on nail dystrophy or psoriatic arthritis. Potential side-effects are hepatitis, hypercholesterolaemia, dry skin, cheilitis and hair loss, among others. Regular monitoring of serum liver and renal function tests and lipids is required, and patients are asked to abstain from alcohol.

Ciclosporin   Ciclosporin, an immunosuppressant, is increasingly used for psoriasis. It is recommended that it is used in short courses to clear the psoriasis and then stopped, although it can be used as a long-term treatment. The main side-effects are hypertension and renal compromise. There also appears to be a small long-term risk of malignancy, in particular lymphoma. It may have some beneficial effect on nail dystrophy and arthritis.

Hydroxycarbamide (Hydroxyurea)   Hydroxycarbamide (hydroxyurea) is used less commonly now for psoriasis, but may be effective.

Other drugs   Various other drugs have been tried for difficult psoriasis, such as mycophenolate mofetil, but can only be prescribed on a named-patient basis. Further research into the causes of psoriasis are likely to identify new therapies in the future.

Dry skin and pruritus

Pruritus is a distressing, common problem in the elderly, affecting at least 50% of those aged 60 and over. The most common cause is excessive dryness of the skin. The ageing process of the skin involves drying, due to loss of sebaceous glands.[10, 11] Women in particular may complain of dry, itchy skin after the menopause. Liberal use of emollients, including bath emollients, will help to reverse this. Soap-based cleansing products further dry and irritate the skin, and therefore should be replaced by emollients. There are several emollients that can be used, which are cheap to buy over-the-counter without the need for patients to buy expensive cosmetic moisturisers. Urea-based emollients or 0.25–0.5% menthol in aqueous cream may be helpful for symptomatic relief. Antihistamines may be effective, in particular the sedating antihistamines if sleep is disturbed. Any degree of eczema should be treated appropriately and infestation with scabies should be excluded.

If pruritus is persistent, not responding to these simple measures, a search should be made for signs of subtle skin disease or underlying systemic causes such as renal failure (uraemia), liver disease, iron-deficiency anaemia, diabetes and hypothyroidism. Malignancy, in particular lymphomas, can present with pruritus. In some cases severe pruritus may herald the onset of bullous pemphigoid, an autoimmune blistering disorder.[12] Treatment of the underlying cause may reduce the pruritus. Severe, intractable pruritus can respond well to phototherapy, also to ciclosporin in addition to the above measures. It is also important to identify psychological problems as pruritus may be difficult to treat until these have been dealt with.

Bullous pemphigoid

Bullous pemphigoid is an autoimmune blistering disorder affecting the elderly.[13] It is unusual for it to present before the age of 60. An auto-antibody is produced to components of the basal layer of the epidermis, resulting in pruritus and erythematous lesions, then blistering which may be extensive (Figure 13.1). The mucous membranes such as the conjunctiva and mouth may be involved. The incidence is estimated to be six to seven cases per million per year in France and Germany.[14] Drugs have been occasionally associated with the onset of bullous pemphigoid, including furosemide (frusemide), sulfasalazine, penicillins, penicillamine and captopril. The majority of patients require systemic treatment, most usually prednisolone, often with azathioprine.

Resistant cases may require methylprednisolone infusions or ciclosporin. The prognosis is related to the extent of involvement, and the general condition of the patient. A fine balance is often required between high enough doses to treat the condition, without causing significant side-effects such as diabetes and cardiac failure. Inpatient therapy is usually required in the acute stages as intensive skin care and nursing are necessary. A few patients die from this condition. Long-term maintenance treatment is usually required for at least 18 months to prevent relapse.

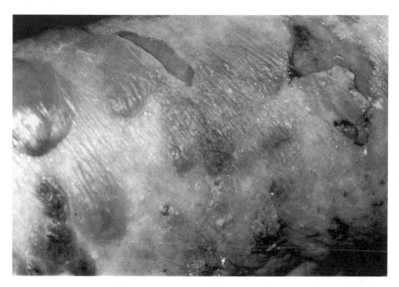

Figure 13.1 Extensive blistering due to bullous pemphigoid. Courtesy of Dr R A Marsden FRCP, physician to the Skin Department, St George's Hospital, London.

Drug eruptions

Drug eruptions are commonly seen in dermatological practice, particularly in the elderly because of reduced organ capacity and increased prescribing in this group. The incidence is difficult to obtain reliably due to significant underreporting but the reaction rate has been estimated at about 2% of prescriptions.[15] The degree of severity can range from a limited maculopapular eruption which causes some discomfort to a widespread, severe eruption which may be life-threatening (Figure 13.2).

Occasionally mucous membranes can be involved, as in Stevens–Johnson syndrome, with blistering of the mouth, conjunctivae and genital mucosa. Rarely, severe blistering occurs generally, as in toxic epidermal necrolysis. Urticaria and angioedema make up 20% of cases.[15]

Treatment is supportive, with topical emollients, moderate- or potent-strength topical steroids and dressing of blistered areas. Severely affected patients will require high-dependency or intensive care. The place of systemic steroids is controversial. An effort should be made to identify and avoid the offending drug, although this may be difficult in patients on multiple drug therapy.

Fixed drug eruption is an often unrecognised cause of recurrent eruptions which recur each time the drug is taken, and has a long list of possible causes.

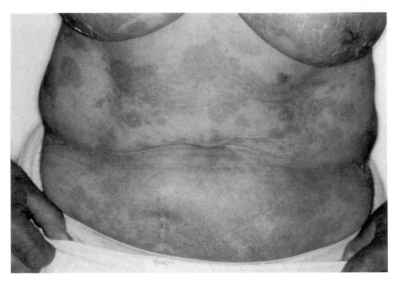

Figure 13.2 Drug eruption due to terbinafine. Courtesy of Dr R A Marsden FRCP, physician to the Skin Department, St George's Hospital, London.

Wound healing in the elderly

More attention has recently been given to the changes in wound healing brought about by age in an effort to find therapies to improve surgical wound healing. However, many aspects are still poorly understood.

Research has shown that wounds contract more slowly with increasing age, epithelialisation is slower and tensile strength of scars is less.[16] The rate of wound dehiscence is two to three times higher in people of more than 60 years of age, and wound-healing complications are generally more prevalent.[17] Scar tissue formation is less in the elderly. With increasing age, the response to injury demonstrates delayed cellular migration and proliferation, a delayed metabolic response and delayed remodelling. Recent research has shown that the inflammatory response during cutaneous wound healing is also altered by the ageing process.[18, 19] Oestrogens appear to have a role in the formation of scar tissue, in part explaining the reduction of scar tissue in the elderly.[20]

Wound dressings

The choice of available wound dressings is enormous and can be bewildering to the inexperienced.[21] It is best to use a few appropriately, and use the invaluable resource of a wound care specialist nurse if available. Table 13.1 gives a summary of dressings discussed below.

The elderly are more likely to develop chronic ulcers, wound healing in general tends to be slow and the skin is fragile, thus it is important to use the most effective dressings. Many of the newer dressings are expensive, and there is a need for controlled trials before

Table 13.1 Wound dressings for different applications

Nature of wound	Type of dressing
All	**Primary** (in direct contact with wound)
Surgical and/or superficial wounds	**Passive dressings (protective only)** e.g. gauze, Mepore, Melolin, N-A Ultra, Mepitel **Active dressings** (interact with wound)
Necrotic tissue	Hydrogel or hydrocolloids, e.g. Granuflex, Intrasite Dry dressings on fingers/toes Surgical debridement Enzymatic agents, e.g. Varidase, larvae
Slough	Surgical debridement Larvae Enzymatic agents Hydrocolloids, Iodosorb for small wounds Alginates, gel-forming polysaccharide dressings for larger exudative wounds Hydrogen peroxide cream for short periods
Granulation tissue	Silicone foam or alginate ribbon for cavities Hydrocolloid paste/gel for small cavity wounds Alginate fibre/hydrocolloid dressings for shallow wounds
Epithelialising wounds	Alginates, hydrocolloids Perforated plastic film such as Melolin, knitted silicone viscose dressings (i.e. primary dressings)
Exudate	Foam dressings, absorbent beads, alginate sheets, cavity dressings, hydrocolloids
Wound infection	Systemic antibiotics Flamazine – *Pseudomonas* spp. infection Metronidazole gel – fungating wounds, Gram-negative organisms Potassium permanganate soaks – moist wounds Medicated tulle dressings, e.g. Bactigras, Sofra-Tulle
Malodour	Charcoal dressings Firm occlusion (not hydrocolloid)
All except small surgical and superficial wounds	**Secondary dressings** (over top of primary dressing) Gamgee, gauze, simple absorbent pads Orthopaedic wadding (Velband, Soffban) Hydrocolloids Foam sheets, e.g. Allevyn

they are used regularly. Extra expense may be justified if dressings need to be changed less often and pain is improved.

Ideal dressings should promote healing, protect the wound, act as a barrier to infection, maintain a moist environment, relieve pain, and should not shed fibres or adhere to the wound. They should also be hypoallergenic, easy to use and dressing changes should be painless and infrequent.

Factors which affect choice of dressings include the depth of the wound, whether the wound is necrotic, sloughy, granulating or epithelialising and the degree of exudate, odour, pain and infection.[22]

Classification

Dressings may be classified into primary – in direct contact with the wound – or secondary – that is, placed over a primary dressing.

Primary dressings may be further classified as active, creating a favourable environment for healing and playing an active part in wound healing, or passive, having a protective function only.

Passive dressings (protective only) should be low adhesive such as Mepore or Melolin, which are often used for surgical and superficial wounds. Non-adherent dressings such as N-A Ultra or Mepitel are useful for ulcerated areas as they do not stick, and allow the skin to granulate. The latter is expensive but can be left in place for up to 2 weeks. Plain gauze can be used as a primary dressing but tends to stick. Paraffin gauze should probably not be used for open wounds as granulation tissue tends to grow through it and is therefore traumatised when the dressing is removed.

Active dressings[21] include alginates, foams, hydrocolloids, hydrogels, hydropolymers, cadexomer-iodine, hydrofibres and graft skin. The choice of dressing depends on the nature of the wound.

Necrotic tissue

Necrotic (dead) tissue should separate spontaneously if a wound is kept moist. If exposed to a dry atmosphere, dead tissue becomes dehydrated, shrinks and becomes green or black in colour. Separation is delayed indefinitely and the wound is painful.[23] The easiest methods of treatment are hydrogel (e.g. Intrasite) or hydrocolloid dressings (e.g. Granuflex) which retain moisture and rehydrate the wound. The only exception would be necrotic peripheral lesions which should simply be protected with dry dressing while awaiting amputation or recovery.

Other options are debridement, which is the quickest, most effective technique, but the patient often requires a general anaesthetic and care needs to be taken if tendons or nerves are exposed in the wound. Debridement with topical anaesthetic may be possible in superficial wounds.

Enzymatic agents may also be useful, for example Varidase, which digests necrotic tissue. It is applied directly to the wound or injected into or under necrotic tissue. Larvae (maggots) have been used in some centres. They are placed directly into the wound and eat only necrotic tissue. Skill is required in their use and they are available from only a limited number of sources.

Slough

Slough is whitish-yellow, moist necrotic tissue. It can be difficult to differentiate from normal fibrinous exudates; however, the latter can easily be lifted from the wound whereas slough is adherent. Slough may delay healing and increases the risk of infection.[24] It can be removed by mechanical debridement – although this may be very painful – larvae, or by enzymatic methods. Debrisan, Iodosorb and hydrocolloid dressings are useful for small, moist sloughy wounds. Wounds producing a greater amount of exudate may be dressed with alginate dressings, or a gel-forming polysaccharide dressing such as Aquacel. Hydrogen peroxide cream may be useful for short periods to loosen slough, but there is a risk of maceration of surrounding skin.

Granulation tissue

Granulating wounds contain vascular tissue essential for the healing process. Cavity wounds should be filled with a silicone foam dressing or with alginate fibre ribbon. Small granulating cavity wounds can be dressed with hydrocolloid pastes or gels. Shallow wounds may be dressed with an alginate fibre dressing or a hydrocolloid dressing depending on the amount of exudate. Overgranulating wounds can be treated with the topical application of Terra-Cortril.

Epithelialising wounds

Epithelialising wounds are in the final stages of healing, and the type of dressing can significantly alter the time taken to complete healing. Both alginates and hydrocolloid dressings are more advantageous than the traditional paraffin gauze. Other alternatives are perforated plastic film dressings such as Melolin and knitted viscose dressings impregnated with silicone.

Wound exudate, infection and malodour

Exudate is wound fluid produced by all open wounds. It plays a vital part in the healing process by keeping the wound moist; however, excessive exudate can macerate the surrounding skin and lead to infection. Many types of products have been developed to manage exudate, including foam dressings, absorbent beads, alginate sheets, cavity dressings and hydrocolloid dressings.[25]

Wound infection may require treatment with systemic antibiotics. Flamazine applied directly to the wound is useful for *Pseudomonas* spp. infection and metronidazole gel may be used for fungating wounds infected with Gram-negative organisms. Potassium permanganate soaks can be useful in a very moist wound as a mild antiseptic and drying agent. Medicated tulle dressings are available (e.g. Bactigras, Sofra-Tulle, Inadine). There is a risk of skin sensitivity and bacterial resistance with topical antibiotics.

Malodorous wounds may be treated with charcoal dressings. A firmly occlusive dressing will also help to reduce odour, but not an occlusive dressing such as DuoDERM/Granuflex because they tend to cause excessive exudate.

Secondary dressings

Finally, the choice of secondary dressing is important, because this influences the control of moisture, the spread of bacteria and the prevention of malodour.[26] Simple absorbent pads are used on heavily exuding wounds over alginate sheets. Gamgee was one of the original absorbent pads, but tends to shed fibres and is less effective than other newer dressings. Gauze and simple absorbent pads (e.g. Surgipad) are still widely used to soak up blood and exudate and provide a barrier to infection.

Orthopaedic wadding (e.g. Velband, Soffban) is used beneath pressure bandages to treat ulcers, and is also useful on other types of wounds to prevent pressure damage. Hydrocolloids may be used as secondary dressings over gels or alginates, particularly where exudate is heavy. Foam sheets (e.g. Allevyn) are useful to absorb exudate and provide protection from trauma. They can also be used over hydrogels and alginates but may preferentially take up moisture.

Leg ulcers

Chronic leg ulcers are a common but neglected subject.[27] The economic burden of ulcers to the National Health Service is immense and there is considerable cost to patients in terms of pain and immobility.

Much of the care of patients with ulcers is undertaken by practice and district nurses, with most of the cost taken up by nursing time. In the past, some of these patients were admitted to hospital, but this should be unnecessary with good care in the community.

It has been demonstrated that time to healing, quality of life and the rate of recurrence of ulcers can be significantly reduced by setting up dedicated leg ulcer clinics in the community, staffed by nurses with specific training, and with good links with relevant hospital specialist services such as vascular surgeons, geriatricians and dermatologists.[28]

The most common causes of leg ulcers are venous disease, arterial disease and diabetes, but many patients will have ulcers of mixed aetiology. Other less common causes[29] include rheumatoid arthritis, and other forms of vasculitis, malignancy, and unusual infections such as deep fungal infections. All patients therefore require assessment with a medical history, simple clinical examination, palpation of peripheral arterial pulses and ankle–brachial pressure index (ABPI) measured by hand-held Doppler, dip-stick urine testing and possibly blood glucose. Any medical problems should be treated. A biopsy should be considered for unusual or persistent ulcers to exclude malignancy.

Venous ulcers

These are the most common type of ulcers, with an overall incidence of about 0.2%,[30] rising with age. They are seen just above the ankle, particularly the medial side. They occur as a result of long-standing venous disease such as varicosities and incompetent valves, resulting in venous hypertension, and are associated with a sedentary lifestyle. Venous hypertension manifests initially as oedema and skin changes, including pigmentation, scar formation, thickening and possibly varicose eczema. The abnormal skin is therefore liable to break down into ulcers after the slightest trauma.

The mainstay of treatment is now compression bandaging, which reverses the effects of venous hypertension and therefore improves the rate of healing. Simple dressings are applied after cleansing, depending on the state of the ulcers. Adherent dressings should be avoided. Dry skin is treated with moisturisers and varicose eczema treated appropriately.[31]

One of the most effective compression regimens is four-layer bandaging.[32, 33] A layer of Velband orthopaedic wadding applied over the dressing followed by a crêpe bandage, Elset and Coban (cohesive compression bandage) was originally used by Charing Cross Hospital. Other multilayer systems are in use. If the patient has evidence of arterial disease, modified versions must be used which do not apply such high compression.

Infection (cellulitis) is a common complication and should be treated with systemic antibiotics.

Bandages can usually be left in place for a week at a time, sometimes longer, reducing valuable nursing time for dressings and lessening pain. The prognosis for healing is related to the length of time ulcers have been present, the size and underlying medical problems. Increasing mobility and avoiding sitting for prolonged periods with the legs down are likely to improve healing.

Once healing has been achieved there is evidence to show that recurrence is less likely when patients wear compression hosiery.[34] Walking is helpful by improving the venous calf pump. Patients with obvious varicosities should be assessed by Doppler ultrasound, as those with only superficial venous disease may be helped by surgery to their veins.[35]

Arterial ulcers

Many patients with mixed venous and arterial disease will do well on the above regimen. Any patients with severe arterial disease should be referred to a vascular surgeon for further assessment. Arterial ulcers typically occur on the feet, particularly the dorsum and toes, and necrosis may be a prominent feature.

Diabetic ulcers

These typically occur on the feet and toes, sometimes on pressure points, and may be very deep. Loss of sensation as well as damage to small arteries, infection and poor healing are all implicated. They are more likely to occur in poorly controlled diabetics or those in whom diabetes may have been undiagnosed for years. Liaison with specialist diabetic nurses, chiropodists and vascular surgeons will be necessary. Attention to the presence of infection, bacterial and fungal, is important. In deep ulcers underlying osteomyelitis should be excluded.[36]

Warts and calluses

Warts

Viral warts (due to the human papillomavirus) are less common in the elderly than in the young, although they do occur, particularly in the immunocompromised, such as renal transplant patients. They are seen on the trunk and limbs rather than the more typical sites of hands and feet. Keratolytics such as salicylic acid compounds may be useful, but the most effective treatments are cryotherapy and surgical methods including curettage and cautery, and excision.

More common in the elderly are seborrhoeic warts or keratoses – raised brown lesions with a stuck-on, warty appearance which may be quite unsightly. They are benign lesions but occasionally cause diagnostic confusion with melanomas. Treatment is usually requested on cosmetic grounds and includes cryotherapy and surgical methods.

Actinic keratoses can look warty, and are often seen in the elderly on sun-exposed sites such as the scalp, face, neck and limbs (Figure 13.3). They are due to long-term sun damage and the majority of cases occur in fair-skinned people exposed to sunlight, with a maximum prevalence in Queensland, Australia.[37] Although they carry a 1% per annum chance of malignant change, these lesions are in general

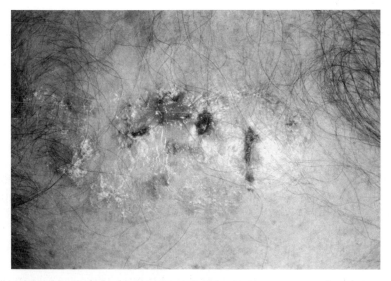

Figure 13.3 Large solar keratosis on a balding scalp. Courtesy of Dr R A Marsden FRCP, physician to the Skin Department, St George's Hospital, London.

benign. They can be treated with topical fluorouracil (Efudix) which causes significant inflammation and destruction of the abnormal skin. Hydrocortisone may be useful to treat inflamed lesions and to reduce the inflammation associated with fluorouracil Efudix. Otherwise, treatment is cryotherapy or surgical methods as above.

All the above lesions can be confused with skin malignancies. If any doubt arises, a biopsy should be performed for pathological diagnosis.

Calluses

Callus formation[38] arises mainly on the toes and plantar surface of the feet, and is common in the elderly. Hard skin is formed over pressure areas as a protective reaction, which eventually becomes pathological. Even when the stimulus is taken away, lumps of hard skin form and these may be very painful. Ill-fitting footwear, arthritis, deformity and uneven gait all predispose to callus formation.

The patient's footwear should be examined, as well as the gait and any deformities, as some predisposing factors may be remediable, for example by giving advice on suitable footwear and arranging for special footwear or inserts in shoes. It is important to identify patients with poor arterial blood supply or diabetes, firstly because the callus may cover an area of necrosis, and secondly because great care must be taken with treatment.

The simplest treatment is the regular application of moisturiser. A urea-containing preparation may be useful, and absorption will be helped by soaking the area in warm water beforehand. Salicylic acid paints or impregnated pads can help to break down hard skin; shaped padding to relieve pressure will also be helpful.

Removal of hard skin with a scalpel may be undertaken for symptomatic relief but usually needs to be done regularly on a frequent basis. In a few cases surgical correction of toe and other deformities may be helpful.

People with diabetics should only be treated by specialist chiropodists, because of the high risk of introducing infection which can be fatal.

Conclusion

In summary, skin disease of the elderly includes a different spectrum of conditions to that seen in younger adults. Alterations in the skin itself, immunity, hormone profile and wound healing all play a part. It is important to remember that the elderly in particular suffer from multiple pathology and that their skin problems may be related to other underlying diseases.

Acknowledgements

I would like to acknowledge the advice given on the text of this chapter by Professor P S Mortimer MD FRCP, physician to the Skin Department and professor in dermatology, and Ms Debra Doherty SRN, clinical nurse specialist in leg ulcer management, St George's Hospital, London.

Photographs are reproduced by kind permission of Dr R A Marsden FRCP, physician to the Skin Department, St George's Hospital, London.

References

1. Fedok F G. The aging face. *Facial Plast Surg* 1996; 12: 107–115.
2. Davies I. The mechanisms of aging. In: Graham-Brown R A C, Monk B E, eds. *Skin Disorders in the Elderly*. Oxford: Blackwell, 1992: 7–33.
3. Kligman A H, Graham J A. The psychology of appearance in the elderly. In: Gilchrest B A, ed. *Geriatric Dermatology. Clinics in Geriatric Medicine*. Philadelphia: W B Saunders, 1989: 213–222.
4. Koblenzer C S. Psychologic aspects of aging and the skin. *Clin Dermatol* 1996; 14: 171–177.
5. Marks R. *Dermatologic Problems in the Elderly*. New York: HP Publishing, 1992: 4–7.
6. Monk B E, Graham-Brown R A C. Eczema. In: Graham-Brown R A C, Monk B E, eds. *Skin Disorders in the Elderly*. Oxford: Blackwell, 1992: 58–71.
7. Burton J L, Holden C A. Eczema, Lichenification and Prurigo. In: Champion R H, Burton J L, Burns D A, Breathnach S M, eds. *Textbook of Dermatology*. Oxford: Blackwell, 1998: 629–680.
8. Camp R D R. Psoriasis. In: Champion R H, Burton J L, Burns D A, Breathnach S M, eds. *Textbook of Dermatology*. Oxford: Blackwell, 1998: 1589–1650.
9. Graham-Brown R A C, Camp R D R. Psoriasis. In: Graham-Brown R A C, Monk B E, eds. *Skin Disorders in the Elderly*. Oxford: Blackwell, 1992: 34–57.
10. Schwindt D A, Wilhelm K P, Miller D L, Maibach H I. Cumulative irritation in older and younger skin: a comparison. *Acta Derm Venereol (Stockh)* 1998; 78: 279–283.
11. Thaipisuttikul Y. Pruritic skin diseases in the elderly. *J Dermatol.* 1998; 25: 153–157.
12. Alonso-Llamazares J, Rogers R S, Oursler J R, Calobrisi S D. Bullous pemphigoid presenting as generalized pruritus: observations in six patients. *Int J Dermatol* 1998; 37: 508–514.

13. Kleinsmith D M, Perricone N V. Common skin problems in the elderly. In. Gilchrest B A, ed. *Geriatric Dermatology. Clinics in Geriatric Medicine*, vol. 5. Philadelphia: W B Saunders, 1989: 193.

14. Wojnarowska F, Eady R A J, Burge S M. Balloon eruptions. In: Champion R H, Burton J L, Burns D A, Breathnach S M, eds. *Textbook of Dermatology*. Oxford: Blackwell, 1998: 1817–1898.

15. Breathnach S M. Drug Relations. In: Champion R H, Burton J L, Burns D A, Breathnach S M, eds. *Textbook of Dermatology*. Oxford: Blackwell, 1998: 3349–3518.

16. Eaglstein W H. Wound healing and aging. In: Gilchrest B A, ed. *Geriatric Dermatology. Clinics in Geriatric Medicine*, vol. 5. Philadelphia: W B Saunders, 1989: 183–188.

17. Partridge C. Influential factors in surgical wound healing. *J Wound Care* 1998; 7: 350–353.

18. Sunderkötter C, Kaldin H, Luger T A. Aging and the skin immune system. *Arch Dermatol* 1997; 133: 1256–1261.

19. Ashcroft G S, Horan M A, Ferguson M W. Aging alters the inflammatory and endothelial cell adhesion molecule profiles during human cutaneous wound healing. *Lab Invest* 1998; 78: 47–58.

20. Ashcroft G S, Dodsworth J, van Boxtel E *et al*. Estrogen accelerates cutaneous wound healing associated with an increase in TGF-β_1 levels. *Nat Med* 1997; 3: 1209–1215.

21. Hansson C. Interactive wound dressings. a practical guide to their use in older patients. *Drugs Aging* 1997; 11: 271–284.

22. Thomas S. A guide to dressing selection. *J Wound Care* 1997; 6: 479–482.

23. Bale S. A guide to wound debridement. *J Wound Care* 1997; 6: 179–182.

24. Tong A. The identification and treatment of slough. *J Wound Care* 1999; 8: 338–339.

25. Thomas S. Assessment and management of wound exudate. *J Wound Care* 1997; 6: 327–330.

26. Thomas S. The importance of secondary dressings in wound care. *J Wound Care* 1998; 7: 189–192.

27. Ruckley C V. Evidence-based management of patients with leg ulcers. *J Wound Care* 1997; 6: 442–444.

28. Stevens J, Franks P J, Harrington M. A community/hospital leg ulcer service. *J Wound Care* 1997; 6: 62–68.

29. Bowman P H, Hogan D J. Leg ulcers: a common problem with sometimes uncommon etiologies. *Geriatrics* 1999; 54: 43–53.

30. Callum M J, Ruckley C V, Harper D R *et al*. Chronic ulceration of the leg: extent of the problem and provision of care. *BMJ* 1985; 290: 1855–1856.

31. Cameron J. Skin care for patients with chronic leg ulcers. *J Wound Care* 1998; 7: 459–462.

32. Fletcher A, Cullum N, Sheldon T A. A systematic review of compression treatment for venous leg ulcers. *BMJ* 1997; 315: 576–579.

33. Carr L, Philips Z, Posnett J. Comparative cost-effectiveness of four-layer bandaging in the treatment of venous leg ulceration. *J Wound Care* 1999; 8: 243–247.

34. Veraart J C J M, Neumann H A M. Effects of medical elastic compression stockings on interface pressure and edema prevention. *Dermatol Surg* 1996; 22: 867–871.
35. Zimmet S E. Venous leg ulcers: modern evaluation and management. *Dermatol Surg* 1999; 25: 236–241.
36. Renwick P, Vowden K, Wilkinson D, Vowden P. The pathophysiology and treatment of diabetic foot disease. *J Wound Care* 1998; 7: 107–110.
37. Mackie R M. Epidermal skin tumours. In: Champion R H, Burton J L, Burns D A, Breathnach S M, eds. *Textbook of Dermatology*. Oxford: Blackwell, 1998: 1651–1694.
38. Booth J, McInnes A. The aetiology and management of plantar callous formation. *J Wound Care* 1997; 6: 427–430.

14

Palliative care in the elderly

Mahesh Sodha

The World Health Organization (WHO) in 1990[1] defined palliative care as:

> The active total care of patients whose disease is not responsive to curative treatment. Control of pain, other symptoms, and of psychological, social and spiritual problems is paramount. The goal of palliative care is achievement of the best quality of life for patients and their families. Many aspects of palliative care are also applicable earlier in the course of the illness in conjunction with anti-cancer treatment.

Cancer in the elderly

Although cancer affects all ages, it is increasingly viewed as a disease of the elderly since some 70% of all new cancers are diagnosed in people over the age of 60. Of course, cancer is not the only disease which requires palliative care. Other major terminal illnesses traditionally cared for by hospices and palliative care teams include acquired immune deficiency syndrome (AIDS) and motor neurone disease (MND). However, since AIDS cannot be considered to be a disease of the elderly, it has been excluded from this chapter. MND has an onset age of between 40 and 60 years and is not particularly considered a disease of the old age. However, some of the symptom control needs of cancer sufferers are shared by patients with MND and the many other ultimately terminal diseases of old age and are discussed in this chapter.

It is clear that the rapid growth and great advances made in palliative cancer management have been largely initiated by the British hospice movement. When Dame Cicely Saunders established St Christopher's Hospice in 1967, the aim was to provide a place not only where effective care could be given to patients, but also where research and teaching could take place. St Christopher's soon became a model for hospice care all over the UK and in the USA. The philosophy of hospice care has now spread to more than 40 countries, breaching political and religious boundaries in doing so.

The philosophy of hospice care is to offer a patient, whether at home, in hospital or in a hospice, palliative rather than curative care with the emphasis on quality rather than length of life. Care is extended to the patient's family and includes emotional and psychosocial support and interventions. Death is recognised as part of life and discussed as openly as the patient wishes. This holistic approach can only be provided by a multidisciplinary team. A pharmacist is regarded as an important member of this team.

The essential components of palliative care are:

- good symptom control, which will allow
- improved communication, in turn leading to
- relevant family support, which can be physical and psychological.

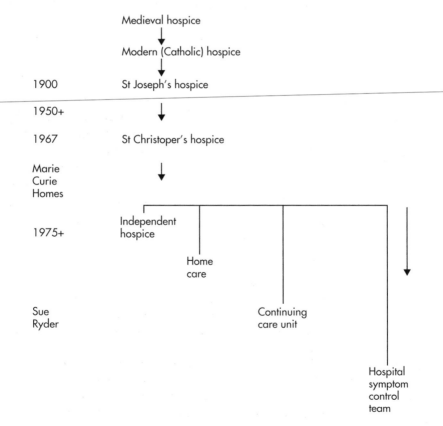

Figure 14.1 Hospice development. Reproduced with permission from Twycross.[2]

A family tree of the modern hospice movement is shown in Figure 14.1.[2] This clearly illustrates that, together with the growth of hospices, whole new areas of palliative care have emerged with the introduction of home care and hospice-based support teams.

Symptom control and care of dying

The chronic nature of terminal pain has been described, with a distinction made from acute pain.[3] This article examines the general principles of palliative care in hospices. More importantly, the treatment of patients as a whole is emphasised, treating not only physical symptoms but taking into account emotional, spiritual and social aspects in palliative care. According to Dame Cecily Saunders:

> The main aim of the professional palliative care team – the increasingly skilled symptom control, the supportive nursing, the social work, and the mobilisation of the community resources – is to enable the dying person to live *until* he/she dies, at his/her own maximum potential, performing to the limit of his physical activity and mental capacity with control and independence wherever possible.[4]

To understand adequately and to be able to intervene in all the physical, psychosocial and spiritual domains requires a range of skills. This is the main reason for the success of the interdisciplinary team in palliative care. Since no one professional can have all the skills, the availability of many team members provides opportunity for support from a number of sources. A multidisciplinary team typically consists of doctors, nurses, pharmacists, physiotherapists, social workers and the clergy. Support often needs to be sought from other specialists such as psychologists, anaesthetists and alternative therapists such as acupuncture and aromatherapy specialists.

A pharmacist's contribution is to:

- offer an efficient and prompt supply of medication
- provide tailored formulation to meet the individual patient needs
- offer advice and support to patients on symptom control
- liaise closely with the other members of the palliative care team on all aspects of pharmaceutical care
- monitor therapy with respect to the patient's liver and renal function
- offer advice to the clinicians and nurses on unusual formulations, routes of administration, dosages, side-effects and adverse drug reactions
- provide educational support in the form of talks to nurses and other members of the team

- attend regular team meetings where each patient is assessed holistically, to contribute to pharmaceutical care plans for the patient
- offer guidance to patients and others in the community on the use of syringe drivers and drugs used in these devices.

Risk–benefit ratio in palliative care

In palliative care, where the life expectancy is short and the emphasis is on quality of life, the whole risk–benefit ratio with respect to side-effects is altered compared with other situations in medical care. There is little point in worrying about a patient developing renal failure over a period of time with the use of high-dose non-steroidal anti-inflammatory drugs, for example if a patient has possibly 3 months to live and this is the only therapy which is able to improve quality of life and enable the patient to live free from pain.

It is this shift in the risk–benefit ratio that helps to explain the number of unlicensed medications and unlicensed doses being advocated in palliative care. From an ethical point of view this is largely justified. From a legal point of view, the current opinion is that any unlicensed medication can be acceptable provided it is agreed that such treatment is accepted as a norm by a body of medical carers in this field.

Clinical aspects of the management of pain

The International Association for the Study of Pain[5] defines pain as: 'an unpleasant sensory and emotional experience associated with actual or potential tissue damage or described in terms of such damage'. However, in simple terms pain is when a patient says it hurts and only the patient is able to assess it. One of the barriers to effective assessment is the failure on the part of health care professionals to believe the patient. Hence the most important first stage in managing pain is a thorough investigation of the nature of the pain.

Pain associated with cancer may result from tumour infiltration of pain-sensitive structures such as nerves, bones and soft tissue, radiotherapy, or from surgery, or from tumour- or radiation-induced vascular occlusion.

It is possible to subdivide pain into three types:

- Somatic pain (nociceptive pain) follows the classical pain pathways (Figure 14.2) initiated by stimulation of nociceptors on the nerve endings in response to such triggers as soft-tissue damage by tumour invasion. Such pain

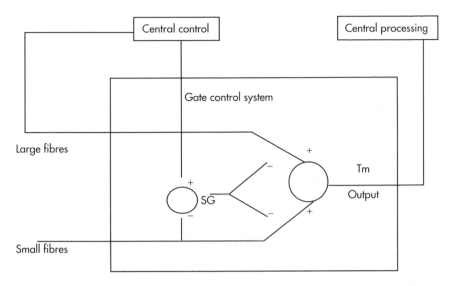

Figure 14.2 Pain pathways. SG = Substantia gelatinosa cell; Tm = spinal cord transmission cell. Adapted with permission from Melzack *et al.*[7]

is almost always responsive to treatment with opioid analgesics. This pain is typically localised and is often described as 'aching' or 'gnawing'.

- Visceral pain, also common in cancer, results from infiltration, compression, distension or stretching of thoracic and abdominal viscera, usually as a result of primary or metastatic tumour growth (e.g. liver metastasis). This type of pain is poorly localised and frequently described as 'deep', 'squeezing' or 'pressure' and may be associated with nausea.

- Neurogenic or neuropathic pain: here the pain is not initiated by stimulation of receptors in the nerve endings but pain impulses are generated as a result of some neuronal dysfunction (e.g. inflammation or nerve damage). Examples of such a variety of pain include trigeminal neuralgia and pains of diabetic neuropathy. This variety of pain responds poorly to opioid analgesics given orally or systemically (it can respond to epidural opioids) but is often successfully treated with tricyclic antidepressants such as amitriptyline at a lower dose than required for its antidepressant action. Another class of effective drugs is the antiepileptics such as phenytoin, carbamazepine and sodium valproate. Flecainide, an antiarrhythmic drug, is also effective in some types of neurogenic pains. In cancer patients, neuropathic pain often occurs as a result of compression of peripheral nerves or the spinal cord. This pain is typically described as shooting or burning and/or tingling in the nerve distribution. Superimposed paroxysms of electrical shock-like sensations sometimes occur.[6] Sometimes it is also described as a constant dull ache with a pressure of 'vice-like' quality.

Having identified the possible cause of the pain and its nature, it is possible to use the WHO analgesic ladder approach (1986).[8] The hospice philosophy is to acknowledge this approach but the patient must be treated holistically and total needs satisfied. The WHO ladder (Figure 14.3) starts with non-opioid analgesics (paracetamol) at level 1 for mild-to-moderate pain, stepped up to a weak opioid (such as codeine and dihydrocodeine) at level 2 when pain is not relieved on level 1. If the effect of the weak opioid and non-opioid is still insufficient to manage pain adequately, the third step of the ladder recommends strong opioids such as oral morphine.

The WHO ladder approach has been tested in a number of studies. One showed that, of 156 cancer patients, 87% ultimately became pain-free using the ladder.[9]

This approach is only suitable for nociceptive pain responsive to opioids. For pain such as that of bony metastasis, which is only partially sensitive to morphine, other adjuvant drugs such as non-steroidal anti-inflammatory agents may be necessary at each stage on the ladder. Antidepressants and antiepileptic agents may be required for neurogenic pain, as described above.

In a few instances, the team fails to achieve adequate symptom control despite the best efforts of the carers. The most difficult cases may be explained by some new theories. There are two varieties of pain, described as paradoxical pain[10] and overwhelming pain,[11] which

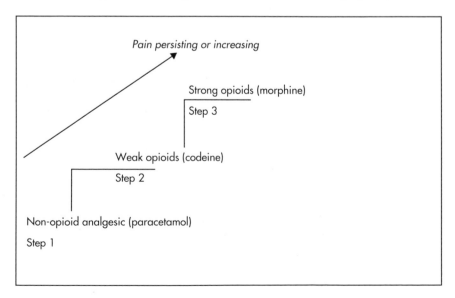

Figure 14.3   World Health Organization three-step analgesic ladder.

remain very difficult to treat. The term 'paradoxical pain' was intro-duced by the Pain Research Institute in Liverpool to describe the nociceptive variety of pain that is normally sensitive to opioids, but which does not respond to even very large doses of morphine and diamorphine and can in some instances get worse on treatment with morphine or diamorphine. This has been explained as follows:[10] morphine is metabolised in the liver to its 3- and 6-glucuronides, both of which bind to opioid receptors in the central nervous system. However, morphine-6-glucuronide is even more potent than morphine itself, while the 3-glucuronide is thought to have antagonistic action at the opioid receptors. Hence the patient's final response to morphine depends on the ratio of the two glucuronides produced. The normal ratio in most patients is 5 : 1 but in patients who exhibit paradoxical pain the ratio is higher, i.e. lesser quantities of the active 6-glucuronide are produced compared to the antagonistic 3-glucuronide.

It is believed that such patients who metabolise morphine un-usually would benefit from treatment with methadone, which is metabolised differently. However, methadone, being a very long-acting drug, is often difficult to use because of accumulation and complex pharmacokinetics. The theory of paradoxical pain is controversial and not universally accepted.

The term 'overwhelming pain' has been used to describe chronic, unrelieved severe cancer pain. Such pain usually responds to adequate doses of morphine with co-analgesics if necessary. However, where large doses of morphine are used, without success, it may be that all the other anxieties of the patient are not addressed. In one instance, a patient with inoperable cancer of the oesophagus was admitted to a hospice, still in pain despite receiving a dose of 12 g of morphine per day orally. He was free of pain a week later with 60 mg of morphine per day orally with 10 mg of diazepam at night. This was achieved with listening, explanation and setting of positive rehabilitation goals.[11]

There are cases where nociceptive pain is resistant to opioids when there is either peripheral or central neural sensitisation causing allodynia or hypersensitivity. Such sensitisation often occurs due to an injured peripheral nerve or an injured part of the central nervous system. Pain associated with inflammation is a good example of peripheral nerve sensitisation and this responds well to non-steroidal anti-inflammatory drugs. Central sensitisation can also occur in the dorsal horn and this requires use of drugs that block N-methyl-D-aspartate receptors (NMDA). Drugs that block these receptors include ketamine and dextromethorphan.[11]

The hospice approach is to combine pharmacological inter-ventions with practical 'tender loving care', aiming to meet not only the patient's needs but also those of the family. This holistic care aims to provide emotional, spiritual and social support to the patient and family to enable living to the full as well as coming to terms with the illness. Even a simple task like enabling patients to make a will can help them to understand the inevitability of death and move towards acceptance. It may at the same time resolve many family anxieties.

Clinical aspects of management of nausea and vomiting

Nausea is a subjective, unpleasant sensation associated with the upper gastrointestinal tract, often accompanied by an urge to vomit (see also Chapter 7). Vomiting is the forceful expulsion of gastrointestinal con-tents through the mouth. It is possible to experience nausea with or without retching for prolonged periods without vomiting. Nausea and vomiting result from the stimulation of the chemoreceptor trigger zone (CTZ) and/or the vomiting centre in the medulla oblongata. The vomiting centre is the final common pathway for the initiation of vomiting from any cause. The vomiting centre is not sensitive to chemical stimulation itself but receives impulses from the CTZ, which is sensitive to many drugs, including opioids and some tumour factors produced in cancer patients by the tumour cells.

The causes of nausea and vomiting in terminally ill patients can be classified into four groups:

- Iatrogenic: drugs such as opioids acting centrally and others such as non-steroidal anti-inflammatory drugs may irritate the gastric mucosa.
- Organic: faecal impaction, bowel obstruction, squashed stomach due to enlarged liver or ascites or raised intracranial pressure.
- Metabolic: raised levels of urea (uraemia) or calcium.
- Psychological: anxiety and fear.

The management of nausea requires careful diagnosis of the cause as the antiemetic drugs act at different receptor sites. It may be possible to manage nausea induced by opioids with dopamine antag-onists since it is the dopamine receptors that are responsible for the stimulation at the CTZ. Although nausea due to opioids does subside after 7–10 days of treatment due to tolerance, humoral factors secreted by tumour cells may continue to contribute to nausea and vomiting. Antihistamine drugs are thought to act directly on the vomiting centre and are useful in treating all nausea and vomiting regardless of the cause. This is often a reason for the choice of cyclizine in the control of nausea in terminally ill patients in whom the cause is not yet determined. In addition, the hospice aim is to treat the patient holistically, looking at both physical and psychosocial causes of nausea and vomiting.

Some causes of nausea (mainly due to obstruction of the gastro-intestinal tract) remain extremely difficult to manage. Partial success has been achieved with the use of octreotide, which reduces the volume of the secretions in the lumen of the intestinal tract, thereby reducing the volume and frequency of the vomit. This palliative effect, while improving the quality of life for the patients, does not entirely relieve the symptom.

Assessment of pain and nausea and vomiting

It is well recognised that pain is a complex experience and four main components of pain are described: nociception, sensation, suffering and behaviour.[12] This model discards the notion of a linear relationship between the amount of noxious input and the intensity of pain experienced. The perception of pain and the level of pain assessed are highly individual in nature, subjective and very difficult to assess objectively. Pain tolerance is influenced by fear, anxiety, previous experience of pain, the significance of pain, cultural attitudes and differences. Various coping mechanisms can be utilised by different people.

Similarly, while the number of episodes of vomiting can be measured objectively, the sensation of nausea can only be assessed subjectively. Again, nausea can be influenced by fear, anxiety, previous experience of nausea and the significance of it to the patient.

Various methods of pain assessment have been researched. Objective measures relying on biochemical indexes, such as changes in plasma hormone levels, are expensive and often inaccurate and unreliable. Subjective methods of assessment include visual analogue scales with pain scores of 1–10, verbal rating scales (where each point in a scale describes the pain sensation as mild, moderate, severe, etc.), and McGarth's faces scale (where random faces depicting 'happy', 'grumpy' etc. are shown to patients so that they select the face that best represents their feelings in relation to pain).[13]

Visual analogue scales have been shown to achieve a reasonably accurate assessment of pain in acute sufferers. Verbal rating scales have a correlation with visual analogue scales but do not have the same sensitivity as numerical rating scales (e.g. from 1 to 10) but, as with visual analogue scales, patients need to be alert, not confused and have a degree of coordination.[14]

However, the main drawback of all unidimensional scales is that they fail to recognise the complexity of the pain experience since pain has a strong emotional or affective component. Attempts have been made to overcome this by using two methods:

- Combination of rating scales where separate scales are used for sensory and reaction components of the pain experienced.
- Multidimensional models: the best known is the McGill Pain Questionnaire,[8] which is a well-established tool that measures pain through three dimensions – sensory, affective and evaluative. It is, however, complex and cumbersome for repeated use.

Another instrument used to assess pain in cancer patients is the Wisconsin Brief Pain Inventory (WBPI) which is designed to evaluate the history, intensity, location and quality of pain experienced and to determine what effect the pain has on the patient's life.[15] The method involves recording pain at its worst, at the usual level and at the time of completing the WBPI on visual analogue scales rated from 0 to 10 (based on nine subdivided questions).

A simple and effective tool for assessment of different symptoms such as pain, nausea, dyspnoea and psychological symptoms has been developed.[16] The Edmonton Symptom Assessment System (ESAS) tool consists of nine visual analogue scales. These include pain, shortness of breath, nausea, depression, activity, anxiety, well-being, drowsiness and appetite. However, more research is necessary to validate and define the accuracy of this tool in patients with cognitive failure, language or neurological deficits, although in cognitively aware patients, ESAS has an acceptable level of validity and reliability.

Management in the elderly

In the elderly, accurate assessment of pain depends largely on good communication skills between the clinician and the patient. Many elderly patients do not like complaining and may not reveal their suffering willingly. Often in these circumstances it is only when the whole palliative care team discuss each case individually that the full nature of the elderly patient's suffering comes to light. It is frequently the careful observations of the nursing staff that enable accurate assessment.

Another very important issue to be considered in the elderly relates generally to the special nature of drug handling in the elderly

(Chapter 2) and to pharmacokinetics of the drugs used. Elderly people with impaired renal function tend to become oversedated easily and careful dose titration and frequent review are necessary. Although morphine is metabolised in the liver by glucuronidation, the metabolites morphine-6-glucuronide and morphine-3-glucuronide are eliminated via the kidneys and the active metabolite morphine-6-glucuronide will accumulate in the presence of impaired renal function.

Similarly, use of dopamine antagonists such as haloperidol, levomepromazine (methotrimeprazine) and metoclopramide warrant caution. These drugs are necessary in palliative care for the control of nausea and vomiting but the elderly are especially susceptible to the extrapyramidal side-effects of these drugs. Of course, these drugs ought not to be prescribed in the elderly cancer patient when Parkinson's disease is present. However, in practice, it is very common for pharmacists to intervene and suggest an alternative such as cyclizine or domperidone in such a patient.

Dyspnoea in terminal illness

The term 'dyspnoea' is used to describe either excessive awareness of breathing or discomfort in the act of breathing, but for the purpose of this chapter dyspnoea is defined as the subjective sensation of breathing difficulty in terminally ill patients with advanced cancer. Non-malignant causes of dyspnoea (for example, chronic obstructive airways disease) are not considered in this chapter.

Prevalence

In hospice practice, dyspnoea is one of the most prevalent symptoms, and is often more difficult to manage than pain. A variety of studies have shown that 29–74% of all terminally patients complain of dyspnoea.[17] It is most common in patients with advanced carcinoma of the lung.

Causes

The causes of dyspnoea are as numerous and varied as are the causes of pain. To treat dyspnoea rationally it is important to be familiar with possible causes, as intervention is on the basis of aetiology in the first instance.

Dyspnoea may result from:

1.   Mechanical factors which stimulate the cerebral cortex and lead to a sensation of 'air deficiency'.
2.   Pain on breathing.
3.   Psychogenic factors such as fear and anxiety.
4.   Impaired diffusion of respiratory gases.

The mechanisms of dyspnoea (Figure 14.4) are complex and poorly understood. Considerable research effort is currently being undertaken in this area. It is clear that the majority of these patients are not oxygen-deficient, having a normal PO_2 even in cases of gross dyspnoea. Stretch

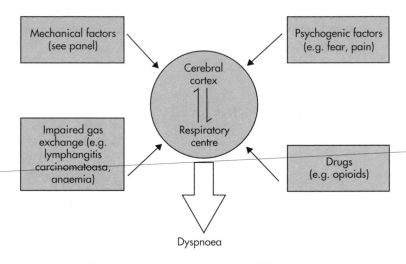

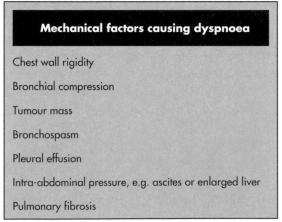

Figure 14.4 Mechanism of dyspnoea in malignant disease.

receptors may be implicated or there may be some other means of perceiving 'stiffness' in the lungs and in some cases there is the inability to draw a deep breath. Compounding the problem of dyspnoea in all patients are the psychological and psychosocial problems it inevitably engenders. Being anxious or frightened is a natural consequence of being unable to breathe properly, and the limitation of mobility it imposes creates another set of problems. In addition, fear and anxiety about the cancer itself and its outcome may focus in the dyspnoea.

Management

Since dyspnoea is a subjective experience it is not always easy to assess its severity and it is best evaluated on the basis of the patient's expression of distress. Patients with dyspnoea are often afraid and fears of suffocation or choking are common. Reassurance and explanation often help, as do other therapies such as massage, relaxation, distraction (for example, music) and increased air movements (open windows, fan). A pleural effusion, if present, may have to be drained and relief of any ascites could also help.

Drug management of dyspnoea

Here only palliative management with drugs is discussed and treatment with cytotoxic agents and radiotherapy is excluded, although such agents may be relevant in palliative management.

Bronchodilators   Many patients may have obstructive airways disease concomitantly with their carcinoma. It must be remembered that most lung cancer sufferers are smokers or ex-smokers and often suffer from other respiratory disease. Since obstructive airways disease is commonly found to coexist with advanced cancer, it seems logical to try bronchodilators in patients with dyspnoea.

Corticosteroids   These agents are indicated for bronchospasm when bronchodilators alone have failed to have an effect. For acute relief the oral or parenteral route is more reliable than the inhaled route, but for maintenance therapy the inhaled route is preferable. Major airways obstruction by tumour can be treated with high-dose corticosteroids (for example, dexamethasone 12 mg/day given as a single dose or divided dose each morning) to reduce the oedema around the tumour. Following such treatment a patient may require radiotherapy or laser or insertion of a stent (an expandable metal stent inserted into the bronchus).[18] Dexamethasone can often then be reduced or stopped.

Respiratory stimulants   Several classes of drugs have a respiratory stimulant action and these include progestogens, methylxanthines, cannabinoids and doxapram. These agents, with the exception of nabilone (see below), a synthetic derivative of tetrahydrocannabinol, have proved to be of little use in dyspnoea.

Respiratory sedatives   These classes of drugs include opioids, benzo-diazepines, phenothiazines and cannabinoids.

Opioids   For many years opioids have been the mainstay of sympto-matic treatment. Morphine suppresses the sensation of dyspnoea at doses of up to 10 mg every 4 h (slow-release morphine tablets 30 mg 12-hourly) over and above the dose needed for pain relief without any evidence of respiratory depression.[19] This would convert to diamorphine 20 mg via subcutaneous infusion over 24 h.

More recently, nebulised diamorphine (or morphine) has been found to be equally if not more effective and can be given in doses of 5–20 mg in 5 ml of normal saline every 4 h or as required.[20] It is best to start with small doses and increase as necessary. Larger doses (15 mg or more) should be started in an inpatient setting. Pharmacokinetic studies have shown that with a 5 mg nebulised dose the absorption is probably about 1.7 mg.[21] This has led to the postulation that morphine probably has a direct pulmonary effect in addition to its central effect. Although nebulised morphine or diamorphine is generally safe, it can in some indi-viduals cause bronchoconstriction, probably due to release of histamine. It is best to give the first dose under supervision, with ready availability of an antihistamine agent. Fentanyl is a short-acting opioid which does not cause histamine release and might be usefully utilised in nebulised form.[22] However there is currently no experience of its use in palliative care.

Lidocaine (lignocaine)   Nebulised lidocaine has also been used but recent trials have not been able to confirm real benefit at the concen-trations tested.[23] However, nebulised saline can help by moistening airways which have been dried out with mouth breathing and medi-cation, and may assist the expectoration of thick secretions.

Benzodiazepines, butyrophenones and phenothiazines   Anxiety is an important factor in some patients' dyspnoea and anxiolytic drugs such as haloperidol (5–15 mg orally or subcutaneously) may be required. Diazepam 5–20 mg is also useful but caution is necessary here because diazepam can reduce respiratory drive, and should only be used in patients with extreme anxiety and low $PaCO_2$. Promethazine is a useful alternative to diazepam. Promethazine appears to reduce breathlessness and improve exercise tolerance without significant depression of respiration and alteration of lung function.[24] The precise mechanism of action of promethazine is not known in this context but, like other phenothiazines, it inhibits dopamine receptors and is also known to block acetylcholine receptors (antimuscarinic effect) in addition to its well-known antihistamine action at H_1 histamine receptors. The combined action is to dry out bronchial secretions, sedate the patient and to antagonise any allergen-induced histamine release. (Some patients may also have reversible obstructive airways disease concomitantly and probably benefit from antihistamines.) Because of its long half-life a single night-time dose of 10–25 mg of promethazine may be adequate. One or two daytime doses of 10–25 mg may be needed in addition.

Nabilone   In patients already on opioids and where promethazine has not been effective it is worth considering nabilone. Nabilone is a synthetic derivative of tetrahydrocannabinol which is one of the active ingredients of marijuana. It is licensed in an oral presentation of 1 mg as an antiemetic for nausea associated with cytotoxic chemotherapy. It is not licensed for management of dyspnoea but may be beneficial. The action of nabilone is thought to be of both a central sedative and stimulant effect together with a combination of adrenergic and anticholinergic effects on the airways. For dyspnoea it is recommended at a dose of 100–200 micrograms every 8 h.[25] These doses are prepared by opening the 1 mg capsules and suspending the contents in xanthan gum, such as Keltrol 1%.

Oxygen therapy   Relatively few patients with advanced cancer suffer from dyspnoea as a result of hypoxia and therefore do not often benefit from oxygen therapy aimed at increasing their PO_2. Some patients however may have been accustomed to oxygen therapy for past chronic obstructive airways disease or may have developed a psychological attachment to it. Hypoxia of recent onset may induce agitation and confusion. In this instance increasing inspired oxygen concentration may help. However, continuous therapy is often a barrier to nursing, especially if a mask is used. The patient has inaudible speech, loses the freedom to drink and often suffers from the drying effects of oxygen, when a humidifier may help. The use of nasal prongs may be better if oxygen use is thought to be essential. Intermittent therapy can be very useful in some patients. Confident management, preferably in a calm, airy and smoke-free environment, together with the use of oral or nebulised opioid and/or promethazine may make it possible gently to wean many of these patients off continuous or even intermittent oxygen therapy.

Cough in terminal illness

Cough in terminally ill patients, like pain and dyspnoea, may or may not be related to the malignancy. Non-malignant causes of cough include respiratory infection, postnasal drip, asthma, gastro-oesophageal reflux and chronic bronchitis. Underlying causes ought to be treated appropriately.

The cough reflex is probably initiated by three types of receptors:

1. Stretch receptors, found mainly in the upper respiratory tract (larynx, trachea and large bronchi) but also located in the pleura, pericardium and diaphragm
2. The small C-fibre endings commonly located in the small airways; these are more sensitive to chemical rather than mechanical stimuli
3. The afferent fibres (myelinated and unmyelinated neurons which synapse in the central cough centre)[26]

Cough is a common symptom in lung cancer patients: an incidence of 70–90% has been reported. A primary lung tumour or lung metastases may stimulate the cough reflex by impinging on receptors. A broncho-oesophageal fistula may admit swallowed liquids into the bronchial tree and, with complete oesophageal obstruction from tumour, saliva over-spill may occur from the pharynx into the trachea. Inhalation pneumonia is a common complication of these problems.

Management of cough

Physiotherapy and a change of the patient's position, especially after giving 5 ml of nebulised normal saline to loosen mucus, is helpful. Opioids are very effective as cough suppressants. Codeine, morphine and methadone are particularly effective by their action on the cough centre. Methadone linctus 2 mg in 5 ml has the advantage of a long half-life and is used at a dose of 2–4 mg every 8 h. However, the disadvantage is that toxic accumulation may occur with repeated doses. The size of the dose or its frequency may be reduced if the patient becomes drowsy. If the patient is already on another strong opioid for pain control, titration of the analgesic dose becomes complicated and control of the cough may well be possible simply by increasing the dose of the original opioid.

For intractable cough nebulised lidocaine (lignocaine) or bupivacaine is also very effective: 5 ml of 2% solution of lidocaine (lignocaine) used at night has been shown to be effective. Care must be taken to ensure that food or fluid does not enter the trachea because of the anaesthetised pharynx.

In the last stages of disease, pooling of secretions in the trachea and pharynx in patients who are in a recumbent position and unable to sit up unaided may produce a loose cough. In this situation, as when there is tracheal overspill of saliva which cannot be swallowed, it is appropriate to use an antimuscarinic drying agent such as hyoscine hydrobromide and mechanical suction may sometimes be necessary. Hyoscine can be given either sublingually as tablets, or transdermally (hyoscine patch), or subcutaneously via a syringe driver at a dose of 0.4–1.2 mg over 24 h. Alternatively, glycopyrronium bromide (Robinul) can be used. This has the advantage of less sedation (does not cross the blood–brain barrier to the same extent) and is less likely to cause blurred vision.

Constipation

Constipation is a common condition in the elderly (Chapter 3) but in terminally ill patients it can be a particularly difficult problem to manage. Specific causes include:

- Drugs such as opioids, tricyclic antidepressants and other anticholinergics
- Those related to the cancer, for example, bowel obstruction, hypercalcaemia
- Lack of hydration due to poor intake of fluids and food
- Lack of mobility and exercise

Opioid-induced constipation is most commonly seen and this is best addressed by means of a stimulant/lubricant laxative such as co-danthramer or co-danthrusate preparations usually given prophylactically at the time of starting patients on strong opioids. Untreated, this can lead to complications such as nausea and vomiting and faecal impaction. That such added distress should be iatrogenic in patients already suffering enough in other ways is a serious failure in care. Overflow diarrhoea can be another complication of faecal impaction. This is best managed by use of arachis oil retention enemas followed if necessary by a phosphate enema.

Bowel obstruction

Having excluded obstruction caused by constipation, a non-stimulant antiemetic such as cyclizine can be given. If intestinal colic is a symptom, hyoscine butylbromide can be used instead. Haloperidol is a useful second-line antiemetic. Other abdominal pain will require opioids and the medication may well need to be combined in a subcutaneous syringe driver. Occasionally, high-dose dexamethasone is given to attempt to relieve the obstruction by reducing peritumour oedema. Octreotide has been found to be an extremely useful drug in many of these patients. It is given via continuous subcutaneous syringe driver in a dose of 600 μg over 24 h. Its main action is to reduce the secretions in the lumen of the gut and hence reduce the frequency and volume of vomit.

Confusion

Confusion can occur in the later stages of terminal illness. It is important to isolate the causes which can also include:

- drugs, including opioids and psychotropic drugs. High plasma levels of phenytoin may also result in confusional states
- biochemical causes, most commonly hypercalcaemia and uraemia
- verebral hypoxia due to cerebrovascular accident or ischaemia
- in the elderly, a change of environment or depression
- primary or secondary tumours in the brain.

Management is best approached by addressing any known cause of confusion, such as oversedation, hypercalcaemia or hypoxia. Although antipsychotic drugs such as haloperidol and chlorpromazine can help, they need to be used with caution, particularly in the elderly. These drugs suppress hallucinations and reduce agitation. In certain circumstances increasing the dose because of persistent symptoms can worsen confusion by inducing disorientation.

Hypercalcaemia and bone pain

Hypercalcaemia can occur in as many as 10% of cancer sufferers but is more common in cancers of the lung, breast and prostate. The main cause is secondary tumours in the bone but can also occur as a result of tumour necrosis factors released by certain tumours. Common symptoms are increased non-specific pain, nausea, vomiting, lethargy, dry mouth, thirst, urinary frequency, confusion and weakness. Many of these symptoms are due to dehydration. Clinically, hypercalcaemia is defined as a serum level greater than 2.6 mmol/l corrected for the albumin level and its treatment requires hospitalisation and rehydration prior to administration of intravenous bisphosphonates. Many cancer sufferers with bone secondaries with or without bony pain and in the presence of normal calcium levels are treated with regular bisphosphonates. Both clodronate and pamidronate have been shown to reduce pathological fractures and may relieve bone pain. Pamidronate infusions need to be repeated every 3–4 weeks. The treatment of choice for patients with localised bone pain is radiotherapy. It is important to remember that there is a time lag of up to 2 weeks before the full effects of the treatment are noticed.

This chapter is dedicated to my late father Mr Nanjibhai Sodha.

Acknowledgements

I would like to express my gratitude to Dr David Frampton, Medical Director, Farleigh Hospice, Chelmsford and consultant in palliative medicine, Mid Essex Hospitals Trust for proof-reading the draft manuscript and for his many valuable suggestions that have been incorporated in this chapter. I would also like to thank my wife Shobhna for her encouragement and support whilst writing this chapter.

References

1. World Health Organization. *Cancer Pain Relief and Palliative Care*. Technical report series 804. Geneva: World Health Organization, 1990.
2. Twycross R G. Hospice care – redressing the balance in medicine. *J R Soc Med* 1980; 73: 475–481.
3. Twycross R G. Relief of terminal pain. *BMJ* 1975; 2: 212–214.
4. Doyle D, Hanks G W C, McDonald N. *Oxford Textbook of Palliative Medicine*. Oxford: Oxford University Press, 1996.
5. International Society for the Study of Pain. Subcommittee on taxonomy of pain terms: a list with definitions and notes on usage. *Pain* 1979; 6: 249–252,
6. Eliott K, Foley K M. Neurologic pain syndromes in patients with cancer. *Pain: Mechanisms Syndromes Neurol Clin* 1989; 7: 333–360.
7. Melzack R, Katz J, Jeans M E. The role of compensation in chronic pain: analysis using a new method of scoring the McGill pain questionnaire. *Pain* 1985; 23: 101–112.
8. World Health Organization. *Cancer Pain Relief and Palliative Care*. Report of World Health Organization expert committee. Geneva: World Health Organization, 1986.

9. Takeda F. Results of field-testing in Japan of the WHO draft interim guidelines on the relief of cancer pain. *Pain Clin* 1986; 1: 83.

10. Bowsher D. Paradoxical pain. *BMJ* 1993; 301: 473–474.

11. Twycross R. Paradoxical pain (letter to the editor). *BMJ* 1993; 306: 793.

12. Fordyce W E. Learning processes in pain. In: *The Psychology of Pain*. New York: Raven Press, 1978: 200.

13. McGarth P A. *Pain in Children: Nature, Assessment and Treatment*. New York: Guildford, 1990.

14. Ohnhaus E E, Adler R Methodological problems in the measurement of pain: a comparison between the verbal rating scale and the visual analogue scale. *Pain* 1975; 1: 379–384.

15. Daut R L, Cleeland C S, Flaney R C. The development of the Wisconsin Brief Pain Questionnaire to assess pain in cancer and other diseases. *Pain* 1983; 17: 197–210.

16. Bruera E, Macmillan K, Hanson J, MacDonald R N. The Edmonton staging system for cancer pain: preliminary report. *Pain* 1989; 37: 203–209.

17. Billings J A. *The Management of Common Symptoms. Outpatient Management of Advanced Cancer*. Philadelphia: JB Lippincott, 1985.

18. Simmonds A K, Irving J D, Clarke S W, Dick R. Use of expandable metal stents in the treatment of bronchial obstruction. *Thorax* 1989; 44: 680–681.

19. Light R W, Muro J R, Sato R I et al. Effects of oral morphine on breathlessness and exercise tolerance in patients with chronic obstructive pulmonary disease. *Am Rev Respir Dis* 1989; 139: 126–133.

20. Young I H, Daviskas E, Keena V A. Effect of low dose nebulised morphine on exercise endurance in patients with chronic lung disease. *Thorax* 1989; 44: 387–390.

21. Chrubasik J, Wust H, Friedrich G, Geller E. Absorption and bioavailability of nebulised morphine. *BMJ* 1988; 61: 228–230.

22. Worsley M H, Macleod A D, Brodie M J et al. Inhaled fentanyl as a method of analgesia. *Anaesthesia* 1990; 45: 449–451.

23. de Conno F, Spoldi E, Caraceni A, Ventafrida A. Does pharmacological treatment affect the sensation of breathlessness in terminal cancer patients? *Palliat Med* 1991; 5: 237–243.

24. Woodcock A A, Gross E R, Geddes D M. Drug treatment of breathlessness: contrasting effects of diazepam and promethazine in pink puffers. *BMJ* 1981; 283: 343–346.

25. Ahmedzai S. Respiratory distress in the terminally ill patient. *Respir Dis Pract* 1988; 5: 20–29.

26. Louie K, Bertolino M, Fainsinger R. Management of intractable cough. *J Palliat Care* 1992; 8: 46–48.

15

Compliance, concordance and polypharmacy in the elderly

Larry I Goodyer

This chapter will address two important issues in therapeutics for the elderly: those resulting when self-medication behaviour tends to deviate from the wishes of the prescriber (compliance) and the problems arising when an individual is prescribed multiple medication. Neither of these is unique to the elderly. In terms of compliance there is little evidence that the elderly are any worse than other age groups, and in some situations they may actually be better. However, there are a few identifiable barriers to compliance in the elderly, e.g. reduced cognitive function, which require specific consideration. Likewise, there are a number of chronic diseases that may result in a younger person requiring multiple medication (polypharmacy), but with advancing years and multiple pathologies the likelihood of polypharmacy is greater.

The term 'compliance' has in recent years been derided as too proscriptive, implying that not carrying out the wishes of the prescriber is a deviant behaviour needing correction. Recently the concept of concordance has emerged,[1] implying a more negotiated outcome where patient and prescriber come to mutual agreement on the regimen to be followed. This concept has yet to be formally studied and widely accepted by the health professions. To date most formal studies in the area have approached the subject from the standpoint of compliance, or at least the somewhat gentler term 'adherence'. Therefore, when referring to the literature and research material the term 'compliance' will be retained throughout the chapter. In terms of addressing the issues around self-medication behaviour, the approach suggested by the concordance model will be used.

The aims of this chapter are to address certain of the issues that contribute to the understanding of compliance and concordance, with an emphasis on those that are more relevant to the elderly. It is also useful to define the extent of the problem and expected levels of compliance in various situations.

There are a number of issues concerning the consequences of reduced compliance, varying from a waste of money to a poor clinical outcome. Assessing the medication-taking behaviour of individuals can also be problematic and the various methods of assessment will also be discussed.

Before devising any sensible strategy to aid elderly patients in their medication taking, it is important to have a clear understanding of those factors that might contribute to a perceived level of compliance. Finally, those strategies a pharmacist can take in helping the concordance process will be discussed, again with a particular emphasis on the issues related to the elderly.

Polypharmacy is a very broad-based subject, essentially implying that the greater the number of drugs taken, the increased chance of an adverse drug reaction (ADR) or interaction. In this chapter only some basic principles as they might apply to the elderly will be discussed. The reader should refer to individual chapters of this book for consideration of the most likely adverse events on the elderly.

There is a vast literature on the subject area of compliance and those particularly related only to the elderly have been identified for this chapter. Therefore, unless otherwise stated, all the quoted studies have been performed in the elderly population.

Defining compliance and concordance

Compliance

A suitable definition of compliance to medication would be: 'the extent to which the patient complies with the directions of the prescriber regarding a prescribed drug regimen'.

Such a definition implies that patients have very little say in the therapy they receive, which is largely out of step with the current concepts regarding patient choice in health care. The inference from this traditional view of compliance is therefore that 'doctor knows best' and that his/her decision is final. In order to move away from this model it has been the vogue to use the term 'adherence' rather than compliance. This implies that, while treatment is dictated by the prescriber, it is accepted that the patient will make a decision as to how closely the regimen is followed. In reality there is little to choose between the two terms and they are used interchangeably.

Although there is a vast research literature, many of the studies are small in nature and/or have some inherent faults in their design. At least part of the problem is the way in which compliance is described and quantified. There can be little debate over the concept of complete non-compliance, when the patient fails to take any of the prescribed medicine or simply does not collect a prescription. When considering partial compliance different approaches have been taken by various researchers. Some may consider the percentage of a medication taken within a particular time frame, whereas others may present the percentage of individuals in a defined population making any errors of a certain type.

This illustrates an important principle: that compliance to a regimen is not just an absolute in terms of the correct numbers of tablets taken per day, but when and how the medication is taken. There is an additional concept of 'drug holidays' where the medication may be taken strictly as prescribed and then omitted for a few days. Consider the patient who is prescribed a diuretic and angiotensin-converting enzyme (ACE) inhibitor for chronic heart failure, and these are to be taken daily. Supposing the medication is omitted for 5 days, which may well result in decompensation and hospital admission; for the whole 30-day period the compliance rate would have been over 80%. However, if the medication had been omitted just 1 day in every week there may have been a different outcome. This brings in the concept of 'drug forgiveness', describing the potential problems caused by occasional dose omissions.

Within these definitions, most observers conclude that patients will take around 50% of medication prescribed. The quoted range of compliance in the elderly is between 40 and 75%[2] and studies on the elderly do not show a universally poor level of compliance. For instance, in one study[3] involving 800 elderly patients just 18% had any compliance-related problems; 14% were taking less medication than prescribed, 2% too much medication and 2% no medication.

In terms of self-medication errors, figures established over the last decade[4] indicate that around 25–50% will make some errors in their medication. In certain situations this is found to represent a serious risk to health in up to 30% of cases. Other studies have shown a much lower incidence of serious outcomes.

In defining the level of compliance the following classification system may be useful:[5]

- Partial compliers: those who take between 40 and 80% of the dose prescribed, representing one-third of patients.

- Satisfactory compliers: those who sometimes take more and sometimes less than that prescribed, representing one-third of patients.
- Poor compliers: those who take less than 40% of prescribed medication at widely varying intervals, representing one-sixth of patients.
- Good compliers: people who seldom miss a dose and only occasionally take extra doses, representing one-sixth of patients.

Other factors which are also important in defining compliance-related problems are medications being taken that are prescribed for others (10%), or not currently being prescribed having intended to be discontinued (20%).[2]

Concordance

In 1995 the Royal Pharmaceutical Society of Great Britain in conjunction with Merck, Sharpe and Dome set up a commission to examine the issues of patient compliance.[1] What emerged was a new perspective on the subject, which acknowledged the importance of patients being allowed to make informed choices. The document *From Compliance to Concordance* describes the new initiative and ways in which this approach could be disseminated. This concept is described as follows:

> Concordance is a new approach to the prescribing and taking of medicines. It is an agreement reached after negotiation between a patient and a health care professional that respects the beliefs and wishes of the patient in determining whether, when and how medicines are to be taken. Although reciprocal, this is an alliance in which the health care professionals recognise the primacy of the patient's decisions about taking the recommended medications.
>
> Consultations between patients and doctors are most often concerned with two contrasting sets of health beliefs. Concordance recognises that the health beliefs of the patient, although different from those of doctor, nurse or pharmacist, are no less cogent, and no less important in deciding the best approach to the treatment of the individual. The Concordance Initiative aims to help patients and prescribers to make as well informed a choice as possible about diagnosis and treatment, about benefit and risk, to collaborate fully in a balanced therapeutic alliance, and so to optimise the potential benefits of medical care.

This model therefore hopes to address the difference in health beliefs between prescriber and patients. The goal is to negotiate a medication regimen with which the patient is most happy, in order to achieve a positive therapeutic goal. Encompassed within such a model is the possibility that the patient may choose to have no treatment, or opt for treatment which current evidence suggests does not produce the best outcome. The central argument to support such an approach is that the final regimen chosen by the patient is acceptable to the prescriber providing that an informed choice has been made.

The elderly, in particular, as the largest group of users of chronic medication, warrant special consideration within this new model. Some potential issues are:

- Attitudes of the elderly to the concept of concordance. It may be hypothesised that previous expectations of the doctor–patient relationship would present barriers to meaningful dialogue, i.e. the patient is unwilling to question the decision of the prescriber.
- The extent to which carers need to be involved in the negotiation of therapy. If the elderly person is largely dependent on others for help with medication, then the carers should also be consulted.
- Problems arising from a decline in cognitive function and the extent to which the patient is perceived as being unable to make an informed decision.

Consequences of poor compliance

There are a number of potential consequences resulting from failure of patients to comply with prescribed therapy.

Reduced therapeutic outcome

This certainly does occur but is hard to quantify in formal studies. In elderly patients with chronic heart failure, for instance, it has been demonstrated that there is a better therapeutic outcome as compliance improves.[6] However, in most cases there are a number of other factors that can contribute to a deterioration in condition or poor outcome to therapy. Also some drugs have a good 'drug forgiveness', where doses can be omitted occasionally[5] with little effect on outcome. An example might be an antihypertensive used to treat an individual with mild hypertension.

It is therefore difficult to demonstrate that undercompliance can be directly related to a patient's condition. In the elderly this may be even more problematic as multiple disease states can all be contributing to ill health. Certainly, very few have been able to relate compliance to therapy with global measures of quality of life. Studies that attempt to quantify the relationship usually rely on a panel of experts making a judgement to identify the consequences of under- or overcompliance in the case of each individual.

Adverse effects

Toxicity as a result of overmedication could be a potential hazard. The exact frequency with which this occurs, i.e. accidental overdose, has not been reported. The increased sensitivity of the elderly to drug toxicity from a variety of causes would make them particularly prone to this type of problem. Indeed, another consideration is that undercompliance at least would tend to protect patients from toxicity problems. Certainly, in the case of polypharmacy it is possible for non-compliance to a particular drug to be of benefit to the patient.

Hospital admission

Admission due to either under- or overdosing gives a more quantifiable outcome, but in the elderly there are frequently a number of interrelating factors resulting in a hospital admission. About 10% of admissions in some studies in the elderly have been found to be due to poor compliance. It has been shown that some types of medication are more likely to be associated with admission due to reduced compliance[7] (Table 15.1). However, in this study compliance was only assessed by patient interview, but note the preponderance of cardiovascular medication implicated.

Pharmacoeconomic

Wastage due to non-compliance to prescribed medication has an obvious economic consequence. The practice of repeat prescribing for those with chronic conditions can lead to hoarding of medication that is never taken.

Table 15.1 Study of reason for admission in 315 consecutive elderly patients[7]

Drugs implicated as contributing to admission due to non-compliance	Number of times cited
Furosemide (frusemide)	12
Theophylline	8
Warfarin	3
Salbutamol	3
Glyceryl trinitrate	3
Isosorbide dinitrate	2
Digoxin	2
Captopril	2
Prednisolone	2

Reproduced with permission from Col *et al.*[7]

It has been observed that even good adherence to placebo can have a positive health outcome.[8] In a coronary drug project 5-year mortality was 15% for good adherers and 28% for poor adherers in the placebo arm. A β-blocker postinfarction study showed 1-year mortality of 3% for good adherers and 7% for poor adherers taking placebo. Lipid prevention trials did not show this effect and the phenomena might have less relevance on disease incidence than established disease. One possible explanation is that good adherence leads to the taking-up of other health practices which result in an improved clinical outcome, e.g. the type of patient adhering closely to a diuretic may be more motivated to eat less salt, improve weight, etc.

It may be that good adherence promotes a more positive attitude or 'activates non-specific or concomitant features of the treatment'.[8] The phenomenon may also be related to inability to cope with illness, which agrees with findings of poor compliance with stressed subjects.[9] This adds weight to the view that good adherence to suboptimal therapy (in the physician's view) may have a better outcome than poor adherence to optimal therapy, i.e. concordance.

Assessment of medication-taking behaviour

When considering the therapeutic outcome it is important to take into account the medication-taking behaviour of the patient. This would include not only absolute compliance in terms of numbers of tablets taken within a particular time frame, but also the times the medication is taken and drug-free intervals. There may be lost effort in changing a particular therapy when an expected outcome is not achieved, when the therapy is simply being taken inappropriately. In the spirit of the concordance approach, it is also important that both prescriber and patient identify the way in which the regimen is currently being taken in order to agree on any changes that may be necessary.

A number of methods are available to assess medication-taking behaviour, none of which is ideal and applicable in all situations. However, some may be of use in the clinical trial situation or when monitoring patients at high risk of compliance problems. These methods are briefly discussed below.

Tablet counts

This is the traditional method for assessing compliance and one of the easiest to arrange; compliance is simply expressed as a percentage of the prescribed medication intended. There are a few inherent limitations and problems with tablet counts:

- It is important to consider the time frame over which the assessment is made. For chronic medication a month is the standard measure.
- Counts are best performed in the patient's own home where all supplies can be located and accounted for. Even in this situation there is the possibility of patients not disclosing all supplies.
- Tablet counts give little impression of timing of doses or drug-free intervals.
- It is possible to underestimate compliance if due regard is not given to the amount of tablets left to a previous prescription. It is best to obtain a baseline tablet count of current medication and then perform a second count after the issue of a new prescription.

Interview

Simply asking patients if they take the medicines as prescribed can give some indication of the medication-taking behaviour. There are some points regarding this approach:

- Undoubtedly this method would yield an overestimate in the level of compliance; those who are not adhering to the regimen are less likely to admit poor compliance. For instance, one study[7] found that 77% of elderly patients claimed to be good compliers, but in 20% of cases prescription records indicated that compliance was poor.
- If patients do admit to incidences of non-adherence, they are likely to be telling the truth.
- It is best to ask patients in a non-threatening manner. The following phrase has been used with some success: 'Some people find it difficult to take their medication as prescribed. Is this true in your case?'

Using the interview approach in the elderly, a non-compliance level of just 14% has been reported; 10% admitted to overcompliance and 4% to undercompliance.[3]

Prescription refills

For this method pharmacy computer systems can be used, ideally to match up medicine prescribed to medicines actually collected. In practice it is possible to use records to identify whether patients collect monthly repeats. The main drawback is that a patient may use more than one pharmacy.

Currently there is no mechanism in the UK for matching prescriptions issued to prescriptions presented for an individual, although electronic prescribing and repeat prescribing schemes may change this situation. However, many patients prescribed medication for chronic conditions will use the same pharmacy. The situation in the USA is somewhat different, where the medical insurance system ensures that a complete record of prescriptions dispensed for a patient is held by the insurance company. Indeed, the prescription record method has become standard in American compliance studies.

The monitored dosage systems (see below) do also allow a useful method of monitoring compliance. These will always be returned to the same pharmacy for refilling, and it is a simple matter for the pharmacist to note any unused medication. Tablet dumping is still a possibility and no indication of regularity of medication taken can be measured.

Blood level monitoring

By taking blood levels of a drug it is possible to detect effectively if medication has been taken. There are three potential drawbacks:

- Assays for many drugs are difficult to arrange
- If a drug of short half-life is to be measured, steady state is achieved relatively quickly, so medication taken just a day or so prior to the visit may indicate adequate compliance
- Patients must give permission for blood tests.

To overcome the first two problems, a method was devised[10] whereby a very small non-therapeutic dose of a drug with a long half-life easily assayed, such as phenobarbital, was given along with regular medication. The method has been successful in defining levels of compliance in a variety of situations.

Electronic devices

These are the only reliable methods for assessing medication-taking behaviour in an individual. An electronic sensor is hidden in the top of a tablet container. Every time the container is opened the date is immediately registered on an internal memory chip, and this is later downloaded on to a computer when the medication is returned.[11] Similar devices are available for inhalers and eye drops.

Patients may choose to open containers without consuming medication, although it would be unlikely that this would be performed to a particular pattern. The ethics of hiding such devices to 'spy' on patients routinely could be questioned. In the spirit of concordance it would sometimes be useful to make patients aware of the device and to use data produced from the computer analysis as a discussion point between health worker and patient. It is the author's experience of such devices[12] that even if patients are aware of the hidden electronics, they make only a temporary change in medication taking, reverting to a more usual pattern after a week or two.

Factors contributing to poor compliance in the elderly

It would be impractical to screen every patient using most of the methods described above for potential compliance problems. Therefore, identifying those patients most at risk would alert health carers and enable them to direct resources to helping higher-risk individuals. Table 15.2 lists most of the risk factors that have been investigated for potential relationships to reduced compliance.

A study[7] identified correlations between some of the areas described in Table 15.2 and the likelihood of admission. These include:

- Poor recall of medication being taken
- Female
- Polypharmacy
- Not having home service
- Cost (medication in the USA only)

Table 15.2 Factors that may contribute to poor compliance

Factor	Strength of relationship to reduced compliance
Advancing age	Weak
Gender	Weak
Transport to pharmacy	Weak
Information/knowledge	Moderate
Disability/physical function	Moderate
Certain therapeutic regimens	Moderate
Lifetime medication need	Strong
Regimen complexity	Strong
Side-effects	Strong
Cognitive function	Strong
Using more than one pharmacy	Strong
Not having home services	Strong
Health and medication beliefs	Strong
Cost (USA only)	Strong
Using more than one doctor (USA only)	Strong

Other studies have failed to demonstrate a strong relationship between these factors and a tendency to poor compliance. These issues, which are of particular relevance to the elderly, will now be discussed.

Age and gender

Contrary to popular belief, advancing age is not necessarily related to reduced compliance. One study[13] found that, out of 36 studies where age had been examined for a relationship with level of compliance, only six identified a correlation with advancing years. Another study[14] found that the over-85s were the best compliers overall. There are two possible explanations for this observation: the likelihood that such patients had a more severe disease and were therefore better motivated, and that such people were more likely to be supported by carers.

Gender is not usually shown to be related to compliance issues, although a few studies[2] have indicated that women may have more problems.

Cognitive function, knowledge and health beliefs

There has been a long-running debate concerning the relationship between information given to improve knowledge regarding medication and whether this has any effect on subsequent medication-taking behaviour, i.e. improves compliance. It would be assumed that those with a better knowledge of the purpose of medication and prescribed regimen would be more likely to comply. Some early studies did indicate such a relationship[2] but this was not borne out by more recent work,[5] where increased knowledge did not correlate or even had a negative correlation with compliance.

Studies do not observe universally poor levels of knowledge amongst the elderly. Quite high levels of knowledge have been found,[15] with 75–80% being aware of name, dose and purpose of medication. However, polypharmacy could potentially lead to an information overload. In one study[16] there was a correlation between reduced understanding and numbers of medicines prescribed.

A declining cognitive function would certainly lead to reduced compliance due to forgetfulness. It is difficult to arrive at figures for the scale of the problem as those with very much reduced function would tend to have carers taking responsibility for their medication. It is not necessarily just cognitive impairment that can lead to forgetfulness; a busy lifestyle or preoccupation with an important event could lead to a disruption in medication-taking routines. In one survey of elderly people only 17% cited forgetfulness as a factor contributing to reduced adherence.[2]

Although cognitive decline with advancing years can be a result of a chronic dementia such as Alzheimer's, there are also many acute situations which can lead to confusion in the elderly (e.g. urinary tract/ respiratory infections) and potentially lead to self-medication errors. Many psychotropic agents can result in confusion and antimuscarinic agents in particular have been associated with memory loss in the elderly.

In all these cases it is a possibility that both under- and overdosing of medication can occur. An often cited example is the use of hypnotics in the elderly. In this scenario a person wakes during the night and, forgetting that a hypnotic has already been taken, inadvertently takes a further dose. This leads to a greater hangover effect the next day, resulting in a general increase in confusion at night, potentially leading to further hypnotic overdose.

These are examples of unintentional non-compliance to a regimen. There are many instances where patients may choose not to comply with a regimen. For instance, they may take more medication in the belief that the condition will resolve faster, or as they start to feel better choose to discontinue or reduce a course of treatment.[2]

The factors that actually motivate individuals are beginning to be extensively studied and are of interest to psychologists. One very popular concept has been the health belief model, which would suggest that those who consider their condition to be the most serious would tend to be better compliers. However, this model in itself is not a particularly good predictor of compliance.

A model has been proposed[17] that accounts for the concerns people have regarding their medication together with the perceived necessity of the prescribed medication. As would be expected, those who appreciated the necessity of their medication were more likely to report higher adherence. Conversely, those who had concerns regarding their medication, e.g. harmful long-term effects, tended to have lower adherence, due to minimising perceived risk by taking less medication. However a third of patients will appreciate the necessity of the medication, but still have concerns over the safety of their medication. This is of particular importance for practitioners of the concordance approach.

One study[9] made some interesting observations regarding correlation with compliance in the elderly, while noting that the level of compliance was not necessarily reduced in this age group. It was observed that compliance was reduced by fear of illness, which is contrary to the health belief model. It could be that higher levels of fear produced denial of illness. It was also observed that compliance was reduced if the patient felt that too much time was spent waiting to see a doctor, possibly because this represents resentment and frustration of dependence being expressed as non-adherence. This study also found a correlation between poor compliance and poor knowledge. These observations demand further investigation and verification.

Physical function

A now well-established cause for medication-taking problems[4, 18] is that due to current UK legislation regarding the use of child-resistant containers (CRCs), which must be used whenever a medicine is dispensed unless specifically instructed otherwise by patient or doctor. This can be achieved in one of two ways: Clic Locks on bottles or strip packs, which present problems in taking medication for frail elderly patients.

CRCs are often left unlocked or the tablets transferred to a different container. It has also been noted that some elderly people even use young children to help them open CRCs. Blister packs are better managed by the elderly, although some will still experience problems. There are reports[18] of elderly patients coming to harm from swallowing cut-up blister packs. The physical manipulations involved in self-administering certain formulations may present considerable problems for the elderly, as listed in Table 15.3. Difficulty in swallowing tablets may require changes to liquid formulations, and inhaler problems may necessitate choosing a more suitable device.

Adverse effects

As has been described in Chapter 2, the elderly are more prone to ADRs. It is therefore not surprising that this is an important contribution to

Table 15.3 Factors representing physical barriers to medication taking in the elderly

Swallowing tablets
Measuring liquids
Using inhalers
Instilling drops
Suppositories/pessary form
Applying creams

reduced compliance in this age group. In one study it was found that 17% of admissions related to ADRs, and of this cohort 18% stated that due to an adverse reaction they had not followed the medication schedule.[7]

Some drug groups would certainly have a tendency to cause ADRs in the elderly, which may lead to them discontinuing medication. Disturbances in sleep caused by psychotropics and the antimuscarinic effects of drugs, particularly constipation, are cited as the most troublesome. Alternatively, the therapeutic effect may lead to an unacceptable disturbance in lifestyle. The restriction imposed by diuretics is a good example where the drug is omitted on the days the patient is away from home. Another potential scenario is an adverse reaction noted by the patient who, due to the presence of polypharmacy, chooses to discontinue a drug which is not actually responsible for the problem. Stewart and Craasos[4] point out that, generally, if medication requires some behavioural change in a patient, compliance is likely to be reduced.

Social factors

For the elderly person support in taking medication can sometimes be essential and it has been demonstrated that living with a relative does have an influence on compliance.[5,9] One study[7] found no relationship with living alone, although it failed to assess whether or not there was some outside help.

Simply being unable to leave the house may present problems to an elderly patient, who would normally lose contact with the community pharmacist. The potential benefits of pharmacist domiciliary visiting schemes have been demonstrated in a number of studies.[19] It is also probably important for a particular pharmacy to be used by those on chronic medication; non-compliance has been estimated as being nearly four times more likely among patients using two or three pharmacies than just a single one.[7] This was one factor behind the National Health Service interest in repeat prescribing schemes where prescriptions for repeats are automatically forwarded to a pharmacy of the patient's choice.

Discharge from hospital also presents particular problems for patients in arranging adequate supplies of the correct medication. Although a 1-week supply of a new regimen may be given by a hospital, it may take much longer for a house-bound patient to arrange supplies through a general practitioner. However, a period in hospital can itself be a motivation to higher levels of compliance, at least initially.[20]

Polypharmacy and regimen complexity

There is good evidence that increasing complexity of a regimen would lead to difficulties with medication taking[4,5] and that drug errors can increase by up to 15-fold when the number of prescribed items increased from one to four drugs. More than two medications per day can lead to a threefold increase in the likelihood of self-reported non-compliance. It also been found that one-quarter of elderly patients were taking an over-the-counter medication for conditions also being treated with prescribed medication. In general the aim is that any single medication is not taken more than twice a day.[5]

Not all studies universally demonstrate this effect; some show no association with numbers of prescribed drugs. It has been shown in a few studies that those with a more complex regimen are better compliers.[20] This may be because those with more severe illness may be prescribed more medications, but are more motivated to take them. This applies more to complexity of regimen to treat a specific condition rather than polypharmacy *per se*. It was observed that patients with more than one glaucoma medication were better compliers, although those on a number of different medications, apart from that used to treat glaucoma, had a poorer compliance overall.[21]

Therapeutic area

If targeting services to patients who may have compliance problems, it would be useful if the pharmacist could identify specific drug groups which are likely to cause problems. Most studies do not show correlation of poor compliance with any particular drug. One study[2] listed the rate of intentional non-compliance to the following groups of drugs:

- Psychotropics: 13%
- Musculoskeletal: 60%
- Antibiotics: 35%
- Gastrointestinal: 18%

Compliance to cardiovascular medication in the elderly, especially diuretics, is often quite high.[20] However, in a study examining digoxin, patients were found to have only been dispensed enough tablets for 111 days in the year. For glaucoma medication[21] 23% did not take any medication in the year and the mean number of days without therapy in the year was 112. Analgesics tend to be associated with an over-compliance that would be expected in this therapeutic area,[5] whereas both bronchodilators and benzodiazipines appear to have the poorest rates of compliance.

Strategies to resolve compliance/concordance issues

In order to embrace the principles of concordance, it is important to approach the issue with the aim of reaching a mutual agreement with the patient. Some of the strategies that have previously been used to improve compliance can also be adopted when negotiating a regimen with a particular patient. As an example, consider the following aspects, which are listed as important:[16]

- give clear information and written instruction
- set clear treatment goals
- avoid polypharmacy
- assist in organising system.

Firstly, the treatment goals should not necessarily be dictated by the prescriber but negotiated with the patient. In theory, if the patient wishes to accept less treatment and clearly understands the potential therapeutic consequences, then that approach should be adopted. The information and written instruction should be of the type and breadth that the patient requests, not necessarily those dictated by the manufacturer or what the prescriber feels to be appropriate. The system used for organising medicines should also be discussed fully with patients, with due attention to that which best fits their lifestyle. Although the overall aim is to minimise polypharmacy, any medication which is discontinued should also be discussed and explained. It may be that an individual is quite happy with a relatively complex regimen.

Involving the patient in medication taking is very much within the spirit of concordance. Self-medication programmes initiated in hospital have been shown to help with adherence postdischarge[22] but a long-term effect has not been fully assessed.

The next sections will consider the processes which the pharmacist should undertake when discussing medication with a patient with a view to negotiating concordance to a regimen.

Patient interview and identification of issue

This is the cornerstone of the concordance process. Taking the time to understand patients' views regarding both their condition and how it is managed will help to decide the most appropriate regimen and devise measures that ensure adherence.

Although it is important to take time to elucidate potential problems, this may be impractical to provide for all patients at risk.

Therefore identifying the highest-risk patients in order to prioritise patients is an essential exercise, and demands further research.

The siting for such an assessment can also be important, as it is necessary to discuss all of the medication currently being taken. For elderly house-bound patients a domiciliary visit may be required, and this is perhaps the best setting for a discussion of concordance issues as it would be expected that the patient would feel less threatened in such an environment. Otherwise a 'brown bag' review could be performed[23] where the patient places all of the medication currently being taken into a bag and attends a medication review at either a pharmacy or health centre. The brown bag review is probably more cost-effective than a domiciliary visit, but may not provide as accurate a picture of the medication taken as patients may fail to bring in their whole supply.

Who should carry out such interviews? The general practitioner may be well placed to negotiate therapy with patients, but most do not have the time to carry out thorough reviews. The pharmacist certainly has the pharmaceutical knowledge, although he/she may be lacking in negotiating and communication skills. The opposite is probably true of the nurse. The best approach would be a partnership of all three health professionals. How this could be achieved in practice has not been well studied. Perhaps the pharmacist should concentrate on gaining a clear picture of the individual's current medication-taking behaviour and devising with the patient an appropriate pharmaceutical care plan. The nurse could discuss the patient's understanding of the illness and fears regarding medication. Both could feed back to the prescriber with suggested changes to a regimen.

Before the interview it is important for the health professional to elucidate the intended treatment, ideally from practice records if available. Due care should be taken that there are no interface issues

Table 15.4 Checklist for patient interview and review

Literacy problems
Recent hospital admissions and attendance at outpatients or day centre
Number of pharmacies used
Number of prescribed and over-the-counter medications
Medications taken more than twice a day
Likely side-effects
Possible interactions and contraindications
Administration problems
Social functioning: can the patient self-medicate?
Packaging and labelling: consider aid
Monitoring outcome

resulting in unintended therapy. A knowledge of the diagnosis is also helpful, although in many cases this can be elucidated from the pre-scribed medication. The interview should cover the various points made in Table 15.4. Some of the interventions that can be taken are con-sidered in the following sections. A scheme of the process following identification of issues is given in Figure 15.1.

Explaining the purpose and other information

Whether or not knowledge of medication actually improves adherence, patients should be in possession of the necessary information if they are to take an active role in discussion regarding their therapy.

Patient information leaflets (PILs) are now available through patient packs produced by manufacturers or other sources. These may be of variable quality and readability; those included in patient packs often contain too broad a range and detailed information in order to satisfy the requirements of the product licence. A further problem for

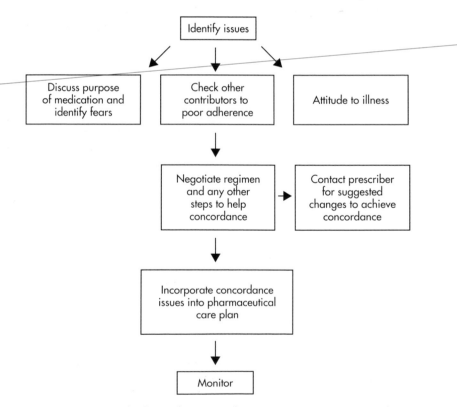

Figure 15.1   Suggested scheme for concordance process.

some elderly patients is the small print of such leaflets. There is certainly a requirement for individualised information sheets for medication. An interesting approach is the use of computer-generated leaflets, as described by Raynor et al.[24] A further possibility is that a web-based service will become available to deliver patient-specific information on medication in a clear and concise manner.

The American Geriatrics Society[16] has described the information it feels should be made available to the elderly regarding their medication, as shown in Table 15.5. This range of information should be presented both written and orally.

In terms of concordance there are probably a few key areas that should be covered. The understanding of the patient's own illness may need to be clarified, and it could be argued that this is not necessarily the province of the pharmacist. However, other important areas may be better discussed with a pharmacist, and these might include: the advantages or disadvantages of particular regimens and medication, the limitations of the medication and likelihood and importance of any adverse reaction or interaction. The aim should be not to persuade the patient to follow any one regimen but for them to make an informed decision. Work is still needed to determine the benefits and feasibility of such an approach.

Simplification of regimen

As has already been discussed, simplification of a regimen to once- or twice-daily medication can improve adherence. A further principle is to ensure that medication taking can fit conveniently into the patient's daily activities. In some cases longer-acting medication may be appropriate, but it must be remembered that those with a longer half-life may have a tendency to accumulate in the elderly.

Table 15.5 Information for patients

Specific information	General information
Name	Not to take another person's medication
Purpose	Unless instructed otherwise, keep taking the
Dose/strength	medication
When to be taken in relation to food/other medicine	Take prescribed dose unless told otherwise
	Do not transfer into an inappropriate
Common side-effects	container
How long to be taken	Avoid taking in the dark
Other warnings	

CODE	PRESCRIPTION/ DESCRIPTION	– USE – OTHER INSTRUCTIONS	TIME OF DAY	NUMBER	Monday	Tuesday	Wednesday	Thursday	Friday	Saturday	Sunday	Monday	Tuesday	Wednesday	Thursday	Friday	Saturday	Sunday	Monday	Tuesday	Wednesday	Thursday	Friday	Saturday	Sunday	Monday	Tuesday	Wednesday	Thursday	Friday	Saturday	Sunday
			BREAKFAST TIME																													
			LUNCH TIME																													
			DINNER TIME																													
			NIGHT																													
			BREAKFAST TIME																													
			LUNCH TIME																													
			DINNER TIME																													
			NIGHT																													
			BREAKFAST TIME																													
			LUNCH TIME																													
			DINNER TIME																													
			NIGHT																													
			BREAKFAST TIME																													
			LUNCH TIME																													
			DINNER TIME																													
			NIGHT																													
			BREAKFAST TIME																													
			LUNCH TIME																													
			DINNER TIME																													
			NIGHT																													
			BREAKFAST TIME																													
			LUNCH TIME																													
			DINNER TIME																													
			NIGHT																													
			BREAKFAST TIME																													
			LUNCH TIME																													
			DINNER TIME																													
			NIGHT																													

Figure 15.2 Diary card.

MEDICINE REMINDER CARD

NAME...

DATE ISSUED..

PLEASE TAKE THIS CARD WITH YOU WHEN YOU GO
TO YOUR DOCTOR OR CHEMIST AND WHEN YOU
COME BACK FOR YOUR NEXT HOSPITAL APPOINTMENT.

TICK OFF EACH DOSE AS YOU HAVE BEEN SHOWN.
IF YOU FORGET, DON'T WORRY – JUST LEAVE THE
SPACE BLANK.

REMEMBER

DO NOT TRANSFER YOUR MEDICINES INTO OTHER
CONTAINERS.

TO THE PHARMACIST

PLEASE MARK EACH CONTAINER WITH THE CORRECT
CODE LETTER.

WHEN ALTERNATIVE DRUG BRANDS ARE DISPENSED
PLEASE AMEND THE DESCRIPTION COLUMN.

Figure 15.2 (continued).

It is always worthwhile checking that the patient is physically able
to administer the medication. Devices such as inhalers may pose particular problems and formulations such as eye drops may also be difficult
to self-administer. Even handling and picking up tablets could be
difficult with arthritic hands.

Carers

A number of studies have been discussed which highlight the importance
of negotiations with a carer, be it relative, friend or other health professional, who is responsible for the patient's medication. For elderly
patients who can take no responsibility for their medication, the concordance process may well have to be undertaken directly with the carer.

Aids to compliance

In order to overcome problems with forgetfulness and other physical
problems with compliance there are a number of strategies that can be
adopted.

List and diaries

It is sometimes found to be helpful to provide patients with a clear written list of their medication in which are stated the name, appearance and dosage to act as 'reminder cards'. A few studies have examined the use of such cards and patients do often find them helpful, particularly when issued on discharge from hospital (Figure 15.2). Sometimes a tablet is physically stuck on to a card, with written instructions beside each one to aid identification. A principal disadvantage is that the list would need updating every time medication is changed and without a formal mechanism for making such alterations, this could contribute to confusion regarding the intended current regimen.

As shown in Figure 15.2, the reminder card may be combined with a diary for the patient to make a record each time the medication is taken. In a study of 150 elderly patients, such a diary actually made little difference to compliance.[25]

Compliance aids and monitored-dosage systems

There is a plethora of devices that claim to help patients in remembering to take medication.[26] However, they are not a panacea for compliance and if patients are to benefit they need proper instruction and support in their correct use. The ideal device would have the following properties:

- easy to manipulate and open
- child-resistant
- not require regular refilling on less than a monthly basis
- maintain the integrity of the medication
- portable

Few can meet all these specifications and a device suiting one individual may not be appropriate for another. Versions of the widely used Nomad and MDS systems are also employed in nursing homes as monitored-dosage systems, which allow accurate records to be kept of whether medication has been removed from a container. These systems also allow some degree of compliance monitoring, as tablets remaining in the system when returned to the pharmacy for refilling can be recorded. Studies regarding long-term stability of medication in such containers are not available, but there is certainly variability in the amount of moisture that may enter these devices, potentially affecting shelf-life.[27]

The Nomad and MDS systems are designed to be refilled by a pharmacist, whereas others such as the Dosette can be filled by a carer.

Table 15.6 Some medication reminder/organiser devices

Product	Description	Comment
Compliapack – domiciliary pack	Blister packing in hot seal cards Four dose intervals per card for 1 week Completely disposable	Two sizes of blisters available Must be prepared in the pharmacy
Dosette box	Box with sliding lids Four dose intervals for 1 week Maxi version has a larger container Braille markings	Some find the lids difficult to open Potential for tablets to fall out if lid slides out too far Can be filled by a carer
Medi planner/medidispenser	Box with pop-up lids Four dose intervals for 1 week Braille markings	Similar to Dosette but some may find lids easier to manipulate
Medidos systems/medimemo	Diary-sized closing box Contains seven separate slips, one for each day of the week, allowing four dosage intervals Box opens by slip cover Individual compartment size may be adjusted Medimax has extra capacity	Some may find it difficult to manipulate Each strip can be removed from the box if travelling away from home Can be filled by carer Options of various carrying cases Tablets could fall out if cover is pulled too far
Mediwheel	Rotating wheel with four compartments Available in a weekly pack of seven	May be filled by carer Designed for use by those who have difficulties opening other types of container
Medsystem	A pouch containing seven trays each with four compartments Easy-to-remove slide-off lid Also available as a single weekly tray	Tablets could fall out if cover is moved too far Somewhat larger than other systems employing a daily removable strip
Nomad controlled-dosage system for home use	Box allowing 7 days of medication with up to six dosage intervals Below slider is a perforated seal to prevent medication falling out if pulled too far	Modified slider available for arthritic patients Must be filled in the pharmacy
Venalink	Cold- or heat-sealed blister packs Variety of sizes of blisters Four dose intervals for 1 week	Completely disposable Must be filled in the pharmacy

Some suppliers stock individual daily reminder boxes that are not included in this table.

However many health authorities have been unhappy to let health or social services workers fill such devices for insurance reasons. This has lead to a few schemes whereby pharmacists provide a domiciliary MDS scheme, which also allows pharmaceutical contact for otherwise house-bound individuals.

A comparison of a range of devices currently available in the UK is shown in Table 15.6. Studies which highlight the various advantages and disadvantages of individual devices are needed, although the Medidose proved the most popular in one survey.[28] The key message when supplying such devices is to ensure that the patient both desires and understands its use and that some follow-up service is provided.

Packaging and labels

There are two important issues here: legibility of labels and the use of child-resistant containers. In terms of labels the advantages of large labels are obvious for those with poor eyesight. In one study[2] up to 60% of elderly patients experienced problems in reading labels. In particular it is important to ensure that the ubiquitous 'as directed' is not inappropriately used.

For child-resistant containers, blister packs do offer a useful alternative which is manageable by most elderly people. As well as the frail elderly, other groups may also experience problems with such containers, including those with arthritis, chronic pain syndromes, tremors and poor eyesight.

Polypharmacy – general principles

In the preceding discussion regarding concordance/compliance, a number of issues relating to polypharmacy have already been identified and discussed. Apart from confusion over dose regimen, the principal reason for avoiding polypharmacy is to reduce potential adverse events and interactions. The rationale is that the fewer drugs prescribed, the less likely the adverse event.

The elderly are particularly prone to polypharmacy due to the chronic, and often multiple, nature of conditions to which they are prone. Also, without adequate medication review those prescribed for acute conditions may remain prescribed long after they are required; analgesics are a notorious member of this category, but hypnotics and medication for 'dizziness' are also often prescribed for longer than necessary.

Table 15.7 The medication appropriateness index criteria and relative weights[29]

Criterion	Relative weight applied to inappropriate ratings
Is there an indication for the drug?	3
Is the medication effective for the condition?	3
Is the dosage correct?	2
Are the directions correct?	2
Are there clinically significant drug–drug interactions?	2
Are there clinically significant drug–disease interactions?	2
Are the directions practical?	1
Is this drug the least expensive alternative compared with others of equal utility?	1
Is there unnecessary duplication with other drugs?	1
Is the duration of therapy acceptable?	1

Reproduced from Hanlon *et al.*[29] with permission.

In terms of adverse reactions to certain medications, there are particular groups that pose special problems for the elderly, as described in other chapters. In particular, those affecting the central nervous system or motor function should be monitored closely, as should any medication lowering blood pressure resulting in a tendency to postural hypotension.

The key to avoiding the problems of polypharmacy lies in regular medication review. It is not an uncommon experience for elderly patients admitted into hospital to be taken off most of their regular medication and benefit greatly as a result. The pharmacist can have a pivotal role in reviewing medication to reduce polypharmacy[29] either in the community setting or on the hospital ward. A useful checklist for reviewing the appropriateness of medication and to reduce polypharmacy is given in Table 15.7.[29] The prime concern when reviewing medication for the elderly should be to identify any medication that is unnecessary, before considering what could further be prescribed.

References

1. *From Compliance to Concordance. Achieving Shared Goals in Medicine Taking.* London: Royal Pharmaceutical Society of Great Britain, 1997.
2. Salzman C. Medication compliance in the elderly. *J Clin Psychiatry* 1995 (suppl. 1): 18–22.
3. Spagoli A, Ostino G, Borg A *et al.* Drug compliance and unreported drugs in the elderly. *J Am Geriatr Soc* 1982; 30: 329–333.

4.   Stewart R B, Craasos G J. Medication compliance in the elderly. *Med Clin North Am* 1998; 73: 1551–1561.

5.   McElnay J C, McCallon C R, Al-Deagi F, Scott M. Self reported medication non-compliance in the elderly. *Eur J Clin Pharmacol* 1997; 53: 171–178.

6.   Goodyer L I, Miskelly F, Milligan P. Does encouraging good compliance improve the patients' clinical condition in heart failure? *Br J Clin Pract* 1995; 49: 173–176.

7.   Col N, Fanale E, Kronholm P. The role of medication noncompliance and adverse drug reactions in hospitalisations in the elderly. *Arch Intern Med* 1990; 170: 841–845.

8.   Horwitz R, Horwitz M. Adherence to treatment and health outcomes. *Arch Intern Med* 1993; 153: 1863–1868.

9.   Lorenc L, Branthwaite A. Are older adults less compliant with prescribed medication than younger adults? *Br J Clin Psychol* 1993; 32: 485–492.

10.   Pullar T, Kumar S, Tindall H, Feely M. Time to stop counting the tablets? *Clin Pharmacol Ther* 1989; 46: 163–168.

11.   Urquhart J. Role of patient compliance in clinical pharmacokinetics. *Clin Pharmacokinet* 1994; 27: 202–215.

12.   Punchak S, Goodyer L I, Miskelly F. Use of an electronic monitoring aid to investigate the medication pattern of analgesics and NSAIDs prescribed for osteoarthritis. *Rheumatology* 2000; 39: 448–449.

13.   Haynes R D. A critical review of the determinants of patient compliance with therapeutic regimens. In: Sacket D L, Haynes R D, eds. *Compliance with Therapeutic Regimens*. Baltimore: Johns Hopkins University Press, 1976: 27–39.

14.   Monane M, Bohn R, Gurwitz J *et al*. Compliance with antihypertensive therapy among elderly Medicaid enrollees: the roles of age, gender and race. *Am J Public Health* 1996; 86: 1805–1808.

15.   Blenkiro J. The elderly and their medication: understanding and compliance in family practice. *Postgrad Med J* 1996; 72: 671–676.

16.   Ennis K J, Reichard R A. Drug compliance in elderly. *Postgrad Med* 1997; 102: 211–224.

17.   Horne R, Weinman J. The Beliefs and Medicines Questionnaire (BMQ): the development and evaluation of a new method for assessing cognitive representations of medication. *Psychol Health* 1999; 14: 1–24.

18.   Sexton J, Gokani R. Pharmaceutical packaging and the elderly. *Pharm J* 1997; 259: 697–700.

19.   Foulsham R, Goodyer L. Referrals made by different health care professionals to community pharmacists for domiciliary visiting. *Int J Pharm Pract* 1999; 7: 86–92.

20.   Monane M, Bohn R, Gurwitz J *et al*. Noncompliance with congestive heart failure therapy in the elderly. *Arch Intern Med* 1994; 154: 433–437.

21.   Gurwitz J H, Glynn R J, Monane M *et al*. Treatment for glaucoma: adherence by the elderly. *Am J Public Health* 1993; 83: 711–716.

22.   Lowe C J, Raynor D, Courtney E A *et al*. Effects of self-medication programme on knowledge of drugs and compliance with treatment in elderly patients. *BMJ* 1995; 310: 1229–1231.

23. Nathan A, Goodyer L, Lovejoy A, Rashid A. 'Brown bag' medication reviews as a means of optimising patients' use of medication and of identifying potential clinical problems. *Family Pract* 1999; 16: 278–282.

24. Raynor D K, Booth T G, Blenkinsopp A. Effects of computer generated reminder charts on patients' compliance with drug regimens. *BMJ* 1993; 306: 1158–1161.

25. Atkin P A, Finnegan T P, Ogle S J *et al.* Are medication cards useful? *Med J Aust* 1995; 162: 300–301.

26. Sprey L. Monitored dosage systems. *Pharm J* 1995; 254: 767–770.

27. Report to the RPSGB. Report of the moisture permeability testing of monitored dosage systems. *Pharm J* 1994; 252: 18–19.

28. Walker R, Mandal A, Daymond T *et al.* Assessment of compliance devices by patients. *Pharm J* 1990; 245 (suppl): R1.

29. Hanlon T, Weinberger M, Samsa G *et al.* Randomised, controlled trial of a clinical pharmacist intervention to improve inappropriate prescribing in elderly outpatients with polypharmacy. *Am J Med* 1996; 100: 428–437.

16

Research in the elderly: ethics, consent and methodology

C Alice Oborne

Scope

Aspects of research which are similar whether young or old subjects are involved have largely been excluded from this chapter. Readers interested in general information on good clinical research practice are directed to the European Community directive on conduct of clinical trials (91/507/EC) and to the International Conference on Harmonisation (ICH) international consolidated Guideline on Good Clinical Practice. Prominence has been given to drug-related research. The intention is to highlight key areas of interest and concern, emphasising ethics of research in elderly human subjects, consent to participate in research and research consent in non-competent or partially competent elderly subjects. Finally, some research tools specific to elderly subjects are outlined. The term 'clinical research' is used in this chapter in its widest sense, to cover research involving both patients and non-patient (healthy) volunteers.

Medication use by the elderly population

Elderly people currently consume three times as many medicines as younger patients.[1] Two-thirds of older people take at least one pre-scribed medicine daily and elderly community-dwelling subjects are pre-scribed a mean of two to four items each.[2-4] People aged 65 years or over currently constitute less than 20% of the UK population, yet this group consumes 45% of all prescribed drugs.[4] The elderly population is expanding and most recent projections estimate that 30% of the UK population will be aged 65 years or over by 2010, with the consequence that elderly persons will consume an even greater proportion of all prescribed drugs.

Physiological changes occurring with increasing age

Significant pharmacokinetic and pharmacodynamic changes occur with increasing age, including reduced drug clearance and differential receptor sensitivity. This frequently results in an altered response to a given dose of drug.[5,6] In general, renal clearance of water-soluble drugs is reduced in ageing subjects to a greater extent than hepatic clearance of lipid-soluble drugs, although knowledge in this area is still incomplete.[7–10] Pharmacokinetics in older persons are discussed fully in Chapter 2.

Pharmacodynamic changes in the interaction between drugs and the β-adrenoceptor appear to cause a decreased response to β-blockers in older subjects, with the result that β-adrenoceptor-blocking drugs reduce blood pressure less effectively in older hypertensives.[7,11] Acute and chronic diseases are more prevalent in older populations; frequently, elderly people have several concurrent conditions. The presence of illnesses, such as heart failure and renal failure, can affect drug handling and drug response at least as much as chronological age.[7,9]

Variability in disease prevalence and outcomes

Most diseases have an age-related prevalence. For example, in the general population the respective prevalences of stroke, hypertension and heart failure increase with increasing age. In patients with non-rheumatic atrial fibrillation (AF), the risk of stroke also correlates with advancing age.[12] On the other hand, the number needed to treat to prevent one ischaemic stroke decreases with increasing age and thus the overall benefits from stroke prophylaxis are greater in the elderly population.[13]

Similar age-associated variability is seen when the risks of drug therapy are considered, with both incidence and severity of adverse drug reactions rising with increasing age.[14] Ninety per cent of fatal gastro-intestinal haemorrhages associated with non-steroidal anti-inflammatory drugs (NSAIDs) reported to the Committee on Safety of Medicines are in people aged 60 years or over. Although this may be related to greater NSAID use by elderly people, altered physiology, comorbid conditions and concurrent prescriptions all appear to increase the risk of NSAID morbidity in older subjects.[15,16]

Health carers attending elderly patients occasionally argue that the benefit from drug therapy in an older person is less than that in younger persons due to reduced long-term survival or an increased risk of adverse events. Although future life expectancy may be less in older individuals, data indicate that the absolute risk of an event is often much higher in older patients, resulting in greater overall treatment benefit in population terms. This was clearly illustrated by a systematic review of studies of hypertension treatment, which found two to four times as many young people as older people need to be treated to prevent an equivalent number of cardiovascular events.[17] Thus, variability in therapeutic risks and benefits mean that conclusions from studies in younger populations cannot reliably be extrapolated to elderly subjects.[18, 19]

A case for inclusion of elderly subjects in clinical trials

Older subjects continue to be excluded from clinical studies.[19, 20] A survey of published original research found a third of studies excluded elderly people without justification.[19] Trials of drug treatments in arthritis have included few older patients and hardly any over the age of 85 years, yet almost 50% of older people report some form of arthritis.[21]

Exclusion of likely drug recipients from early clinical trials led to problems in the 1980s when the NSAID benoxaprofen was marketed as having a favourable adverse effect profile and disease-modifying properties in rheumatoid and osteoarthritis. It was withdrawn 18 months later after reports of skin and liver toxicity, particularly in elderly recipients. This heightened toxicity in elderly people was not identified before marketing because investigation in elderly subjects was abandoned at an early stage of drug development.[22, 23]

The need for drug safety and efficacy data in older subjects is tempered by likely greater risks of pharmacotherapy in frail elders with comorbidities. Concurrent drug therapies and multiple pathologies may cause investigators concern about introduction of bias, or make interpretation of results more difficult because the greater heterogeneity in elderly subjects results in more variable data.[24] Securing informed consent is often more time-consuming and complicated in elderly subjects.

The benoxaprofen case demonstrates that clinical trials should involve all the expected recipients of the drug under investigation. Application of the results of studies which excluded elderly patients to the management of elderly people is inappropriate and possibly dangerous.[18–20] World Health Organization (WHO) guidelines strongly support this notion and some advocates argue that the (potentially greater) risks of drug therapy in elderly subjects are best investigated in the rigorous setting of a clinical trial. Further, risk–benefit evaluations applied to elderly patients should assess overall benefit and risk reduction from baseline event risk in elderly populations.

Areas for drug research in elderly people

Premarketing (phase II and III) clinical trials

After phase I clinical studies (involving 50–100 healthy volunteers) have provided sufficient data to merit continued development of a new chemical entity, phases II and III trials are initiated.[25] Currently, few of the 200–400 carefully selected patients in phase II studies are elderly, whether or not the disease being treated occurs in elderly people. Risks associated with investigational compounds in elderly patients are often perceived to be too great at this stage. However, when the disease is almost unknown in younger patients, e.g. dementia, phase II studies do include large numbers of older subjects. Phase III studies usually involve 3000 or more patients and older individuals may be recruited.

Postmarketing (phase IV) studies

At the time of licensing, a new drug may have been administered to as few as 3500 individuals. Premarketing clinical trials cannot hope to recognise every one of a drug's adverse effects, or identify all populations at greater risk of adverse effects (e.g. NSAIDs in elderly patients).[25] To test drug safety and efficacy in common clinical practice, drug manufacturers usually organise a programme of phase IV (postmarketing) studies. These studies often use observational cohort and case-controlled designs where drug recipients and matched controls are identified from the general population, rather than the more scientifically rigorous placebo-controlled double-blind designs of earlier phases. Most phase IV studies involve collection of clinical data after the decision has been made to prescribe the drug and so the ethical question concerning inclusion of elderly subjects in phase IV surveys is not whether to include them, but whether omission is unethical. It can be argued that these patients are a useful source of data not already collated in premarketing studies.

Additional phase II and phase III trials may also be conducted after the initial product licence is granted. These studies in new patient groups or for different indications may include elderly patients.[25]

The Medicines Control Agency Yellow Card spontaneous reporting scheme may also provide postmarketing safety data for elderly recipients.

Other drug-related research

Additional drug-related studies recruiting elderly subjects include pharmacoepidemiological surveys of prescribing or drug consumption by elderly people[1-3, 26] and major outcome studies such as comparisons between drug classes in specific diseases. Qualitative research methodologies encompass interviews, observation and focus groups and are rich sources of descriptive information. As the views, drug beliefs and experiences of young people cannot be reliably extrapolated to elderly people, qualitative techniques may be used in elderly populations.[3]

Ethical considerations of research in elderly populations

Ethical research codes: World Medical Association codes

Ethical aspects of clinical research on human subjects are governed by international and national regulations. The first internationally accepted ethical guidelines, the Nuremberg Code, agreed in 1949, were a direct result of atrocities in the name of research during the Second World War.

The World Medical Association was founded in 1947 and has produced a number of ethical guidelines, including a modernised Hippocratic oath called the Declaration of Geneva (updated in Stockholm, 1994).[27] An International Code of Medical Ethics is based upon the Declaration of Geneva. The World Medical Association also adopted the Declaration of Helsinki (DH) in 1964. The DH is the most widely accepted guidance worldwide on the conduct of clinical research involving human subjects and was most recently revised in Edinburgh in 2000.[27] National guidelines governing human biomedical research in the UK have their foundations in the DH. These include the Association of British Pharmaceutical Industry Guidelines, Royal College of Physicians of London Guidelines, ICH Guideline on Good Clinical Practice, the UK Department of Health Guidelines and the European Commission Guidelines for Good (Research) Clinical Practice for Trials on Medicinal Products (GCP).

Both the GCP guidelines and DH state: 'the purpose of biomedical research must be to improve diagnostic, therapeutic and prophylactic procedures and the understanding of the aetiology and pathogenesis of disease'. They also recognise that research is necessary for medical advancement: 'medical progress is based upon research which ultimately must rest in part upon experimentation involving human subjects'.

These clinical practice and research codes emphasise the subject's rights, interests, dignity and welfare and consideration of subjects' wishes. The codes also identify a number of ethical principles central to the conduct of human research. These are:

- benefice, relating to the risk–benefit of research
- justice, which requires that the risks of research be equally distributed
- respect for persons, relating to autonomy and consent.

Risk–benefit of research

Research into ageing and diseases common in older people holds the key to addressing the health problems of the elderly population, thus it appears unethical not to research potentially treatable diseases.[27–31] However, the likely benefit of research must be weighed against possible risks, burden or distress to the subject and estimating these risks may be difficult. Some have proposed a sliding-scale relationship between the likelihood and extent of any distress or hazard to the research participant, and ethical concern. Thus, merely noting patient details causes no distress and a blood test may mean minor distress, but no hazard. Some research procedures have clear potential for the subject to benefit (e.g. randomised drug trials), but a different scenario to consider would be where there is no possibility of direct clinical benefit to the individual, such as investigations of disease pathology or phase I drug studies. The DH specifies that the benefits and risks of a new treatment should be assessed against the best current choice of treatment.

Distribution of risk

The DH also states that the risks associated with research are only justified if there is a reasonable likelihood that the population in which the research is carried out stand to benefit from the results of the research. Elderly subjects are currently under-represented in many studies. However, it would appear unethical to assess a treatment in, for example, terminally ill elderly patients, simply because any adverse event was unlikely to affect remaining life expectancy.

Informed consent

In the context of medical care and clinical research, consent is required in order to preserve and protect an individual's freedom. Cardozo summed up the meaning of consent in what has become a classic statement of civil liberties:[28]

> Every human being of adult years and sound mind has a right to determine what shall be done with his own body and a surgeon who performs an operation without his patient's consent commits an assault for which he is liable in damages.

Informed consent consists of three parts. Firstly, the individual has freedom of choice and consent to participate must be voluntary. Secondly, sufficient information must be provided in a way that is clearly understandable to the subject concerned. The DH specifies that information provided during the consent process should encompass an overview of the trial protocol, anticipated benefits and risks of the study and discomfort it may entail. Thirdly, the subject must be sufficiently competent to appreciate what is being explained and to weigh up the position before reaching a decision.[27, 32, 33] Most guidelines dictate that written consent is obtained for all research and is recorded in patients' case notes. They also specify that if only verbal consent is given, it should be formally witnessed and documented. Many research codes also recommend that information that has been disclosed in order to obtain consent is documented.[27–30, 32–36]

Incompetent subjects

Estimates of dementia range from 1.4% in people aged between 65 and 70 years to 20% in those aged over 80 years.[37] This condition contributes to the increased prevalence of mental incapacity in aged populations. Although persons incompetent to give informed consent are still valuable subjects for medical research, by definition they cannot give informed consent to research.

Competence depends upon context and there is a distinction between different competencies.[32–35] An older person may be incompetent with respect to property. Another sense of incompetence, termed incompetence with respect to the person, is a patient's ability to make or act upon rational decisions. These people may not be able to determine whether they would like tea or coffee, or receive a medical intervention. Although an elderly person may be competent in one aspect but not the other, there is a regrettable tendency of some health carers to assume that a person who is incompetent in the sense of not being able to manage the daily business of life is also incompetent to make decisions concerning medical treatment options. The failure to distinguish between these two different kinds of incompetence means that subjects who are incompetent with regard to property only, but who still possess a clear conception of the self as well as the ability to make sensible choices concerning treatment, may be deprived of their moral right to make decisions concerning their own fate.

Decision-making by doctors, researchers or carers acting on behalf of the subject is not appropriate for subjects who are incompetent only with respect to property. A balance must be sought between respecting the autonomy that remains and protecting patients from undesirable harm or risk.

To complicate the issue of competence, cognitive function may fluctuate over short time intervals, making subjects inconsistently competent, or cognitive impairment may develop gradually over time, e.g. in the dementias. Variability or deterioration in cognition and therefore competency during participation in research raises difficult questions concerning the subject's continued consent to participate.

The DH provides that 'for a research subject who is legally incompetent, physically or mentally incapable of giving consent ... the investigator must obtain informed consent from the legally authorised representative in accordance with applicable law. These groups should not be included in research unless the research is necessary to promote the health of the population represented and this research cannot instead be performed on legally competent persons'. Thus, informed consent should be obtained from the incompetent elderly person's legal guardian or a responsible relative, in accordance with national legislation.[27-30] Unfortunately, this legislation is lacking in the UK and those involved in the conduct of research using elderly patients who can no longer exercise autonomy have to fall back upon common law and ethical principles.[27,32-36] Literature from the British Medical Association highlights that, except in cases where a legal guardian has been appointed, no individual or office holder has legal authority to consent to treatment being given to an adult who is mentally incapable of making a decision.[36]

One solution to the problem of consent to participate in research is agreement of an enduring power of attorney.[38] The linchpin of this solution is the assignment of a durable power of attorney in the early stages of mental deterioration, before the patient loses the capacity to give informed consent. At present these agreements are rarely seen in UK research recruits.

Often carers or family members act as the patient's advocate. Although this is considered fair because family members are likely to know the patient best and can thus act in his or her best interests, the law does not deal with this fully and it has not been tested legally in the research context.

Admission to hospital under a section of the Mental Health Act 1983 does not necessarily indicate inability to consent, as patients' right to give or withhold consent to treatment for a physical condition is not lessened by the fact of their compulsory detention under the Act.[36]

Testing for competence

Whilst competence is often regarded as within the sphere of legal judgement, clear legal standards are lacking for determining when a person is not competent to make medical decisions. Adults are simply presumed competent unless found to be otherwise by a court of law.[28–30] In clinical practice, it is rare to find either the courts or guardians legally appointed by them to be involved in making this decision. Rather, current procedures dictate that health carers identify those individuals whose competence is in doubt. Several decision-making models have emerged, all of which assess mental status by measuring consciousness, orientation and memory. In the UK the mini-mental state examination and Alzheimer's Disease Assessment Scale (cognitive subscale) are frequently used.

Some argue that a general mental status assessment is not appropriate and the prospective subject's appreciation of the project must be evaluated. A US National Institute of Health panel concluded that 'a key factor on potential participants' decision-making is their appreciation of how the study applies to them ... in the context of their lives'.[39] This panel endorses a sliding-scale approach to decisional capacity in the research setting, requiring an increasing level of appreciation as study risks increase and potential benefit for the subject decreases. The panel similarly suggests that many prospective research subjects incapable of independent research decision making remain capable of selecting a research proxy, as the capacity required to designate a proxy is far less than the capacity required to understand a detailed protocol.

Research ethics committees

All clinical research which involves human subjects must be submitted to a specially appointed research ethics committee for advice, consideration and comments. Local research ethics committees (RECs) in individual UK health authorities and multicentre RECs acting for a whole health region perform this function. RECs have a predefined composition of medical and lay representatives, intended to ensure a broad general consensus to govern the ethical acceptability of research.[40] RECs are responsible for ensuring that all research projects involving human subjects are morally justifiable, that the highest standards of practice are maintained, that participants' rights are safeguarded and to give advice on other ethical aspects.[27,28]

Elderly people in nursing homes and residential homes

The institutionalised elderly population represents the extremes of frailty, cognitive impairment and multiple illnesses. A dichotomy arises: many diagnoses lead to higher drug use, yet frailty means that therapy is particularly hazardous. Unfortunately, drug research in nursing and residential homes is frequently very difficult, as informed consent may not be obtainable, relatives may be difficult to contact or health carers reluctant to allow access due to concerns about confidentiality.[41]

Paternalism

Medicine has a long history of paternalism and it is only since the 1960s that issues of patient autonomy and informed consent were thrust into the forefront.[34] Old habits, however, die hard, so many older physicians and older patients are more accustomed to a paternalistic style of medical care that emphasises the health carer as the decision maker rather than the patient. Today's elderly patients, long accustomed to paternalistic medical practice, may be bewildered when told that they must contribute to making the decision to participate in research.

Methodological considerations: tools used in elderly subjects

Although design and conduct of clinical studies are frequently similar whether young or old subjects are involved, it is of interest to highlight selected research tools used specifically in older subjects.

The frailty of elderly patients requires research instruments that do not trouble subjects too much, yet are sensitive enough to detect change. In recognition of the insensitivity of traditional tools to changes in elderly subjects' functional status or quality of life in the research setting, novel cognitive, functional (e.g. activities of daily living) and global tools have been developed. This was driven in part by the European Medicines Evaluation Agency and by the Food and Drug Administration in the USA. These bodies required that both cognitive improvement and measurable clinical benefit (e.g. function) were demonstrated before considering licensing drugs for the treatment of Alzheimer's disease in Europe and the USA. Some commonly used tools are described below. Results of some tests may be affected by the examiner's cultural background, presence or absence of family members or by short-term fluctuations in cognitive function.[29]

Cognitive tests

The mini-mental state examination is a brief, physician/researcher-administered structured examination of cognitive function. It was developed as a screening tool but is often used as a secondary measure of cognitive function in clinical trials. This 30-point test includes an assessment of orientation (year, season, town), naming (pencil, watch) and praxis (ability to perform an action).[42]

The Alzheimer's Disease Assessment Scale cognitive subscale (ADAS-cog) was developed to measure drug effects on cognition objectively. It is widely used and assesses memory, orientation, language, construction, praxis, drawing and naming (e.g. scissors, comb).[43] ADAS-cog is more comprehensive than the mini-mental state examination, taking up to one hour to complete.

Global interview-based scales

Global assessments are overall, subjective independent ratings of the patients' total condition by a clinician experienced in the management of patients with Alzheimer's disease. Although global assessments are less reliable than objective measures, they are frequently used in trials of Alzheimer's disease drugs to validate the results of objective tests. The Food and Drug Administration Clinician's Interview-Based Impression of Change (CIBIC) scale rates change from baseline, on a scale of 1 (very much improved) to 7 (very much worse). It takes about 10 minutes and can be conducted without (CIBIC) and with the patient's carer present (CIBIC-plus).[44] Clinician's Global Impressions (CGI) assess Severity (CGIS) or Change (CGIC), also using a 1–7 scale.[45] Several variations have been developed.

The Clinical Dementia Rating (CDR) uses a structured interview to assess several domains, including cognition, function, language, affect and impulse control, resulting in an overall score from 0 to 18.

Activities of daily living

Activities of daily living (ADL) assessments frequently rely upon the reports of carers in close and regular contact with the subject. These tools may be used to evaluate drug-related change in everyday functioning. The Barthel functional ADL index evaluates basic self-care, including continence, mobility, dressing, bathing and feeding, with a maximum score of 21.[46] Instrumental ADL tools assess shopping, cooking, doing laundry, handling finances, using transportation, driving and telephoning.[47]

Behaviour scales

Behavioural problems such as delusions, hallucinations and agitation often occur in dementia syndromes. The ADAS-noncognitive subscale is essentially limited to the behaviour the patient exhibits during test-taking. Scores range from 50 (most severe) to zero. Many other behavioural assessments are available, including the Nursing Home Behaviour Problem scale.[48]

Tools to evaluate prescribing

Both subjective and objective tools have been developed to assess the quality of prescribing for elderly subjects. Some tools assess patients clinically, for which subjects must give consent (with associated difficulties in elderly subjects), whilst others use only information documented in individual patients' notes to evaluate prescribing.[26, 49] Such audit tools do not require interaction with or clinical assessment of subjects, obviating the need for consent.

Work in elderly hospitalised and nursing home populations has resulted in a set of objective, evidence-based measures of prescribing quality.[26, 49] These prescribing indicators use drug indications and contraindications documented in individual patients' notes to evaluate prescribing appropriateness. An example is shown in Figure 16.1. Elderly subjects are more sensitive to benzodiazepines, with more frequent and more pronounced adverse effects. Although benzodiazepines may be appropriate in specific conditions, initiation as a hypnotic should generally be avoided in elderly patients.[5, 49, 50]

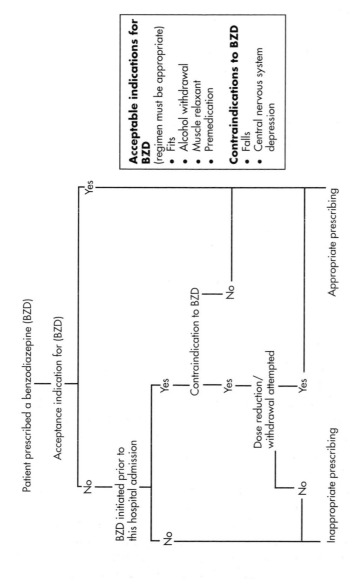

Figure 16.1 Algorithm to assess appropriateness of benzodiazepine prescribing for elderly patients. Reproduced with permission from Oborne et al.[26] and Batty et al.[49]

Conclusion

Improving the health and well-being of older people will be amongst the greatest medical challenges of this century. Despite the current emphasis on evidence-based practice, therapeutic decision making which is supported by reliable data is frequently difficult due to the scarcity of data from elderly populations. People aged 65 years and over are major users of medication, yet extrapolation of data from younger populations may be invalid.

Medical research is an integral part of medical progress. Indeed, a lack of such experimentation could be regarded as morally indefensible. Whilst it is recognised that the risk of untoward effects is potentially higher in older subjects, study design should be optimised to minimise these risks and so that essential risk–benefit data can be obtained for elderly people. Furthermore, study populations should be stratified to include sufficient older people to permit valid conclusions for subgroups of the elderly population.

Investigators are responsible for the promotion of patient welfare, autonomy, rights and adherence to ethical guidelines in all research collaboration.

References

1.   Chrischilles E A, Foley D, Wallace R *et al*. Use of medications by persons 65 and over: data from the established populations for epidemiologic studies of the elderly. *J Gerontol* 1992; 47: M137–M144.
2.   Rumble R H, Morgan K. Longitudinal trends in prescribing for elderly patients: two surveys four years apart. *Br J Gen Pract* 1994; 44: 571–575.
3.   Cartwright A, Smith C, eds. Prescribed medicines taken and kept by the elderly people. In: *Elderly People, their Medicines, and their Doctors*. London: Routledge, 1988: 15–74.
4.   Anon. Medication for older people. Summary and recommendations of a report of a working party of the Royal College of Physicians. *J R Coll Physicians Lond* 1997; 31: 254–257.
5.   Bertz R J, Kroboth P D, Kroboth F J *et al*. Alprazolam in young and elderly men: sensitivity and tolerance to psychomotor, sedative and memory effects. *J Pharmacol Exp Ther* 1997; 281: 1317–1329.
6.   Jennings P E. Oral antihyperglycaemics. Considerations in older patients with non-insulin-dependent diabetes mellitus. *Drugs Aging* 1997; 10: 323–331.
7.   Tregaskis B F, Stevenson I H. Pharmacokinetics in old age. *Br Med Bull* 1990; 46: 9–21.
8.   Woodhouse K W, James O F W. Hepatic drug metabolism and ageing. *Br Med Bull* 1990; 46: 22–35.

9. Kinirons M T, Crome P. Clinical pharmacokinetic considerations in the elderly: an update. *Clin Pharmacokinet* 1997; 33: 302–312.

10. Zoli M, Magalotti D, Bianchi G *et al*. Total and functional hepatic blood flow decrease in parallel with ageing. *Age Ageing* 1999; 28: 29–33.

11. Messerli F H, Grossman E, Goldbourt U. Are beta-blockers efficacious as first-line therapy for hypertension in the elderly? A systematic review. *JAMA* 1998; 279: 1903–1907.

12. Wolf P A, Abbott R, Kannel W B. Atrial fibrillation: a major contributor to stroke in the elderly. The Framingham study. *Arch Intern Med* 1987; 147: 1561–1564.

13. SPAF II investigators. Warfarin versus aspirin for prevention of thromboembolism in atrial fibrillation: stroke prevention in atrial fibrillation II study. *Lancet* 1994; 343: 687–691.

14. Walker J, Wynne H. Review: the frequency and severity of adverse drug reactions in elderly people. *Age Ageing* 1994; 23: 255–259.

15. Committee on Safety of Medicines. Nonsteroidal anti-inflammatory drugs and serious gastrointestinal adverse reactions 1. *BMJ* 1986; 292: 614.

16. Griffin M R, Ray W, Schaffner W. Nonsteroidal anti-inflammatory drug use and death from peptic ulcer in elderly persons. *Ann Intern Med* 1988; 109: 359–363.

17. Mulrow C D, Cornell J A, Herrera C R *et al*. Hypertension in the elderly: implications and generalizability of randomised trials. *JAMA* 1994; 272: 1932–1938.

18. Bell J A, May F E, Stewart R B. Clinical research in the elderly: ethical and methodological considerations. *Drug Intell Clin Pharm* 1987; 21: 1002–1007.

19. Bugeja G, Kumar A, Banerjee A K. Exclusion of elderly people from clinical research: a descriptive study of published reports. *BMJ* 1997; 315: 1059.

20. Bayer A, Tadd W. Unjustified exclusion of elderly people from studies submitted to research ethics committee for approval: descriptive study. *BMJ* 2000; 321: 992–993.

21. Rochon P A, Fortin P R, Dear K B G *et al*. Reporting of age data in clinical trials of arthritis: deficiencies and solutions. *Arch Intern Med* 1993; 153: 243–248.

22. Anon. Benoxaprofen. *BMJ* 1982; 285: 459.

23. Halsey J P, Cardoe N. Benoxaprofen: side effect profile in 300 patients. *BMJ* 1982; 284: 1365–1368.

24. Bene J, Liston R. Clinical trials should be designed to include elderly people. *BMJ* 1998; 316: 1905.

25. Gruer P J K. Post-marketing surveillance. In: International Drug Safety Department, Glaxo Group Research (UK) (eds) *Drug Safety: A Shared Responsibility*. Edinburgh: Churchill Livingstone, 1991: 27–36.

26. Oborne C A, Batty G M, Maskrey V *et al*. Development of prescribing indicators for elderly medical inpatients. *Br J Clin Pharmacol* 1997; 43: 91–97.

27. World Medical Association. *Handbook of World Medical Association Policy*. http://www.wma.net/e/policy.html

28. Dyer C, ed. *Doctors, Patients and the Law*. Oxford: Blackwell Scientific Publications, 1992.

29. Elford R J, ed. *Medical Ethics and Elderly People*. Edinburgh: Churchill Livingstone, 1987.

30. Mason J K, McCall Smith R A. *Law and Medical Ethics*, 3rd edn. London: Butterworths, 1991.

31. Hodes R J, Cahan V, Pruzan M. The National Institute on Ageing at its twentieth anniversary: achievements and promise of research on ageing. *J Am Geriatr Soc* 1996; 44: 204–206.

32. Seltzer H, Duncan J, eds. *Legal and Healthcare Ethics for the Elderly*. Washington: Taylor and Francis, 1996.

33. Lowe D. *Planning for Medical Research: A Practical Guide to Research Methods*. Cheshire, UK: Astraglobe, 1993.

34. Waymack M H, Taler G A. *Medical Ethics and the Elderly: A Case Book*. Chicago: Pluribus Press, 1988.

35. Finch J D. *Aspects of Law Affecting the Paramedical Professions*. London: Faber and Faber, 1984.

36. British Medical Association. *The Handbook of Medical Ethics*. London: BMA, 1984.

37. Jones R W. Dementia. *Scott Med J* 1997; 42: 151–153.

38. Dukoff R, Sunderland T. Durable power of attorney and informed consent with Alzheimer's disease patients: a clinical study. *Am J Psychiatry* 1997; 154: 1070–1075.

39. National Bioethics Advisory Committee, eds. Informed consent and limitations on decision making capacity. In: *Research Involving Persons with Mental Disorders that may Affect Decision Making Capacity*. National Bioethics Advisory Commission: http://bioethics.gov/capacity/TOC.htm, 1998: 1–12.

40. Royal College of Physicians. *Guidelines on the Practice of Ethics Committees in Medical Research involving Human Subjects*. London: Royal College of Physicians of London, 1990.

41. Ratzan R M. The experiment that wasn't: a case report in clinical geriatric research. *Gerontologist* 1981; 21: 297–302.

42. Folstein M F, Folstein S E. Minimental state: a practical method for grading the cognitive state of patients for the clinician. *J Psychiatr Res* 1975; 12: 189–198.

43. Mohs R C. The Alzheimer's disease assessment scale. *Int Psychogeriatr* 1996; 8: 195–203.

44. Knopman D, Knapp M J, Gracon S I, Davis C S. The clinician interview-based impression (CIBI): a clinician's global change rating scale in Alzheimer's disease. *Neurology* 1994; 44: 2315–2321.

45. Guy W, ed. Clinical global impressions (CGI). In: *ECDEU Assessment Manual for Psychopharmacology*. Rockville, MD: US Department of Health and Human Resources, Public Health Service, Alcohol Drug Abuse and Mental Health Administration, NIMH Psychopharmacology Research Branch, 1976: 218–222.

46. Mahoney F I, Barthel D W. Functional evaluation: the Barthel index. *Maryland State Med J* 1965; 14: 61–65.

47. Royal College of Physicians Research Unit and British Geriatrics Society. *Standardised Assessment Scales for Elderly People*. London: Royal College of Physicians, 1992.

48. Ray W A, Taylor J, Lichtenstein M, Meador K G. The Nursing Home Behavior Problem Scale. *J Gerontol* 1992; 47: M9–M16.
49. Batty G M, Oborne C A, Swift C G, Jackson S H D. Development of an indicator to identify inappropriate use of benzodiazepines in elderly medical inpatients. *Int J Geriatr Psychiat* 2000; 15: 892–896.
50. Morgan K, Clarke D. Longitudinal trends in late-life insomnia: implications for prescribing. *Age Ageing* 1997; 26: 179–184.

Index

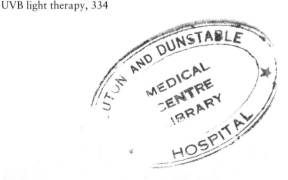